# Recent Advances in Drug Discovery and Development

# Recent Advances in Drug Discovery and Development

Edited by Lisa Torres

AMERICAN
MEDICAL PUBLISHERS
www.americanmedicalpublishers.com

American Medical Publishers,
41 Flatbush Avenue,
1st Floor, New York,
NY 11217, USA

Visit us on the World Wide Web at:
www.americanmedicalpublishers.com



ISBN: 978-1-63927-550-2



**Cataloging-in-Publication Data**

Recent advances in drug discovery and development / edited by Lisa Torres.
p. cm.
Includes bibliographical references and index.
ISBN 978-1-63927-550-2
1. Drugs—Design. 2. Drug development. 3. Pharmaceutical chemistry. I. Torres, Lisa.
RS420 .R43 2022
615.19--dc23

# Table of Contents

# Preface

In my initial years as a student, I used to run to the library at every possible instance to grab a book and learn something new. Books were my primary source of knowledge and I would not have come such a long way without all that I learnt from them. Thus, when I was approached to edit this book; I became understandably nostalgic. It was an absolute honor to be considered worthy of guiding the current generation as well as those to come. I put all my knowledge and hard work into making this book most beneficial for its readers.

A pharmaceutical drug or a medication is used to diagnose, cure, treat or prevent a disease. Drug therapy depends on the science of pharmacology for research and on pharmacy for proper management. Drug development is the process of identifying a therapeautically useful compound through drug discovery, with the help of which a new drug is brought to the market. It is undertaken by pharmaceutical companies, academic scientists, and governments. Drug discovery and development includes pre-clinical research, clinical trials and obtaining regulatory approval to market the drug. This book contains the different approaches, evaluations, methodologies and advanced studies in the field of drug discovery and development. It is a compilation of chapters that discuss the most vital concepts and emerging trends in the field. This book is a vital tool for all researchers and students in this field.

I wish to thank my publisher for supporting me at every step. I would also like to thank all the authors who have contributed their researches in this book. I hope this book will be a valuable contribution to the progress of the field.

**Editor**

# 1

# Challenges of Patient Selection for Phase I Oncology Trials

Mark Voskoboynik and Hendrik-Tobias Arkenau

## 1. Introduction

The modern era of oncology has seen an enormous increase in the number of therapeutic agents being tested on cancer patients with a broad variety of mechanisms of action, indications and rationale for their use. For an oncology drug to gain approval by the relevant government drug authority such as the United States Food and Drugs Administration (FDA) or the European Medicines Agency (EMA) it must demonstrate adequate safety and efficacy as well as have a favourable risk-benefit profile. As a result, all new oncology drugs must go through a process of investigation, usually beginning with pre-clinical laboratory and animal testing all the way through to the required clinical trials. The average time taken for a new drug to progress through clinical testing until the time it is approved is approximately 7.6 years [1]. The costs of drug development are large, estimated at up to $1 billion per approved drug and ever-increasing, placing an increasing burden on health care services [2, 3]. This has tremendous impacts on the cost of health-care provision with novel anticancer drugs often coming with a large price tag of more than $10,000 per month of treatment [4, 5]. Offsetting these costs are the tremendous improvements in patient outcomes that have been made in recent times with targeted therapies such as imatinib, trastuzumab and crizotinib to name just a few [6-8]. Patient selection for early phase oncology trials is of utmost importance because of the cascading effects it has on subsequent drug development and a drug's ultimate success as a safe, beneficial and cost-effective treatment.

## 2. Oncology clinical trials — Background

New drugs are developed in a sequential and rationale manner from the moment of their discovery in the pre-clinical phase through the various phases of clinical trials hopefully leading to their ultimate approval and availability for patients.

### 2.1. Clinical trial phases

Drugs are developed through several phases of clinical trials with each phase designed to answer specific questions and meet various endpoints (Figure 1). Each clinical trial phase can take a variable period of time to complete depending on the treatment setting, particular indication, trial drug and overall patient accrual rates. Each trial phase has specific challenges although a detailed discussion with regards to phase II and III trials is beyond the scope of this chapter.

Phase I trials, including first-in-human (FIH) trials, focus on a small group of patients to attempt to define the safety and tolerability of a particular treatment as well as the optimal dose, usually called the maximum tolerated dose (MTD).

Phase II trials use the information garnered from the Phase I trial, particularly in terms of appropriate dosing and sometimes with regards to patient selection, and a particular treatment is investigated on a larger number of patients, often with more specific disease characteristics than in Phase I patients. Increasingly so, phase II trials have multiple arms and the focus of these trials is on demonstrating a signal for treatment efficacy and consolidating the early safety data yielded from the phase I trial.

If a strong signal for the effectiveness of the trial treatment is obtained from the phase II trial, an even larger phase III trial is then conducted. Phase III trials are designed to establish the efficacy, or lack thereof, a trial treatment. As a result, a larger patient population is required and the trial treatment is compared with an established standard-of-care treatment or placebo if there is no standard treatment available to the particular patient group. Usually, it is the data and results from this study that will be relied upon to gain drug approval.

### 2.2. Phase I clinical trials

The primary aim of a phase I oncology clinical trial is to identify the maximum-tolerated dose (MTD) of a particular drug, defined as the dose level where greater than one-third of patients treated experience a dose-limiting toxicity (DLT). This allows the identification of the optimal and safe drug dose to take forward for further drug development – this is called the recommended phase II dose (RP2D). For cytotoxic drugs, the RP2D is usually the highest dose that can be delivered without exposing patients to unacceptable levels of toxicity. For targeted drugs, the dose of the drug that causes a treatment response and clinical activity may be very different to the MTD [9]. An important component of phase I trials is to provide patients with a safe treatment at doses that are as close to therapeutic as possible. There are often multiple secondary endpoints in phase I trials including the tolerability, response to treatment, pharmacokinetics of the study drug(s) and pharmacodynamics.

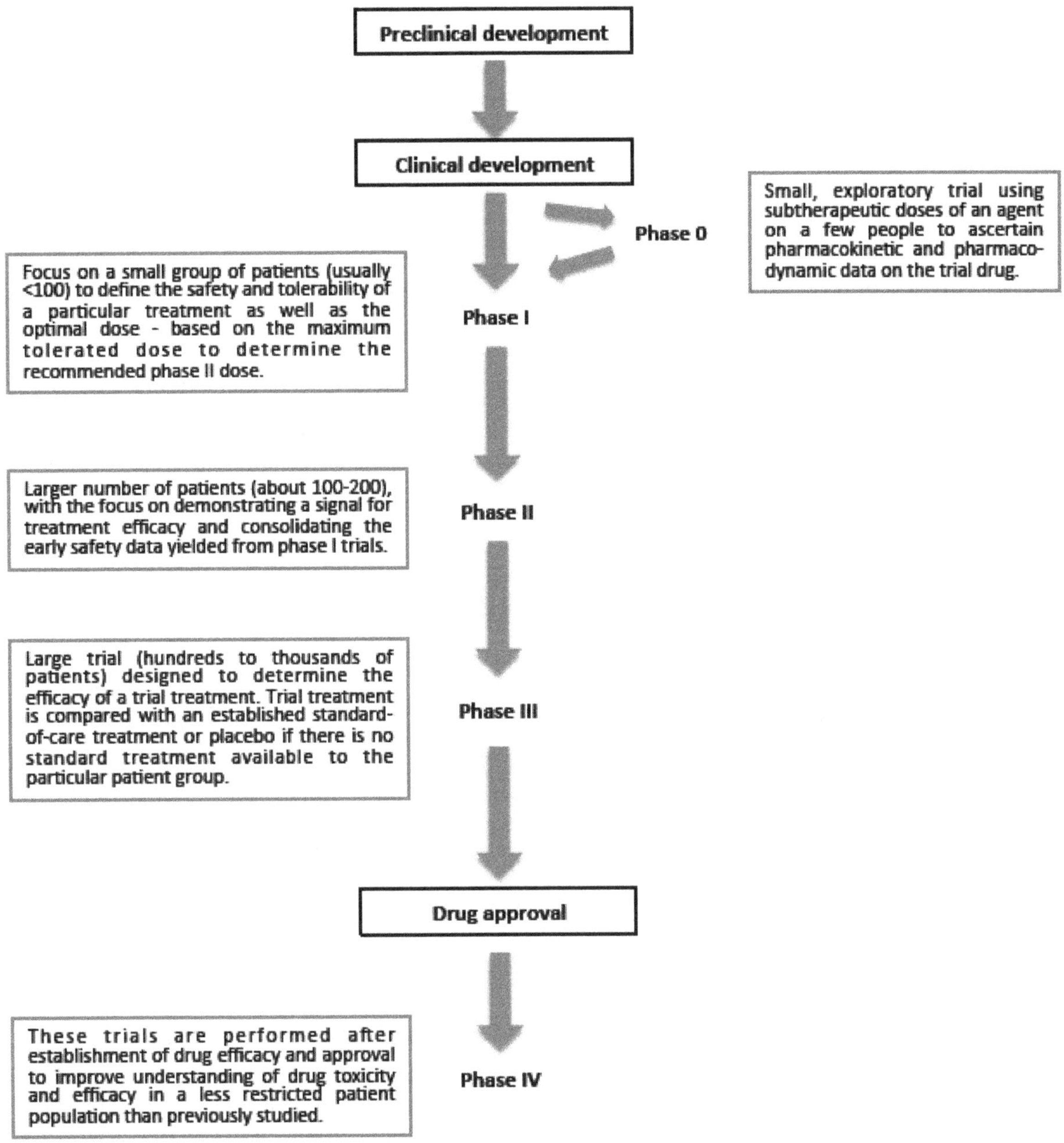


**Figure 1.** The standard pathway for oncology drug development, including the various clinical trial phases.

The aims of phase I oncology trials clearly impact significantly upon trial design. The intention of phase I trial design is to minimise the number of patients exposed to either sub-therapeutic drug doses or severe treatment-related toxicity. With phase I trial design there is a basic tension between escalating drug doses too quickly, exposing more patients to toxicity, and escalating too slowly, exposing patients to doses of treatment that are sub-therapeutic and ineffective [10]. The design of phase I trials is therefore critical in order to minimise the risk of a negative outcome for each individual patient and at the same time controlling the number of patients required for trial enrolment in order to accomplish the aims of the trial.

The traditional design incorporating the '3+3' method of dose escalation is still the most widely used. This involves treating 3 patients at a time at each dose-level. The dose level should be increased for each subsequent group of 3 patients until at least 1 dose limiting toxicity (DLT) occurs in a group of 3 patients. If only 1 of 3 patients have a DLT, a further 3 patients are treated at the same dose level. If 2 or more DLTs occur per dose level, the dose escalation is stopped and occasionally a further 3 patients are treated at the dose level below. The highest dose level (where ≤1 out of 6 patients had a DLT) below the maximally administered dose had a DLT is considered the MTD and the RP2D. Dose levels are traditionally defined using a Fibonacci dose escalation whereby dose is increased by increments of 100%,67%, 50%, 40% followed by 33% for all subsequent levels.

Novel designs include accelerated titration designs, continual reassessment method and adaptive trial designs [11]. Accelerated titration phase I trial designs attempt to make phase I trials more efficient and more accurate when determining the RP2D. A group of proposed accelerated titration designs were developed by Simon and colleagues in 1997 [12]. The key features of these designs are rapid dose escalation, intra-patient dose escalation and the ability to analyse trials using a dose-toxicity model [11]. The most popular of these designs, 'design 4', starts with an initial accelerated phase that doubles the dose at each dose level, comprising of single patients. When the first DLT is experienced, the cohort for that particular dose level is expanded to include 3 patients and subsequent to this, standard phase I dose escalation and design is employed. This design also allows intra-patient dose escalation if a particular patient has no toxicity at their current dose. By use of a simulated phase I trial, as presented by Simon and colleagues in this paper, there was a significant reduction in the number of patients that were treated at sub-therapeutic doses, without a significant increase in the proportion of patients exposed to significant treatment toxicity. Other adaptive trial design methods exist, including the continual reassessment method (CRM) introduced by O'Quigley and colleagues in 1990 [13].

The potential benefits of novel designs are that fewer patients are treated with sub-therapeutic or nontherapeutic doses however they do not seem to have the reduced the number of patients that are enrolled onto trials. By adapting these novel trial designs, the most appropriate recruitment structure can be used for the particular drug under investigation.

## 3. Patient selection for clinical trials

### 3.1. Estimation of prognosis in oncology

Selecting the appropriate patient for early phase clinical trials is a fundamental component of any clinical trial design. A key component, in particular for phase I trials, but probably true for all phases of drug development, is the assessment of an individual patients prognosis. Many patients being considered for enrolment onto a phase I oncology trial have had progressive metastatic disease through all standard lines of treatment and often have a limited life expectancy. Standard trial eligibility criteria have been designed largely with the intention of minimising the number of patients enrolled onto these studies that have a poor prognosis and a greater potential for toxicity.

Estimating prognosis is inherently challenging for a clinician and estimates are often made based on intuition and experience rather than in a scientific or an evidence-based manner. Physicians' often make inaccurate estimates of a patient's prognosis, usually by being optimistic and overestimating survival. Various studies have shown that overestimation of the prognosis of terminal patients can be up to 5 times longer than their actual survival, exemplifying just how difficult making these estimates are [14-16].

Routine trial eligibility criteria include good performance status, adequate organ function (including haematological, kidney and liver etc.), and typically an anticipated life expectancy of greater than 12 weeks. Performance status is most commonly assessed using the Eastern Cooperative Oncology Group (ECOG) performance status score that is a score graded 0-5 [17]. It is a validated assessment of a patients ability to perform routine activities of daily living. A performance status (PS) of 0 indicates that the patient is fully active, ambulant and able to carry all activities without restriction whereas a PS of 5 is applied to a patient that is deceased. Most trials would permit a patient with a PS of between 0 and 1 or 2 (partially restricted in physical activity (PS = 1) and unable to carry out work activities but remain ambulatory and self-caring (PS = 2)). Another commonly used assessment score for performance status is the Karnofsky Performance Status (KPS) score which has more specific gradations between 0% (dead) and 100% (asymptomatic without complaints) in 10% increments [18, 19].

It is well documented that patients with a poorer performance status have an inferior prognosis overall when using either the KPS or ECOG PS [20-23]. It has been shown that an ECOG PS of 3 indicates a prognosis of less than 3 months and a PS of 4 of less than 1 month.

A number of other factors can be used to predict the prognosis of oncology patients. For example, the primary malignancy impacts greatly on the prediction of patient survival. For instance, patients diagnosed with metastatic carcinoid tumours often survive for a number of years compared to patients with metastatic pancreatic cancer who have a median overall survival of less than 12 months even with the best treatment currently available [24, 25]. Various laboratory data has also been associated with a poor prognosis such as hypoalbuminaemia, raised inflammatory markers (including leukocytosis, raised C-reactive peptide (CRP), lymphopenia and certain metabolic abnormalities such as hypercalcaemia [26, 27].

A number of tumour-specific prognostic scores have been developed to help stratify patients into various treatments based on their risk. A good illustrative example of this is the Memorial Sloan-Kettering Cancer Center (MSKCC) risk criteria for metastatic clear cell renal cell carcinoma. These criteria, published by Motzer and colleagues in 1999, were developed with five pre-treatment features that were associated with a shorter patient survival [28]. The five prognostic factors were low performance status (KPS <80%), high serum lactate dehydrogenase (>1.5 times upper limit of normal), low haemoglobin (< lower limit of normal), high corrected serum calcium (>10 mg/dL) and absence of prior nephrectomy. Patients with three or more risk factors were considered to be in a 'poor risk' category with a median survival time of 4 months compared to the 'favorable-risk category containing patients with zero risk factors and a median survival of 20 months.

A large number of molecular tests have been shown to have prognostic value in various malignancies. Examples of molecular results that confer a poorer prognosis in advanced cancers include BRAF mutations in colorectal cancer and melanoma, human epidermal growth factor receptor 2 (HER2) positivity in breast cancer and phosphatidylinositol-3,4,5-triphosphate 3-phosphatatse (PTEN) deficiency in prostate cancer to name a few [29-32]. Interestingly, recent developments in targeted therapies have led to the use of newer agents directed against some of these molecular or genetic abnormalities, in some cases resulting in significant improvements in prognosis and overcoming the negative prognostic implications of the result in the first place.

In addition to various clinical, molecular and genetic factors, circulating tumour cells (CTCs) can be used and have been shown to be prognostics in a variety of malignancies. CTCs are shed from solid tumours in to the circulation. Recent improvements in technology has led to a variety of laboratory methods that are able to effectively detect and isolate these CTCs which are usually very rarely found in the circulation. The CellSearch System® (Janssen Diagnostics, Inc) is the most frequently used and is the only FDA cleared device for measuring CTCs as an aid for clinicians treating patients with prostate, breast and colon cancers. A series of key studies conducted approximately 10 years ago showed that patients with higher levels of CTCs in the circulation had a poorer prognosis. For example, patients with castrate refractory prostate cancer and a CTC count lower than 5 / 7.5mL had a median overall survival of 21.7 months compared to patients with a CTC count greater than 5 that had a survival of 11.5 months [33]. Similar results were seen in patients with breast and colon cancer whereby a particular cut-point of CTC counts could be used to clearly differentiate patients with a favourable prognosis from those patients with an unfavourable prognosis [34, 35]. Although there are currently limitations with the technology and its implementation into routine clinical practice, this field is developing rapidly and will likely play a part in patient selection in the future.

Overall, the prediction of a patient's individual prognosis is challenging, complex and involves a variety of factors related to their clinical situation, the characteristics of the cancer, the molecular biology of the cancer as well as other factors including circulating tumour cells (Figure 2).

### 3.2. Phase I patient selection criteria

A number of prognostic scores have been published in recent times with the aim of improving patient selection for phase I clinical trials [36-40]. Probably the most important of these scores and the only one that has been prospectively validated is the Royal Marsden Hospital (RMH) score (see Table 1).

Arkenau and colleagues initially performed a retrospective analysis of 212 patients that were enrolled onto phase I trials and reviewed their demographic data as well as a number of clinical and analytic variables [38]. Using a multivariate analysis model, three independent variables

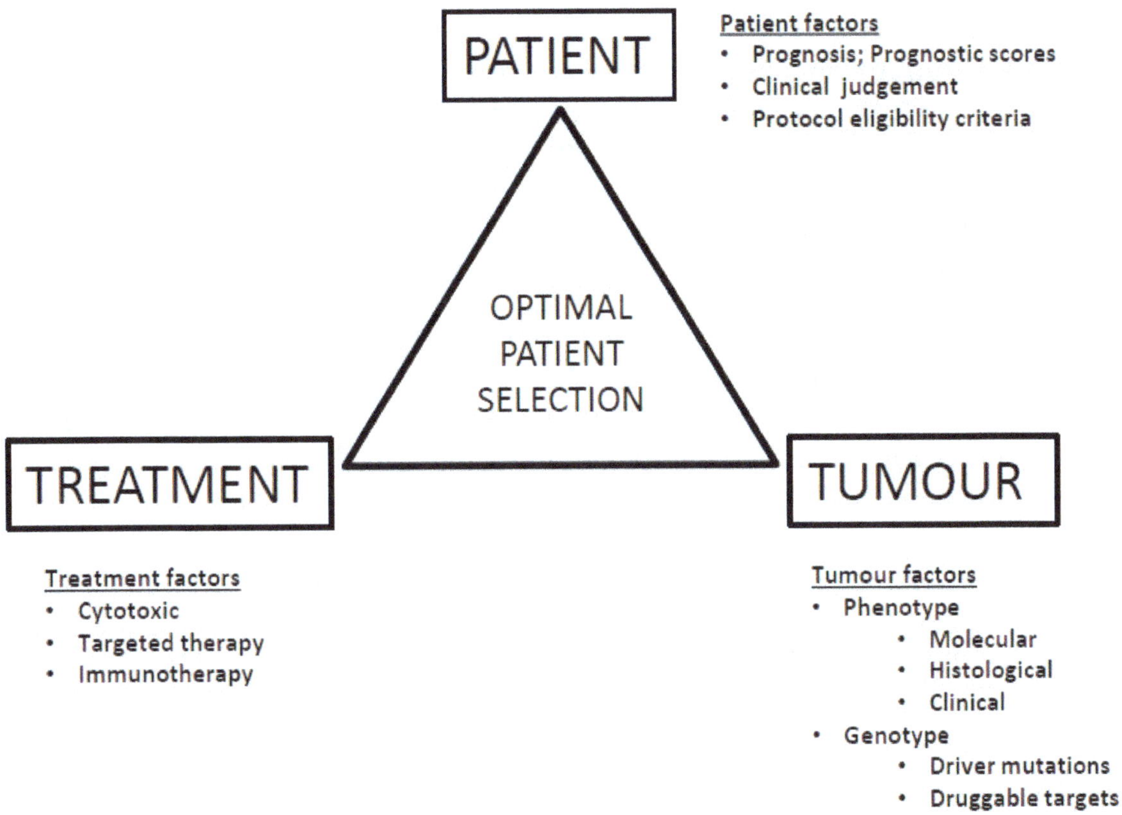


**Figure 2.** Factors impacting on optimal patient selection for phase I clinical trials in oncology.

were determined to be associated with a poor overall survival – an elevated lactate dehydrogenase [LDH] (above the upper limit of normal [ULN]), low albumin (< 35 g/L), and more than two sites of metastases. Using these variables, a score was developed that could separate these patients broadly into two groups, those patients with a good prognosis (RMH score 0 to 1) and those with a poor prognosis (RMH score 2 to 3). This retrospective analysis subsequently led to the prospective validation of this score in a separate publication by the same group. In this validation study, 78 prospective patients that were treated within one of 19 phase I trials were evaluated [36]. 95% of patients had an ECOG performance score of 0 to 1 and were mostly treated with new biologic agents (68%) with a minority (32%) receiving cytotoxic-based treatment. The patients had a broad range of malignancies with over 80% having gastrointestinal, breast, gynecologic, sarcoma or urologic cancers. All patients were required to have evidence of disease progression before study entry. Five patients had a partial response to their treatment (7.5%) and fourteen (17.9%) achieved stable disease at three months as per the Response Evaluation Criteria in Solid Tumours (RECIST). The median overall survival for the entire study population was 27.1 weeks with an OS of 33.0 weeks for patients with a score of 0 to 1, compared to an OS of 15.7 weeks with a score of 2 to 3 (P=0.036). These findings represent the first prospectively validated prognostic score that might assist in the optimal selection of patients for entry into phase I trials.

The RMH prognostic score was further validated at the MD Anderson Cancer Center in their Phase I trials patients [41]. They retrospectively reviewed 229 consecutive patients with lung, pancreatic and head and neck tumours that were treated on 57 phase I trials. They applied the RMH score to these patients and found that the patients with a good RMH prognostic score had a longer median survival than those with a poor prognostic score (33.9 weeks vs 21.1 weeks, P<0.0001). The authors of this study therefore showed that the RMH prognostic score can be accurately applied to patients treated at a separate institution across a range of malignancies treated in a range of trials.

Stavraka and colleagues used a multivariate approach to attempt to identify variables that predicted survival in patients referred to the phase I oncology unit at their institution to devise the Hammersmith Score (HS) [37]. Analyses were carried out on 118 patients with 52 patients (44%) treated in one of 7 phase I trials. Of these patients that actually entered a study, only 1 (2%) had a partial response and 15 (28%) had stable disease. The median OS in patients that entered a study was 22 weeks compared to 11 weeks in those patients that did not enter a study. The multivariate analysis identified four independent negative predictive factors for OS – albumin <35 g/dL (P=0.01), LDH >450 IU/dL (P<0.001), sodium <135 mmol/dL (P=0.06) and ECOG PS≥2 (P=0.04). Based on three of these variables, excluding ECOG PS, a scoring system was devised to stratify patients into either low-risk (HS score 0 to 1) or high-risk groups (HS score 2-3). Patients in the low risk group had a median OS of 31.2 weeks compared to a median OS of 8.9 weeks in the high-risk group (P<0.001).

Chau and colleagues from the Princess Margaret Hospital in Toronto, Canada, assessed 17 potential clinical characteristics in 233 patients enrolled in phase I trials to create their own risk score – the Princess Margaret Hospital Index (PMHI) [39]. In their cohort of patients, the median overall survival was 320 days, significantly longer than the 27 weeks reported by Arkenau for the Royal Marsden group. In the multivariate analysis they found that high LDH (p=0.001), > 2 metastatic sites (p=0.004) and ECOG PS > 0 (p=0.05) were significantly associated with OS. They found that 3 variables were associated with 90-day mortality – albumin <35g/L (p=0.008), > 2 metastatic sites (p=0.02) and ECOG >1 (p=0.001). A single point was assigned to each of these variables and patients with a PMHI score of 0-1 had lower 90-day mortality rate compared to patients with a score of 2-3 (7% and 37% respectively).

A large, European, multicenter study was designed to generate and validate a prognostic model for 90-day mortality which is a common eligibility criterion in phase I oncology trials [42]. Data from 2,232 patients enrolled in phase I trials across 14 oncology units was evaluated. The median overall survival was 38.6 weeks with a 90-day mortality rate of 16.5%. Two prognostic models were derived using a variety of variables including ECOG performance status, albumin, LDH, alkaline phosphatase, number of metastatic sites, lymphocytes, white cell count and time per treatment index (TPTi). TPTi is a log ratio of the time interval between diagnosis of advanced / metastatic and phase I trial entry over the number of lines of systemic treatment. The most predictive combination of variables includes albumin, LDH with ECOG PS or number of metastatic sites – similar to the RMH score. When compared to the RMH score using receiving operator characteristic (ROC) curves, there were no statistically significant differences seen. When the two models derived in this study (models A and B) were applied to patients with PS 0 to 1, patients with higher scores identified patients with OS of less than 11 weeks. When the RMH score was used to define the poorest risk group, their median OS was 14.6 weeks. The prognostic score (derived from model B – 'European score B') was assessed for its performance on a group of 200 patients that were eligible for phase I trials (PS 0-1) and it reduced the 90-mortality by half and the total number of patients recruited by 20%. This score performed almost identically to the RMH score when applied to the same population of patients.

Along a similar but distinct line, prediction models have been devised to try to identify patients at particularly high risk of drug toxicity. In one additional attempt to improve prediction of a patients risk for serious drug-related toxicity (SDRT), a nomogram was developed by Hyman and colleagues [43]. The data from 3,104 patients treated in 127 trials sponsored by the National Cancer Institute Cancer Therapeutics Evaluation Program (CTEP) between 2000 and 2010 was used for the derivation of a nomogram that could potentially estimate a patient's risk for developing serious toxicity. Data was from a large, prospectively maintained database. Trials that were evaluating cytotoxic or molecularly targeted agents were included. Standard phase I eligibility criteria were used to select appropriate patients. SDRT was defined as a grade ≥ 3 non-haematologic or grade ≥ 4 haematologic toxicity attributed to study treatment which is similar to the definition of a dose-limiting toxicity used by the majority of phase I trials. 728 patients (23.5%) experienced a SDRT and a total of 13 (0.4%) patients died as a result of drug related toxicity. Several factors were found to be reliable ($p<0.10$) predictors of serious drug-related toxicities in cycle one of trial treatment. Using a variety of statistical methods, a nomogram was built incorporating ECOG PS, WBC, creatinine clearance, albumin, aspartate transaminase (AST), number of study drugs and agent type (biologic or nonbiologic). This nomogram was independently validated using an independent data set of 234 patients. The authors concluded that by using their nomogram, improvements can be made in patient selection for phase I trials, in particular by prospectively identifying patients at high risk for drug toxicity.

There are a number of older retrospective series published and in a systematic review, Ploquin and colleagues summarised the published literature regarding prognostic models for life expectancy of patients enrolled in phase I trials up till the end of 2009 [44]. Nine publications were identified with all of them being retrospective analyses, except for the RMH score by Arkenau and colleagues in 2009 as described previously [36, 45-51]. Most of these studies fairly consistently identified that patients at greatest risk of death included those with a poorer performance status and greatest tumour volume (for example: increased number of metastatic sites, raised LDH). A consistent limitation of these studies, with one notable exception, is the use of retrospective data almost all were from single centre series which limits the generalizability of these studies.

One of the standard inclusion criteria in clinical trials is a life expectancy of greater than 12 weeks so it would be interesting to see how these scores might apply for this particular inclusion criterion. The RMH score shows that patients in the good prognosis group have a survival of 33 weeks, exceeding this particular criteria but even the median survival of the poor prognosis group exceeds the 12-week threshold (15.7 weeks). The patients in the high-risk group as defined by the HS, albeit retrospectively, had a survival shorter than 12 weeks (8.9 weeks) so potentially patients that fall into this category can be excluded from phase I trials.

With a number of scores now published it is unclear which of these is superior in predicting patient survival and this would require a separate prospective trial to clarify this question. As it currently stands, the RMH score is the only score that has been prospectively validated and therefore has the strongest evidence supporting its use. This is reflected in its more widespread use however further research is required to validate its utility in sites outside the Royal Marsden Hospital and indeed across other countries and across a broad cross-section of patient populations.

| **Score** | **Prospective validation** | **Parameters** | **Overall Survival (weeks)** | **P-value** | **HR** |
|---|---|---|---|---|---|
| Royal Marsden Hospital Score [36]<br>Arkenau 2008 | Yes | LDH (>ULN) = 1<br>Albumin (<35 g/L) = 1<br>> 2 sites of metastases = 1 | Score 0-1: 33.0<br>Score 2-3: 15.7 | 0.036 | 1.4 |
| Hammersmith Score [37]<br>Stavraka 2014 | No | LDH >450 IU/dL = 1<br>Albumin <35 g/dL = 1<br>Sodium <135 mmol/dL = 1 | Score 0-1: 31.2<br>Score 2-3: 8.9 | <0.001 | |
| Princess Margaret Hospital Index [39]<br>Chau 2011 | No | High LDH<br>>2 metastatic sites<br>ECOG PS > 0 | | | |
| European Model B [42]<br>Olmos 2012 | No | Albumin <35 g/dL = 1<br>LDH (>ULN) = 1<br>≥ 3 sites of metastases = 1<br>Low TPTi (<24 weeks/treatment) = 1<br>Increased ALP (>ULN) = 1<br>Low lymphocyte count (<18%) = 1<br>High WBC (>10,500/uL) | Score 0: 141<br>Score 1: 61<br>Score 2: 54<br>Score 3: 37<br>Score 4: 29<br>Score 5: 21<br>Score 6: 11<br>Score 7: 10 | 0.036 (log-rank) | -<br>2.00<br>2.54<br>3.24<br>4.57<br>6.20<br>14.1<br>14.1 |

Abbreviations: LDH = lactate dehydrogenase; PS = performance status; TPTi = time per treatment index, a log ratio of the time interval between diagnosis of advanced / metastatic and phase I trial entry over the number of lines of systemic treatment; ULN = upper limit of normal; WBC = white blood cell count

**Table 1.** Key publications of prognostic scores for phase I oncology trial patients.

# 4. Challenges

## 4.1. Impact of novel agents — Targeted therapies

Conducting phase I oncology trials has a number of inherent challenges. Traditionally, patients enrolled into these trials have exhausted all prior standard available therapies and by virtue of them having an incurable malignancy and very limited future treatment options, have a shortened life expectancy. There has therefore existed a paradoxical situation whereby the ideal patient has an advanced and often heavily pre-treated cancer but requires a prognosis that is suitable for the exposure of a novel investigational drug. The landscape in this field has shifted over recent years with phase I trials increasingly investigating targeted, biological agents as opposed to cytotoxic agents. The result of this change is that patients are being enrolled into phase I trials earlier in their disease course, including in the first line setting. The implications of these changes in practice will in some ways make the task of predicting a patient's prognosis slightly more straightforward as they are earlier in their disease course. On the other hand, predicting the prognosis of treatment-naïve patients might be more unpredictable as the natural history of their cancer has not been allowed enough time to be established.

Further complicating the situation is the advent of targeted agents that have rapid and significant responses. Examples of this include crizotinib in ALK-rearranged metastatic lung adenocarcinoma, vemurafenib in metastatic melanoma harbouring BRAF V600 mutations, EGFR inhibitors such as gefitinib and erlotinib in EGFR mutated lung cancer and idelalisib, a PI3K-delta inhibitor, for indolent lymphomas [7, 52-54]. These new agents increasingly have biomarkers that strongly predict for a response to treatment that can be quite rapid. The presence of these predictive biomarkers might mean that patient selection could potentially be relaxed because of the higher likelihood of a response. An illustrative example of this is the use of EGFR inhibitors in non-small-cell lung cancer. In the initial, large phase III trial of erlotinib, an EGFR inhibitor, compared to placebo in previously treated metastatic non-small-cell lung cancer, an unselected group of patients were treated [55]. The objective response rate in the erlotinib group was only 8.9% although it did result in an improved overall survival in this group of patients. This was an important trial but it certainly did not represent a large step forward for this group of patients. At the same time as these EGFR inhibitors were being developed, it was becoming apparent that the presence of an EGFR mutation, either a base-pair deletion at exon 19 or a point mutation at exon 21 (L858R) predicted for a good response to these targeted agents [56]. Mok and colleagues subsequently published a trial comparing another EGFR inhibitor, gefitinib, to chemotherapy in patients with metastatic adenocarcinoma [54]. In this trial, patients found to be harbouring an EGFR mutation had a 71% response rate to gefitinib, far higher than the 8.9% response rate seen in an unselected group of patients.

The advent of these targeted agents and their improved response rates and often improved safety profiles means that the traditional paradigm of patient selection will need be adapted and should evolve with this change in therapeutic agents. A potential consequence of more clearly defining the patient selection criteria for phase I trials is that the criteria could become too selective. If patients that are entered onto phase I trials are 'super-selected' for the best prognostic population, the toxicity that would be seen might not be entirely reflective of the general population. This might mean that the resulting maximum tolerated dose (MTD) and therefore the recommended phase II dose (RP2D) of the trial drugs would be too high and would potentially create more drug toxicity in the phase II and phase III patients. As we have expressed previously, the cascading effects of an increased rate of drug toxicity due to overly aggressive calculation of MTD could impact on drug development and trial costs and could ultimately have a bearing on the success or failure of that drug [57].

### 4.2. Impact of novel agents — Immunotherapies

Another major advance in the treatment of advanced malignancies has been the development of so-called 'immune-checkpoint inhibitors'. Modern immunotherapy agents include CTLA-4 inhibitors such as ipilimumab and tremelimumab which block the CTLA-4 molecule which is important for down-regulating T-cell activation, thereby enhancing immune activation. Inhibition of the programmed cell death 1 (PD-1) receptor and its primary ligand (PD-L1) with an ever growing number of drugs such as nivolumab, lambrolizumab and pembrolizumab improves the anti-tumour T-cell immune response in a more specific mode of action than CTLA-4 inhibitors. This class of compounds have provided significant improvements in patient outcomes with gains being made in tumour responses and most importantly in patient survival in a broad range of malignancies such as melanoma, renal cell carcinoma and lung cancer amongst others [58-60].

These immunotherapies, in particular the PD-1 and PD-L1 inhibitors, seem to be largely well tolerated, particularly when compared to chemotherapy, and can induce deep tumour responses that are durable [61]. From the initial trials of these agents there appear to be a significant minority of patients that have very prolonged durations of response, far greater than would otherwise be expected with 'traditional' treatments or previous standards of care. For example, patients with metastatic melanoma that were treated with Ipilimumab, a CTLA-4 inhibitor, of the approximately 10% of patients that achieved a response to treatment, many of these continued to have a response more than 12-24 months (median 19.3 months) after treatment was commenced. This is in sharp contradistinction to the patients treated in the 'standard' therapy arm with chemotherapy (dacarbazine) where the median duration of response was 8.1 months [62]. It is not entirely clear how the above patient selection such as the RMH and PMH scores would perform for this class of agents and whether they are applicable. Further research is required to determine the applicability of the phase I prognostic scores to patients enrolled onto trials using these immunotherapies.

## 5. Future of trial design

With the enormous number of novel therapeutic agents being developed and studied in phase I trials, the future for oncology patients seems bright. With the new immunotherapies, including combination therapies, the concept of curing patients with advanced malignancies has even been considered [61]. Adapting trial eligibility criteria and optimising patient selection is vital for the future of a safe and cost-effective drug development process. It is clear that determining the appropriateness of a particular patient for a particular phase I trial is more complex than applying a variety of scores or nomograms. When studying treatments that are personalised for a particular tumour or biomarker or even a mutation it is also important to individualise patient selection. The tendency and temptation is have an easily generalisable patient selection criteria because of its simplicity and reproducibility. The reality is that the behaviour of malignancies differ not only between organ of origin (for example prostate cancer compared to pancreatic cancer) but also within the same cancer type based on its phenotype (for example oestrogen receptor positive breast cancer compared with oestrogen / progesterone / HER-2 negative breast cancer) or genotype (for example BRAF mutated compared to BRAF wild type melanoma).

Given the complexity of patient selection described above, patients should be rationally selected with consideration given to tumour characteristics, patient factors as well as the investigational agents being assessed. Importantly, a degree of flexibility is essential when designing phase I trials for unselected populations to allow for the often extensive inter-patient and inter-tumour variability. The best way forward for optimizing patient selection is to rapidly adapt, in an evidence-based way, to the ever-evolving drug classes being developed as well as the ongoing financial pressures of drug development and not least of all patient expectations and the need for ongoing patient safety.

## Author details

Mark Voskoboynik[1,2] and Hendrik-Tobias Arkenau[1,3]

*Address all correspondence to: tobias.arkenau@hcahealthcare.co.uk

1 Sarah Cannon Research Institute UK, London, UK

2 Department of Medical Oncology, Guy's Hospital, London, UK

3 University College London, London, UK

## References

[1] Kaitin KI, DiMasi JA. Pharmaceutical innovation in the 21st century: new drug approvals in the first decade, 2000-2009. Clinical pharmacology and therapeutics. 2011;89(2):183-8. Epub 2010/12/31.

[2] Kantarjian HM, Fojo T, Mathisen M, Zwelling LA. Cancer drugs in the United States: Justum Pretium--the just price. J Clin Oncol. 2013;31(28):3600-4. Epub 2013/05/08.

[3] Goozner M. The $800 million pill: The truth behind the cost of new drugs: Univ of California Press; 2004.

[4] Smith TJ, Hillner BE. Bending the cost curve in cancer care. N Engl J Med. 2011;364(21):2060-5. Epub 2011/05/27.

[5] Fojo T, Grady C. How much is life worth: cetuximab, non-small cell lung cancer, and the $440 billion question. J Natl Cancer Inst. 2009;101(15):1044-8. Epub 2009/07/01.

[6] Demetri GD, von Mehren M, Blanke CD, Van den Abbeele AD, Eisenberg B, Roberts PJ, et al. Efficacy and safety of imatinib mesylate in advanced gastrointestinal stromal tumors. N Engl J Med. 2002;347(7):472-80. Epub 2002/08/16.

[7] Shaw AT, Kim DW, Nakagawa K, Seto T, Crino L, Ahn MJ, et al. Crizotinib versus chemotherapy in advanced ALK-positive lung cancer. N Engl J Med. 2013;368(25): 2385-94. Epub 2013/06/04.

[8] Piccart-Gebhart MJ, Procter M, Leyland-Jones B, Goldhirsch A, Untch M, Smith I, et al. Trastuzumab after adjuvant chemotherapy in HER2-positive breast cancer. N Engl J Med. 2005;353(16):1659-72. Epub 2005/10/21.

[9] Postel-Vinay S, Arkenau HT, Olmos D, Ang J, Barriuso J, Ashley S, et al. Clinical benefit in Phase-I trials of novel molecularly targeted agents: does dose matter? Br J Cancer. 2009;100(9):1373-8. Epub 2009/04/30.

[10] LoRusso PM, Boerner SA, Seymour L. An overview of the optimal planning, design, and conduct of phase I studies of new therapeutics. Clin Cancer Res. 2010;16(6): 1710-8. Epub 2010/03/11.

[11] Ivy SP, Siu LL, Garrett-Mayer E, Rubinstein L. Approaches to phase 1 clinical trial design focused on safety, efficiency, and selected patient populations: a report from the clinical trial design task force of the national cancer institute investigational drug steering committee. Clin Cancer Res. 2010;16(6):1726-36. Epub 2010/03/11.

[12] Simon R, Freidlin B, Rubinstein L, Arbuck SG, Collins J, Christian MC. Accelerated titration designs for phase I clinical trials in oncology. J Natl Cancer Inst. 1997;89(15): 1138-47. Epub 1997/08/06.

[13] O'Quigley J, Pepe M, Fisher L. Continual reassessment method: a practical design for phase 1 clinical trials in cancer. Biometrics. 1990;46(1):33-48. Epub 1990/03/01.

[14] Christakis NA, Lamont EB. Extent and determinants of error in doctors' prognoses in terminally ill patients: prospective cohort study. BMJ. 2000;320(7233):469-72. Epub 2000/03/04.

[15] Vigano A, Dorgan M, Bruera E, Suarez-Almazor ME. The relative accuracy of the clinical estimation of the duration of life for patients with end of life cancer. Cancer. 1999;86(1):170-6. Epub 1999/07/03.

[16] Glare P, Virik K, Jones M, Hudson M, Eychmuller S, Simes J, et al. A systematic review of physicians' survival predictions in terminally ill cancer patients. BMJ. 2003;327(7408):195-8. Epub 2003/07/26.

[17] Oken MM, Creech RH, Tormey DC, Horton J, Davis TE, McFadden ET, et al. Toxicity and response criteria of the Eastern Cooperative Oncology Group. American journal of clinical oncology. 1982;5(6):649-55. Epub 1982/12/01.

[18] Karnofsky D, Burchenal J. The clinical evaluation of chemotherapeutic agents in cancer. In: Evaluation of chemotherapeutic agents.. New York Columbia University Press; 1949.

[19] Schag CC, Heinrich RL, Ganz PA. Karnofsky performance status revisited: reliability, validity, and guidelines. J Clin Oncol. 1984;2(3):187-93. Epub 1984/03/01.

[20] Yates JW, Chalmer B, McKegney FP. Evaluation of patients with advanced cancer using the Karnofsky performance status. Cancer. 1980;45(8):2220-4. Epub 1980/04/15.

[21] Mor V, Laliberte L, Morris JN, Wiemann M. The Karnofsky Performance Status Scale. An examination of its reliability and validity in a research setting. Cancer. 1984;53(9): 2002-7. Epub 1984/05/01.

[22] Reuben DB, Mor V, Hiris J. Clinical symptoms and length of survival in patients with terminal cancer. Archives of internal medicine. 1988;148(7):1586-91. Epub 1988/07/01.

[23] Miller RJ. Predicting survival in the advanced cancer patient. Henry Ford Hospital medical journal. 1991;39(2):81-4. Epub 1991/01/01.

[24] Conroy T, Desseigne F, Ychou M, Bouche O, Guimbaud R, Becouarn Y, et al. FOLFIRINOX versus gemcitabine for metastatic pancreatic cancer. N Engl J Med. 2011;364(19):1817-25. Epub 2011/05/13.

[25] Zuetenhorst JM, Taal BG. Metastatic carcinoid tumors: a clinical review. The oncologist. 2005;10(2):123-31. Epub 2005/02/15.

[26] Ralston SH, Gallacher SJ, Patel U, Campbell J, Boyle IT. Cancer-associated hypercalcemia: morbidity and mortality. Clinical experience in 126 treated patients. Annals of internal medicine. 1990;112(7):499-504. Epub 1990/04/01.

[27] Al Murri AM, Bartlett JM, Canney PA, Doughty JC, Wilson C, McMillan DC. Evaluation of an inflammation-based prognostic score (GPS) in patients with metastatic breast cancer. Br J Cancer. 2006;94(2):227-30. Epub 2006/01/13.

[28] Motzer RJ, Mazumdar M, Bacik J, Berg W, Amsterdam A, Ferrara J. Survival and prognostic stratification of 670 patients with advanced renal cell carcinoma. J Clin Oncol. 1999;17(8):2530-40. Epub 1999/11/24.

[29] Richman SD, Seymour MT, Chambers P, Elliott F, Daly CL, Meade AM, et al. KRAS and BRAF mutations in advanced colorectal cancer are associated with poor progno-

sis but do not preclude benefit from oxaliplatin or irinotecan: results from the MRC FOCUS trial. J Clin Oncol. 2009;27(35):5931-7. Epub 2009/11/04.

[30] Long GV, Menzies AM, Nagrial AM, Haydu LE, Hamilton AL, Mann GJ, et al. Prognostic and clinicopathologic associations of oncogenic BRAF in metastatic melanoma. J Clin Oncol. 2011;29(10):1239-46. Epub 2011/02/24.

[31] Slamon DJ, Clark GM, Wong SG, Levin WJ, Ullrich A, McGuire WL. Human breast cancer: correlation of relapse and survival with amplification of the HER-2/neu oncogene. Science. 1987;235(4785):177-82. Epub 1987/01/09.

[32] McMenamin ME, Soung P, Perera S, Kaplan I, Loda M, Sellers WR. Loss of PTEN expression in paraffin-embedded primary prostate cancer correlates with high Gleason score and advanced stage. Cancer Res. 1999;59(17):4291-6. Epub 1999/09/15.

[33] de Bono JS, Scher HI, Montgomery RB, Parker C, Miller MC, Tissing H, et al. Circulating tumor cells predict survival benefit from treatment in metastatic castration-resistant prostate cancer. Clin Cancer Res. 2008;14(19):6302-9. Epub 2008/10/03.

[34] Cristofanilli M, Hayes DF, Budd GT, Ellis MJ, Stopeck A, Reuben JM, et al. Circulating tumor cells: a novel prognostic factor for newly diagnosed metastatic breast cancer. J Clin Oncol. 2005;23(7):1420-30. Epub 2005/03/01.

[35] Cohen SJ, Punt CJ, Iannotti N, Saidman BH, Sabbath KD, Gabrail NY, et al. Relationship of circulating tumor cells to tumor response, progression-free survival, and overall survival in patients with metastatic colorectal cancer. J Clin Oncol. 2008;26(19):3213-21. Epub 2008/07/02.

[36] Arkenau HT, Barriuso J, Olmos D, Ang JE, de Bono J, Judson I, et al. Prospective validation of a prognostic score to improve patient selection for oncology phase I trials. J Clin Oncol. 2009;27(16):2692-6. Epub 2009/04/01.

[37] Stavraka C, Pinato DJ, Turnbull SJ, Flynn MJ, Forster MD, O'Cathail SM, et al. Developing an objective marker to optimize patient selection and predict survival benefit in early-phase cancer trials. Cancer. 2014;120(2):262-70. Epub 2014/01/09.

[38] Arkenau HT, Olmos D, Ang JE, de Bono J, Judson I, Kaye S. Clinical outcome and prognostic factors for patients treated within the context of a phase I study: the Royal Marsden Hospital experience. Br J Cancer. 2008;98(6):1029-33. Epub 2008/03/20.

[39] Chau NG, Florescu A, Chan KK, Wang L, Chen EX, Bedard P, et al. Early mortality and overall survival in oncology phase I trial participants: can we improve patient selection? BMC cancer. 2011;11:426. Epub 2011/10/07.

[40] Fussenich LM, Desar IM, Peters ME, Teerenstra S, van der Graaf WT, Timmer-Bonte JN, et al. A new, simple and objective prognostic score for phase I cancer patients. Eur J Cancer. 2011;47(8):1152-60. Epub 2011/03/01.

[41] Garrido-Laguna I, Janku F, Vaklavas C, Falchook GS, Fu S, Hong DS, et al. Validation of the Royal Marsden Hospital prognostic score in patients treated in the Phase I

Clinical Trials Program at the MD Anderson Cancer Center. Cancer. 2012;118(5): 1422-8. Epub 2011/08/09.

[42] Olmos D, A'Hern R P, Marsoni S, Morales R, Gomez-Roca C, Verweij J, et al. Patient selection for oncology phase I trials: a multi-institutional study of prognostic factors. J Clin Oncol. 2012;30(9):996-1004. Epub 2012/02/23.

[43] Hyman DM, Eaton AA, Gounder MM, Smith GL, Pamer EG, Hensley ML, et al. Nomogram to predict cycle-one serious drug-related toxicity in phase I oncology trials. J Clin Oncol. 2014;32(6):519-26. Epub 2014/01/15.

[44] Ploquin A, Olmos D, Ferte C, Cassier PA, Kramar A, Duhamel A, et al. Life-expectancy of patients enrolled in phase 1 clinical trials: a systematic review of published prognostic models. Critical reviews in oncology/hematology. 2012;83(2):242-8. Epub 2012/01/10.

[45] Janisch L, Mick R, Schilsky RL, Vogelzang NJ, O'Brien S, Kut M, et al. Prognostic factors for survival in patients treated in phase I clinical trials. Cancer. 1994;74(7): 1965-73. Epub 1994/10/01.

[46] Yamamoto N, Tamura T, Fukuoka M, Saijo N. Survival and prognostic factors in lung cancer patients treated in phase I trials: Japanese experience. Int J Oncol. 1999;15(4):737-41. Epub 1999/09/24.

[47] Bachelot T, Ray-Coquard I, Catimel G, Ardiet C, Guastalla JP, Dumortier A, et al. Multivariable analysis of prognostic factors for toxicity and survival for patients enrolled in phase I clinical trials. Ann Oncol. 2000;11(2):151-6. Epub 2000/04/13.

[48] Han C, Braybrooke JP, Deplanque G, Taylor M, Mackintosh D, Kaur K, et al. Comparison of prognostic factors in patients in phase I trials of cytotoxic drugs vs new noncytotoxic agents. Br J Cancer. 2003;89(7):1166-71. Epub 2003/10/02.

[49] Penel N, Vanseymortier M, Bonneterre ME, Clisant S, Dansin E, Vendel Y, et al. Prognostic factors among cancer patients with good performance status screened for phase I trials. Investigational new drugs. 2008;26(1):53-8. Epub 2007/09/25.

[50] Wheler J, Tsimberidou AM, Hong D, Naing A, Jackson T, Liu S, et al. Survival of patients in a Phase 1 Clinic: the M. D. Anderson Cancer Center experience. Cancer. 2009;115(5):1091-9. Epub 2009/01/24.

[51] Penel N, Delord JP, Bonneterre ME, Bachelot T, Ray-Coquard I, Blay JY, et al. Development and validation of a model that predicts early death among cancer patients participating in phase I clinical trials investigating cytotoxics. Investigational new drugs. 2010;28(1):76-82. Epub 2009/02/12.

[52] Gopal AK, Kahl BS, de Vos S, Wagner-Johnston ND, Schuster SJ, Jurczak WJ, et al. PI3Kdelta inhibition by idelalisib in patients with relapsed indolent lymphoma. N Engl J Med. 2014;370(11):1008-18. Epub 2014/01/24.

[53] McArthur GA, Chapman PB, Robert C, Larkin J, Haanen JB, Dummer R, et al. Safety and efficacy of vemurafenib in BRAF(V600E) and BRAF(V600K) mutation-positive melanoma (BRIM-3): extended follow-up of a phase 3, randomised, open-label study. The lancet oncology. 2014;15(3):323-32. Epub 2014/02/11.

[54] Mok TS, Wu YL, Thongprasert S, Yang CH, Chu DT, Saijo N, et al. Gefitinib or carboplatin-paclitaxel in pulmonary adenocarcinoma. N Engl J Med. 2009;361(10):947-57. Epub 2009/08/21.

[55] Shepherd FA, Rodrigues Pereira J, Ciuleanu T, Tan EH, Hirsh V, Thongprasert S, et al. Erlotinib in previously treated non-small-cell lung cancer. N Engl J Med. 2005;353(2):123-32. Epub 2005/07/15.

[56] Inoue A, Suzuki T, Fukuhara T, Maemondo M, Kimura Y, Morikawa N, et al. Prospective phase II study of gefitinib for chemotherapy-naive patients with advanced non-small-cell lung cancer with epidermal growth factor receptor gene mutations. J Clin Oncol. 2006;24(21):3340-6. Epub 2006/06/21.

[57] Voskoboynik M, Arkenau HT. Improving patient selection for phase I oncology trials. J Clin Oncol. 2014;32(28):3198-9. Epub 2014/07/30.

[58] Hamid O, Robert C, Daud A, Hodi FS, Hwu WJ, Kefford R, et al. Safety and tumor responses with lambrolizumab (anti-PD-1) in melanoma. N Engl J Med. 2013;369(2): 134-44. Epub 2013/06/04.

[59] Hodi FS, O'Day SJ, McDermott DF, Weber RW, Sosman JA, Haanen JB, et al. Improved survival with ipilimumab in patients with metastatic melanoma. N Engl J Med. 2010;363(8):711-23. Epub 2010/06/08.

[60] Bailey A, McDermott DF. Immune checkpoint inhibitors as novel targets for renal cell carcinoma therapeutics. Cancer J. 2013;19(4):348-52. Epub 2013/07/23.

[61] Eggermont AM, Kroemer G, Zitvogel L. Immunotherapy and the concept of a clinical cure. Eur J Cancer. 2013;49(14):2965-7. Epub 2013/07/31.

[62] Robert C, Thomas L, Bondarenko I, O'Day S, M DJ, Garbe C, et al. Ipilimumab plus dacarbazine for previously untreated metastatic melanoma. N Engl J Med. 2011;364(26):2517-26. Epub 2011/06/07.

# 2

# The Small Molecule Inhibitor of Protein Kinase Revolution for the Treatment of Rheumatoid Arthritis

Charles J. Malemud

## 1. Introduction

Targeted medical intervention for the treatment of rheumatoid arthritis (RA) has significantly revolutionized clinical outcomes for this autoimmune disease. Until the development of biological drugs which have the capacity to block the activity of most of the critical pro-inflammatory cytokines involved in RA as well as a host of immune cell-mediated events, the medical therapy of RA was limited to the use of first-line treatments including, non-steroidal anti-inflammatory drugs, sulphasalazine, and several immunosuppressive agents, such as glucocorticoids, prednisone and dexamethasone, methotrexate, and anti-malarial drugs (e.g. hydroxychloroquine) [1-5]. Agents that blocked the proliferation of T-lymphocytes, such as leflunomide, abatacept and/or B-lymphocytes (e.g. rituximab) were also employed, but mainly as second-line therapies [6-9].

The momentous development of additional biological drugs for RA arose through the identification of those pro-inflammatory cytokines that were intimately involved in initiating and perpetuating the RA process. Thus, blocking tumor necrosis factor-$\alpha$/tumor necrosis factor-$\alpha$ receptor, interleukin-1β (IL-1β) IL-1β receptor and IL-6/IL-6 Receptor/gp130 signaling pathways with either monoclonal antibodies or engineered fusion proteins prominently entered into the armamentarium for the medical therapy of RA [10-15].

However, what does all of this mean for the future development of additional novel therapies for this chronic and debilitating synovial joint disease? For one thing the revolution in new drug development implies that although additional cellular targets including vascular endothelial growth factor (VEGF), adhesion molecules (e.g. vascular cell adhesion molecule-1; VCAM-1; CD106) and chemokines (e.g. CXC, C, CX3C and their corresponding receptors, CXCR, CCCR, CR and CX3CR) [16-26] which fit securely into a system of well-orchestrated RA pathophysiologic processes in man have been validated through *in vitro* studies as well as from impressive clinical results and *ex vivo* cell analyses with rodent models of human RA. Although none of the CC chemokine receptor antagonists have thus far yielded drugs effective in a rheumatology clinical practice, there are CXCR4 small drug antagonists in clinical trials for cancer, human immunodeficiency virus and the rare WHIM immunodeficiency condition [27].

One aspect in the study of human RA progression revolves around successfully translating from "hypothesis" to experimental validation and then going forward to drug development. This advancement has occurred by recognizing the crucial role played by signal transduction pathways in perpetuating the inflammatory state of RA. Thus, signal transduction has also been identified as the crucial cellular pathway that can cause "apoptosis-resistance" resulting in the aberrant survival of activated T-lymphocytes, B-lymphocytes and synoviocytes in RA synovial tissue [28, 29]. Signal transduction has also been identified as playing a role in the elevated frequency of apoptotic chondrocytes in RA articular cartilage [30, 31]. In that regard, blocking the phosphorylation of specific protein kinases involved signal transduction was explored as a mechanism to not only restore the appropriate balance between cell survival and cell death, which is skewed towards cell survival in RA, but also for blocking those protein kinases involved in up-regulating pro-inflammatory cytokine and matrix metalloproteinase (MMP) gene expression that is so integral to perpetuating inflammation and therefore, the destruction of synovial joints in RA [32-36].

Over the past 8 years or so, we have extensively detailed the genesis of interest in, and the extent to which, kinase activity of mitogen-activated protein kinases (MAPK) and the phosphatidylinositide-3-kinase/AKT/mammalian target of rapamycin (mTOR) (PI3K/AKT/mTOR) pathways influence MMP gene expression and cell survival, respectively [37-41]. We and others have also focused attention on the Janus Kinase/Signal Transducers and Activators of Transcription (JAK/STAT) pathway which was identified and targeted for drug development in RA because JAK/STAT signaling was found to play a major role in RA by promoting pro-inflammatory cytokine gene expression and abnormal cell survival [42-48]. Thus, this latter research focus resulted in the first JAK3-selective small molecule inhibitor (SMI), tofactinib, for use in the treatment of RA [reviewed in 49, 50].

This chapter will critically analyze the current state of drug development for novel protein kinase SMIs for RA, including a brief update and perspective on newer JAK SMI, besides tofacitinib, which are likely to be the targets for future drug development as well as additional protein kinase targets for RA.

## 2. Newer JAK SMIs

There are 4 members of the JAK family: JAK1, JAK2, JAK3 and Tyk2 [51]. JAK1 and JAK3 bind constitutively to the cytoplasmic region of the common gamma chain of cytokine receptors. This domain is the common subunit for many cytokines involved in T-cell and natural killer cell development in addition to B-cell activation making JAK1/JAK3 pertinent targets for intervention in RA [47, 52]. In addition to the JAK3-selective SMI, tofacitinib [54], several other

JAK SMIs, with activity towards JAK 1 and JAK2, including baricitinib [55], CEP-33779 [55], INCB028050, PF-956980 [56, 57], filgotinib (INCB-039110), decernotinib, ruxolitinib, pefcitinib, ABT-494, INCB 047986 and AC-410 [58] are currently in various stages of preclinical testing and/or clinical assessment for altering the clinical course of RA, organ transplant rejection and psoriasis [59].

It has been widely held that JAK1 and JAK3 are essentially regulated by specific tyrosine sites within their respective activation loops [60], including the $NH_2$-terminal kinase domain [45]. As such the activity of both JAK1 and JAK3 need be blocked to ensure inhibition of IL-2-induced STAT5 activation [47]. This assertion is bolstered by evidence that JAK1 has a dominant role over JAK3 [61] likely making selective ATP-competitive JAK3 inhibitors less effective by themselves at the cellular level. Thus, the targeting of suppressor of cytokine signaling as a means to suppress JAK/STAT signaling [45, 62, 63] is also being investigated for its potential to block cytokine-mediated STAT activation.

## 3. Update on tofacitinib — 2014

The approval of tofacitinib by the United States Food & Drug Administration in 2012 for the treatment of moderate-severe RA has paved the way for the development of other JAK inhibitor compounds [64, 65]. The clinical data emerging from 4 Phase II and 4 Phase III RA clinical trials involving tofacitinib was recently summarized [Malemud CJ: Submitted]. In the Phase III RA trials where tofacitinib was compared to placebo a significant American College of Rheumatology-20 (ACR20) response was consistently demonstrated in the tofacitinib arm together with an improvement in the Health Assessment Questionnaire Disability Index and ACR50 response after 3 months of treatment with tofacitinib [66]. Most critically, these Phase III trials demonstrated that the clinical efficacy of tofacitinib was similar to the clinical responses achieved with the TNF inhibitor, adalimumab. Several common adverse events observed in these clinical trials were associated with the tofacitinib group and raised some concerns. This included an increase in the incidence of infections, infestations and creatinine along with an increase in the LDL-cholesterol/HDL-cholesterol ratio and decreased neutrophil counts. However, a recent meta-analysis of various RA clinical trials involving tofacitinib concluded that the frequency of adverse events was not increased by tofacitinib [67].

In another clinical trial where the clinical efficacy of tofacitinib was compared to methotrexate [68], 3 cases of confirmed lymphoma in 5 patients receiving tofacitinib compared to 1 subject in the methotrexate arm was reported. However, the ACR70 response was greater in the tofacitinib group compared to methotrexate, but the mean change in number of bone erosions in both the tofacitinib and methotrexate groups was modest. Importantly the subjects receiving tofacitinib had less cartilage loss at 6, 12 and 24 months of treatment.

Malemud and Blumenthal [50] recently reviewed the variety of cellular mechanisms that have been shown to be altered by tofacitinib which likely contributed to the clinical efficacy of the drug in human RA clinical trials, including the relative selectivity of tofacitinib for JAK1 and JAK3 over JAK2 in ameliorating the severity of arthritis in the rat-adjuvant model [69] as well as data showing that multiple cytokines and signaling pathways in addition to JAK/STAT were inhibited by tofacitinib at effective clinical doses which was distinct from conventional disease-modifying antirheumatic drugs [70].

Although it is expected that the efficacy of tofacitinib in rheumatology clinical practice will have to be continuously monitored, tofacitinib will likely emerge as an important option for RA patients who inadequately respond to low-dose glucocorticoids, methotrexate and the several biologic drugs that are now routinely prescribed for the management of moderate-to-severe RA [50, 71, 72].

## 4. Selective JAK inhibitors in development

### 4.1. Baricitinib

Baricitinib (alternatively known as 1187594-09-7; INCB028050; UNII-ISP444213Y; LY3009104; LY-3009104 (Figure 1) [72] is a novel orally administered JAK inhibitor compound with relative selectivity for JAK1 and JAK2 [74]. In a study conducted among normal volunteers, baricitinib showed a dose-linear and time variant pharmacokinetics with low oral-dose clearance (i.e. 17L/h) and minimal systematic accumulation. Baricitinib also inhibited STAT3 phosphorylation in whole blood *ex vivo*, the results of which correlated with plasma concentrations of the drug. Although baricitinib was well-tolerated with negligible adverse events, the expected reduction in neutrophil counts was also recorded [75].

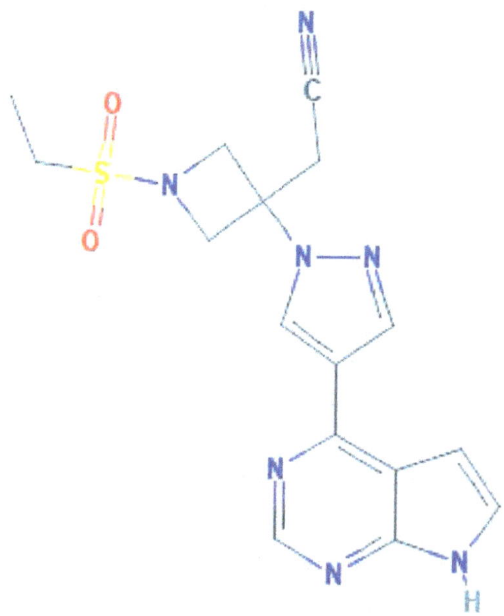

**Figure 1.** The chemical structure (IUPAC Name) of 2-[1-ethylsulfonyl-3-[4-(7H-pyrrolo[2,3-d]pyrimidin-4-yl)pyrazol-1-yl]azetidin-3-yl]acetonitrile (Baricitinib) [73]

## 4.2. Decernotinib

Decernotinib (Figure 2) alternatively known as VX-509, is an orally administered selective JAK3 inhibitor compound which is being evaluated for the possible medical management of RA [58, 76]. In a recently completed study the results of which were reported at the 2014 European League Against Rheumatism (EULAR) annual meeting, the pharmacologic activity of decernotinib was compared to tofacitinib, filgotinib (GLPG 0634) and baricitinib with reference to the blockade of several cytokine signaling pathways in whole blood cell cultures from normal subjects. The cytokine pathways evaluated were the type I and type II interferon (i.e. INF$\alpha$ and INF$\gamma$) pathways, the common $\gamma$ chain cytokine pathways involving IL-15 and IL-21, and the IL-6 and IL-27-mediated signaling [77]. Although the results of this study showed that each of the JAK inhibitor compounds were relatively similar to each other in terms of their ability to block INF$\alpha$ and INF$\gamma$, IL-15, IL-21, IL-6 and IL-27 signaling, tofacitinib and baricitinib were more potent than decernotinib and filgotinib. Of note, these JAK inhibitor compounds exhibited lesser activity towards IL-10, IL-12, IL-23 and erythropoietin, which also signal via JAK/STAT [45]. Moreover, the results of the *ex vivo* studies evaluating the effect of these JAK inhibitor compounds on inhibition of cytokine signaling showed that they had markedly similar activities at clinically relevant doses.

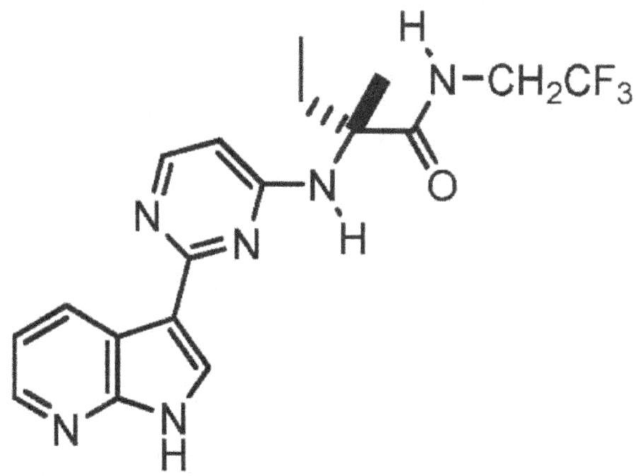


**Figure 2.** The chemical structure (IUPAC Name) of disodium N2-[2-(1H-Pyrrolo[2,3-pyridin-3-yl)pyrimidin-4-yl]-N-(2,2,2-trifluoroethyl)-D-isovalinamide (Decernotinib) [76]

A recently completed 24-week randomized, placebo-controlled, double-blind, phase II study compared 4 dosing regimens of orally administered decernotinib given to 358 active RA patients, measured by increased C-reactive protein levels and in RA patients with at least 6 swollen and 6 tender joints who had an inadequate clinical response to methotrexate [78]. After 24 weeks, the clinical response to decernotinib was statistically significant by ACR20, ACR50 and ACR70 criteria and by positive changes in the Disease Activity Score-28 outcomes measure. However, the percentage of patients with any adverse event was higher in the decernotinib arm relative to placebo (i.e. a stable dose of methotrexate) which led to 9.1% of patients in the decernotinib group and 8.5 patients in the placebo group, respectively, to discontinue treatment. Of note, safety profiles were comparable across all dosage levels of decernotinib.

## 5. Compounds that inhibit TyK2

Tyrosine kinase-2 (TyK2) is the fourth member of the Janus kinase family. However, the development of TyK2-selective SMIs has lagged significantly behind the development of SMIs with activity against the other 3 members of the JAK family [79, 80]. Thus, this remains an ongoing controversy for developing additional small compounds for RA despite the purported critical importance of TyK2 in driving IL-12-related cytokine IL-23 signaling which plays a key role in RA [81, 82].

In RA IL-23 is widely recognized as a key cytokine because of its role in perpetuating the inflammatory response as well as its involvement in the development of the IL-17-producing $T_H17$ T-cell subset, the latter developing as a distinct T-cell lineage apart from the cytokine-producing $T_H1$ and $T_H2$ T-cells [82]. Although the IL-23 receptor was the initial potential target for intervention in RA, inflammatory bowel disease, psoriasis and multiple sclerosis [83], a few laboratories focused on designing and synthesizing diamino 1, 2, 4 triazole compounds which could potentially demonstrate differential inhibition of TyK2 and JAKs 1-3 [81] or small molecule compounds such as APY0201 which was reported to directly inhibit IL-23 production [84].

Until recently, there were no patents filed for the design or production of selective TyK2 inhibitors. In that regard, both tofacitinib and one other small molecule compound, CMP6, failed to markedly inhibit TyK2. However, results with another small molecule compound, Cmpd1, showed some promise in preclinical analyses [85, 86]. For example, Qi et al. [87] recently demonstrated in human cervical cancer HeLa cells that apoptosis was enhanced after incubation of these cells with TNF-$\alpha$ but only if TNF-$\alpha$-induced heat shock protein (HSP)27 phosphorylation was suppressed by Cmpd1, or by MAPKAPK2 knockdown or by overexpression of a non-phosphorylatable HSP27 mutant, HSP27-3A. Thus, these results reported for Cmpd1 could indicate a role for TyK2 inhibition as influencing apoptosis in HeLa which may be useful to "cure" the apoptosis-resistance characteristic of RA synovial tissue [88]. However, in that study, HSP27 phosphorylation also facilitated TNF-$\alpha$ ubiquitination and phosphorylation of TAK1 as well as activation of p38 MAPK and ERK, the TAK1 pro-survival pathway downstream of p38 MAPK and ERK. Therefore, the extent to which further development of TyK2 small molecule inhibitor compounds such as Cmpd1 go forward will likely depend on its capacity to alter arthritis severity in rodent animal models of RA which will be solely dependent on the design and successful synthesis of selective TyK2 SMIs.

## 6. The spleen tyrosine Kinase (SyK) inhibitor, fostamatinib

SyK and the $\zeta$-chain associated protein-70 (ZAP-70) are non-receptor kinases which are preferentially produced by hemopoietic cells of the spleen, mast cells, polymorphonuclear leukocytes and macrophages [89]. In the context of adaptive immunity relevant to RA, Syk and ZAP-70 are major components in T-cell and B-cell receptor signaling [90]. Based on those findings, Syk was considered to be a promising target for RA primarily because of its involvement in regulating, not only T-cell and B-cell proliferation as well as those proliferating cells with the F$\gamma$-activating receptor, but also in mediating immunoreceptor signaling by inflammatory cells and in signaling pathways regulated by immune complexes [91, 92].

Several years ago, Pine et al [93] showed that R788, which is the prodrug of the novel SyK SMI, R406, suppressed the severity of arthritis in collagen-induced arthritis (CIA), a well-validated mouse model of human RA. In addition to the finding that R788 showed significant clinical efficacy in mouse CIA, several surrogate molecules known to play important roles in inflammatory arthritis, namely the CXCR2 ligand KC-GRO-$\alpha$, macrophage chemoattractant protein-1, IL-1 and IL-6 were also reduced in mice with CIA treated with R788 compared to the vehicle control. Of note, the release of cartilage oligomeric matrix protein (COMP), a biomarker of extracellular matrix degradation in articular cartilage, was also suppressed by R788 suggesting a possible chondroprotective effect of R788.

More recent studies have been conducted to assess the pharmacokinetic/pharmacodynamic (PKPD) of R788, alternatively known as Fostamatinib disodium; R935788; R 935788 sodium; FosD, tamatinib fosdium (Figure 3) [94]. Results of these studies revealed that the converted form of the drug, R406, exhibited a PKPD relationship with changes in blood pressure [95]. Thus, the PKPD analysis revealed a concentration-dependent increase in blood pressure with increasing concentrations of R406. Nevertheless Baloum et al. [96] showed that R406 was rapidly absorbed with a terminal $t_{1/2}$ of 12-21 hrs. Furthermore, the solid dosage forms of fostamatinib provided a drug administration regimen whereby fostamatinib could be administered once daily or twice daily to achieve therapeutic levels of the drug.

What additional parameters of adaptive immunity were found to be altered by fostamatinib? Although R406 reduced the responsiveness of dendritic cells to immune complexes administered to mice, R406 did not reduce specific CD4$^{+}$T-cell proliferation in these mice after immunization with these immune complexes [97]. However, R406 did reduce the interactions that occur between dendritic cells and antigen-specific CD4$^{+}$T-cells. This resulted in reduced proliferation of these antigen-specific CD4$^{+}$T-cells compared mice treated with the vehicle control. This change in antigen-specific CD4$^{+}$T-cell proliferation in response to R406 was also characterized by a reduction in the level of several T-cell co-stimulatory biomarkers, namely, inducible T-cell co-stimulator and PD-1 as well as diminished production of the pro-inflammatory cytokines, INF-$\gamma$ and IL-17. Taken together, these *ex vivo* results provided additional support for the indication that inhibiting SyK activity with fostamatinib could be an effective drug therapy to eliminate FcR-driven CD4$^{+}$T-cells responses in RA.

So how did fostamatinib fare in RA clinical trials? The results of several RA clinical trials assessed the clinical efficacy of fostamatinib [98, 99]. Thus, Taylor et al. [98] reported that treatment of moderate-severe RA subjects with fostamatinib improved the DAS-28/C-reactive protein (CRP) score from baseline versus placebo injection at 6 wks at 2 dosage regimens: 100 mg twice daily for 24 wks plus placebo injection every 2 wks and 100 mg twice daily for 4 wks, followed by 150 mg once daily up to wk 24. However, DAS-28/CRP failed to improve when

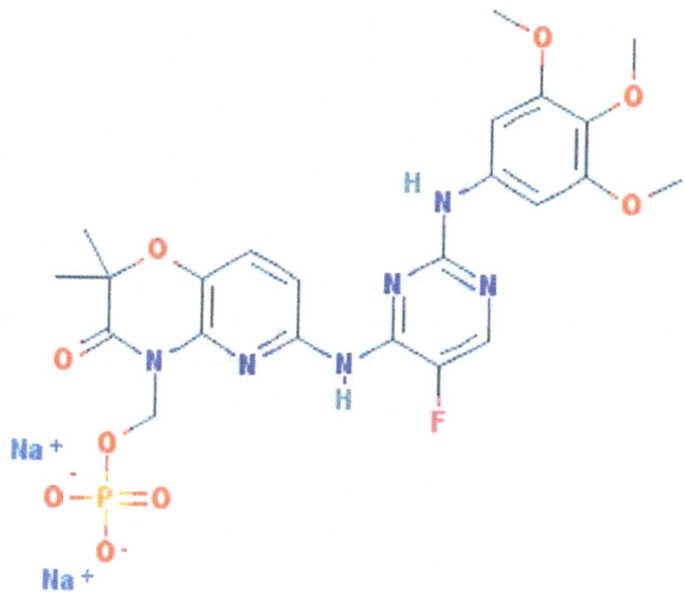

**Figure 3.** The chemical structure (IUPAC Name) of [6-[[5-fluoro-2-(3,4,5-trimethoxyanilino)pyrimidin-4-yl]amino]-2,2-dimethyl-3-oxopyrido[3,2-b][1,4]oxazin-4-yl]methyl phosphate (Fostamatinib Sodium) [94]

fostamatinib was administered at 100 mg twice daily for 4 wks, then 100 mg once daily up to wk 24. Most critically, in a comparator analysis, fostamatinib was less effective than the TNF-$\alpha$ blocker, adalimumab, at wk 24 based on the DAS-28/CRP criteria. The most common adverse effects of fostamatinib in this clinical trial were similar to those previously reported which included increased hypertension and diarrhea. Thus, although fostamatinib demonstrated significant clinical efficacy when employed as a monotherapy using DAS-28/CRP criteria at 6 wks, fostamatinib was inferior to adalimumab at wk 24.

Three additional RA clinical trials measured the effectiveness of fostamatinib on subchondral bone erosions using the modified total Sharp score as an indicator of whether inhibition of SyK retarded the destruction of subchondral bone over a period of 6 months. ACR response criteria were also measured [99]. Once again, hypertension was the most relevant adverse event affecting 40% of fostamatinib-treated subjects with other common negative responses, including, diarrhea, neutropenia and increased hepatic enzyme levels. Some of the fostamatinib-treated RA subjects also developed infections. Most critically, although RA subjects treated with fostamatinib showed a positive clinical response by ACR criteria, none of the 3 clinical trials revealed any significant effects on erosive bone damage over the 6 months of treatment.

Although SyK was shown to play an influential role in regulating the aberrant proliferation of several immune cell types critical to the RA process *in vitro* and *ex vivo*, the results of several RA clinical trials with fostamatinib were not impressive enough to warrant further development of this SyK SMI for RA.

## 7. A perspective on the future development of protein kinase SMIs for RA

The current state of affairs regarding the future development of additional protein kinase small molecule compounds for the treatment of RA should arise from the paradigm employed that ultimately led to the US FDA approving tofacitinib for moderate-to-severe RA. An assessment of the extent to which tofacitinib would be regularly prescribed for the treatment of RA recently concluded that most-marketing surveillance data will ultimately determine the extent to which tofacitinib will only be used to treat RA patients with inadequate responses to conventional DMARDs and/or the several types of biologic drugs now available to treat RA or whether tofacitinib will be employed as a first-line therapy for RA [50]. Although this assertion appears to have some validity based on the current thinking by rheumatologists regarding the use of tofacitinib, decisions must be made by the biopharmaceutical industry as to whether to develop other JAK SMIs for future therapy of autoimmune diseases. Some of these newer small molecule compounds were shown to inhibit JAK1 and JAK3, whereas others may be designed to selectively inhibit JAK2. In that respect, the structure of the JAK3 enzyme may be instructive (Figure 4). It was recently pointed out that tofacitinib was originally introduced as a JAK3-selective SMI, but in reality tofacitinib also inhibits JAK1 and JAK2 [100]. In addition, Chrencik et al. [101] indicated that computational analysis comparing tofacitinib with the TyK2 SMI, CMP-6, showed that kinome-selectivity will be a challenge as a consequence of the overall similarities in structure between JAKs 1-3 and TyK2, as well as the fact that the JAK3 SMI binds to the ATP-binding cavities in an orientation which is similar to JAK1 and JAK2. Therefore, the jury is still out, so to speak, as to whether or not immune-mediated inflammation and other pathophysiologic abnormalities associated with aberrant JAK/STAT signaling in RA can be regulated by focusing on developing a JAK SMI specific for a single member of the JAK family or whether small molecule compounds which are designed to inhibit more than one JAK form would be a more effective RA therapy.

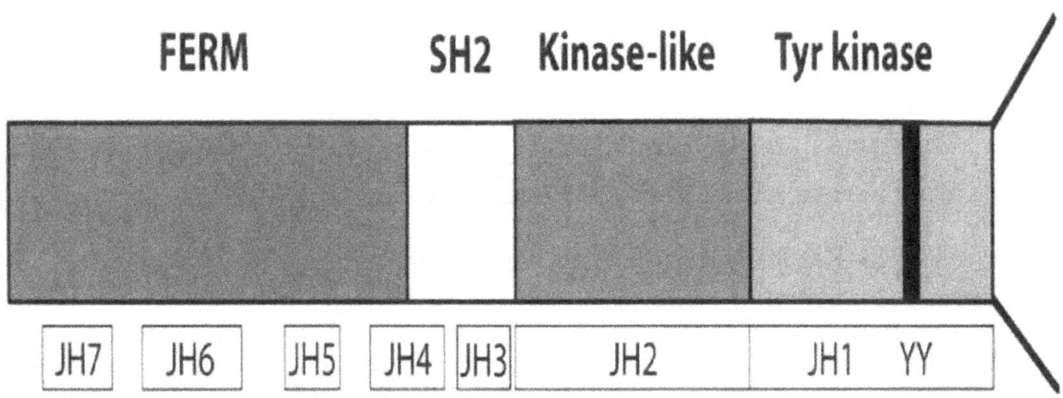


**Figure 4.** The JH domains and phosphorylation sites of JAK3 [45]

The drug armamentarium for treating RA now include, immunosupressants such as methotrexate, as well as immunomodulatory drugs which block TNF-$\alpha$, anti-IL-1, and T-and B-cell activation among other pathways. Therefore the extent to which JAK and/or SyK inhibitors will be employed with equal footing to these well-established drugs with clinical efficacy for RA remains to be determined.

Then there is a host of data that supports a role for other protein kinases in the RA process. However, it can be stated at this time that the results of preclinical and RA clinical trials analyses are more compelling for developing small molecule compounds to inhibit TyK2 than SyK.

Recently, we pointed out that in addition to JAK, TyK2 and SyK, it may be prudent for investigators to consider the role that abnormalities play in other signal transduction pathways associated with RA as future targets for therapeutic intervention [40]. The data supporting a robust level of "cross-talk" between several signaling pathways that contribute to cytokine, matrix metalloproteinase, pro-apoptosis and anti-apoptosis gene expression is well-proven [28, 29, 35, 40, 41] and should be taken into account. In that regard, aberrations found in RA in the PI3K/Akt/mTOR pathway, transforming growth factor kinase-1, bone marrow kinase, nuclear factor κB-inducing kinase and Bruton's tyrosine kinase could become a focus of future small molecule inhibitor drug development.

## Author details

Charles J. Malemud*

Address all correspondence to: cjm4@cwru.edu

Department of Medicine, Division of Rheumatic Diseases, Case Western Reserve University, School of Medicine, Cleveland, Ohio, USA

## References

[1] Feely MG, Erickson A, O'Dell JR. Therapeutic options for rheumatoid arthritis. Expert Opin Pharmacother 2009 10(13) 2095-2106.

[2] Upchurch KS, Kay J. Evolution of treatment for rheumatoid arthritis. Rheumatology (Oxford) 2012; 51 Suppl 6 vi28-vi36.

[3] Taherian E, Rao A, Malemud CJ, Askari A. The biological and clinical activity of anti-malarial drugs in autoimmune disorders. Curr Rheum Rev 2013 9(1) 45-62.

[4] Braun J. Methotrexate: optimizing the efficacy in rheumatoid arthritis. Ther Adv Musculoskelet Dis 2011; 3(3) 151-158.

[5] Kumar P, Banik S. Pharmacotherapy options in rheumatoid arthritis. Clin Med Insights Arthritis Musculoskelet Disord 2013; 6 35-43.

[6] Finckh A, Dehler S, Gabay C. The effectiveness of leflunomide as a co-therapy of tumor necrosis factor inhibitors in rheumatoid arthritis; a population-based study. Ann Rheum Dis 2009; 68(1) 33-39.

[7] Meier FM, Frerix M, Hermann W, Müller-Ladner U. Current immunotherapy in rheumatoid arthritis. Immunotherapy 2013; 5(9): 955-974.

[8] Gibbons LJ, Hyrich KL. Biologic therapy for rheumatoid arthritis; clinical efficacy and predictors of response. Biodrugs 2009; 23(2) 111-124.

[9] Östör AJ. Abatacept: a T-cell co-stimulation modulator for the treatment of rheumatoid arthritis. Clin Rheumatol 2008; 27 (11) 1343-1353.

[10] Astry B, Harberts E, Moudgil KD. A cytokine-centric view of the pathogenesis and treatment of autoimmune arthritis. J Interferon Cytokine Res 2011; 31(12) 927-940.

[11] Mertens M, Singh JA. Anakinra for rheumatoid arthritis: a systematic review. J Rheumatol 2009; 36(6) 1118-1125.

[12] Tanaka T, Kishimoto T. Immunotherapy of tocilizumab for rheumatoid arthritis. J Clin Cell Immunol 2013; S6 001

[13] Malemud CJ. Targeted drug development for rheumatoid arthritis. Future Med Chem 2012; 4(6) 701-703

[14] Taylor PC. Pharmacology of TNF blockade in rheumatoid arthritis and other chronic inflammatory diseases. Curr Opin Pharmacol 2010; 10(3) 308-315.

[15] Geyer M, Müller-Ladner U. Actual status of antiinterleukin-1 therapies in rheumatic diseases. Curr Opin Rheumatol 2010; 22(3) 246-251.

[16] Giatromanolaki A, Sivridis E, Athanassou N et al. The angiogenic pathway 'vascular endothelial growth factor/flk-1(KDR)-receptor' in rheumatoid arthritis. J Pathol 2001; 194(1) 101-108.

[17] Malemud CJ, Reddy SK. Targeting cytokines, chemokines and adhesion molecules in rheumatoid arthritis. Curr Rheum Rev 2008; 4 219-234.

[18] Agawal SK, Brenner MB. Role of adhesion molecules in human synovial inflammation. Curr Opin Rheumatol 2006; 18(3) 268-276.

[19] Szekanecz Z, Koch AE. Vascular endothelium and immune responses: implications for inflammation and angiogenesis. Rheum Dis Clin North Am 2004; 30(1) 97-114.

[20] Lee DM, Kiener HP, Agarwal SK et al. Cadherin-11 in synovial lining formation and pathology in arthritis. Science 2007; 315(5814) 1006-1010.

[21] Haringman JJ, Kraan MC, Smeets TJM, Zwinderman KH, Tak PP. Chemokine blockade and chronic inflammatory disease: proof of concept in patients with rheumatoid arthritis. Ann Rheum Dis 2003; 62(8) 715-721.

[22] Haringman JJ, Gerlag DM, Smeets TJM et al. A randomized controlled trial with anti-CCL2 (anti-monocyte chemotactic protein-1) monoclonal antibody in patients with rheumatoid arthritis. Arthritis Rheum 2006; 54(8) 2387-2392.

[23] Liu J, Merritt JR. CC chemokine receptor small molecule antagonists in the treatment of rheumatoid arthritis and other diseases: a current view. Curr Top Med Chem 201; 10(13) 1250-1267.

[24] White GE, Iqbal AJ, Greaves DR. CC chemokine receptors and chronic inflammation—therapeutic opportunities and pharmacological challenges. Pharmacol Rev 2013; 65(1) 47-89.

[25] Ellingsen T, Hansen I, Thorsen J et al. Upregulated baseline plasma CCL19 and CCR7 cell-surface expression on monocytes in early rheumatoid arthritis normalized during treatment and CCL19 correlated with radiographic progression. Scand J Rheumatol 2014; 43(2) 91-100

[26] Antonelli A, Ferrari SM, Giuggioli D, Ferrannini E, Ferri C, Fallahi P. Chemokine (C-X-C motif) ligand (CXCL) 10 in autoimmune diseases. Autoimmun Rev 2014; 13(3) 272-280.

[27] Debnath B, Xu S, Grande S, Garofalo A, Neamati N. Small molecule inhibitors of CXCR4. Theranostics 2013; 3(1) 47-75.

[28] Wylie MA, Malemud CJ. Perspective: Deregulation of apoptosis in arthritis by altered signal transduction. Int J Clin Rheumatol 2013; 8(4) 483-490.

[29] Malemud CJ. Intracellular signaling pathways in rheumatoid arthritis. J Clin Cell Immunol 2013; 4 160.

[30] Korb A, Pavenstädt H, Pap T. Cell death in rheumatoid arthritis. Apoptosis 2009; 14(4) 447-454.

[31] Malemud CJ, Sun Y, Pearlman E, Ginley NM, Awadallah A, Wisler BA et al. Monosodium urate and tumor necrosis factor-$\alpha$ increase apoptosis in human chondrocyte cultures. Rheumatology (Sunnyvale) 2012; 2 113.

[32] Chang L, Karin M. Mammalian MAP kinase signaling cascades. Nature 2001; 410(6824) 37-40.

[33] Burrage PS, Mix KS, Brinckerhoff CE. Matrix metalloproteinases : role in arthritis. Front Biosci 2006; 11 529-543.

[34] Wu T, Mohan C. The AKT axis as a therapeutic target in autoimmune diseases. Endocr Metab Immune Disord Drug Targets 2009; 9(2) 145-150.

[35] Malemud CJ. The discovery of novel experimental therapies for inflammatory arthritis. Mediators Inflamm 2009; 698769.

[36] Malemud CJ. Regulation of chondrocyte matrix metalloproteinase gene expression. 2014; In: Dhalia NS, Chakraborti S (Editors) Role of Proteases in Health and Disease. Springer Science, UK.

[37] Malemud CJ. Small molecular weight inhibitors of stress-activated and mitogen-activated protein kinases. Mini Rev Med Chem 2006; 6(6) 689-698.

[38] Malemud CJ: Inhibitors of stress-activated/mitogen-activated protein kinase pathways. Curr Opin Pharmacol 2007; 7(3) 339-343.

[39] Malemud CJ. Defining novel targets for intervention in rheumatoid arthritis: An overview. Curr Rheum Rev 2008; 4 214-218.

[40] Malemud CJ. Dysfunctional immune-mediated inflammation in rheumatoid arthritis dictates that development of anti-rheumatic disease drugs target multiple intracellular signaling pathways. Anti-Inflammatory Anti-Allergy Agents Med Chem 2011; 10(2) 78-84.

[41] Wisler BA, Dennis JE, Malemud CJ. New organ-specific pharmacological strategies interfering with signaling pathways in inflammatory disorders/autoimmune disorders. Curr Signal Transduct Ther 2011; 6 279-291.

[42] Yokota A, Narazaki N, Shima Y et al. Preferential and persistent activation of the STAT1 pathway in rheumatoid synovial fluid cells. J Rheumatol 2001; 28(9) 1952-1959.

[43] Kasperkovitz PV, Verbeet NL, Smeets TJ et al. Activation of the STAT1 pathway in rheumatoid arthritis. Ann Rheum Dis 2004; 63(3) 233-239.

[44] Walker JG, Ahern MG, Coleman M et al. Characterisation of a dendritic cell subset in synovial tissue which strongly expresses Jak/STAT transcription factors from patients with rheumatoid arthritis. Ann Rheum Dis 2007; 66(8) 992-999.

[45] Malemud CJ, Pearlman E. Targeting JAK/STAT signaling pathway in inflammatory diseases. Curr Signal Transduct Ther 2009; 4 201-221.

[46] Malemud CJ. Differential activation of JAK enzymes in rheumatoid arthritis and autoimmune disorders by proinflammatory cytokines – potential drug targets. Int J Interferon Cytokine Mediator Res 2010; 2 97-111.

[47] Malemud CJ. Suppression of pro-inflammatory cytokines via targeting of STAT-responsive genes. 2013; In: El-Shemy H (Editor), Drug Discovery. InTech, Croatia.

[48] Laurence A, Pesu M, Silvennoinen O, O'Shea J. JAK kinases in health and disease. An update. Open Rheumatol J 2012; 6 232-244.

[49] Malemud CJ. Inhibitors of JAK for the treatment of rheumatoid arthritis: Rationale and clinical data. Clin Invest 2012; 2 39-47.

[50] Malemud CJ, Blumenthal DE: Protein kinase small molecule inhibitors for rheumatoid arthritis: Medicinal chemistry/Clinical perspectives. World J Orthopedics: 2014; 5(4) 496-503.

[51] Cutulo M, Meroni M. Clinical utility of the oral JAK inhibitor tofacitinib in the treatment of rheumatoid arthritis. J Inflamm Res 2013; 6: 129-136.

[52] Thoma G, Nuninger F, Falchetto R, Hermes E, Tavares GA, Vangrevelinghe E et al. Identification of a potent Janus kinase 3 inhibitor with high selectivity within the Janus kinase family. J Med Chem 2011; 54(1) 284-288.

[53] Smolen JS, van der Heijde D, Machold KP, Aletaha D, Landewé R. Proposal for a new nomenclature of disease-modifying antirheumatic drugs. Ann Rheum Dis 2014; 73(1) 3-5.

[54] Vafadari R, Weimar W, Baan CC. Phosphospecific flow cytometry for pharmacodynamic drug monitoring: analysis iof the JAK-STAT signaling pathway. Clin Chim Acta 2012; 413(17-18) 1398-1405.

[55] Stump KL, Lu LD, Dobrzanski P, Serdikoff C, Gingrich DE, Dugan BJ et al. A highly selective, orally active inhibitor of Janus kinase 2, CEP-33779, ablates disease in 2 mouse models of rheumatoid arthritis. Arthritis Res Ther 2011; 13(2) R68.

[56] Fridman JS, Scherle PA, Collins R, Burn TC, Li Y, Covington MB et al. Selective inhibition of JAK1 and JAK2 is efficacious in rodent models of arthritis: preclinical characterization of INCB028050. J Immunol 2010; 184(9) 5298-5307.

[57] Migita K, Izumi Y, Torigoshi T, Satomura K, Izumi M, Nishino Y et al. Inhibition of Janus kinase/signal transducer and activator of transcription (JAK/STAT) signalling pathway in rheumatoid synovial fibroblasts using small molecule compounds. Clin Exp Immunol 2013 174(3) 356-363.

[58] Norman P. Selective JAK inhibitors in development for rheumatoid arthritis. Expert Opin Investig Drugs 2014; 23(8) 1067-1077.

[59] Hsu L, Armstrong AW. JAK inhibitors: treatment efficacy and safety profile in patients with psoriasis. J Immunol Res 2014; 2014 283617.

[60] Liu KD, Gaffen SL, Goldsmith MA, Greene WC. Janus kinases in interleukin-2 mediated signaling: JAK1 and JAK3 are differentially regulated by tyrosine phosphorylation. Curr Biol 1997; 7(11) 817-826.

[61] Haan C, Rolvering C, Raulf F, Kapp M, Drückes P, Thomas G et al. Jak1 has a dominant role over Jak3 in signal transduction through $\gamma$c-containing cytokine receptors. Chem Biol 2011; 18(3) 314-323.

[62] O'Sullivan LA, Liongue C, Lewis RS, Stephenson SE, Ward AC. Cytokine receptor signaling through the Jak-Stat-Socs pathway in disease. Mol Immunol 2007; 44(10) 2497-2506.

[63] Himpe E, Kooijman R. Insulin-like growth factor-1 receptor signal transduction and the Janus Kinase/Signal Transducer and Activator of Transcription (JAK-STAT) pathway. Biofactors 2009; 35(1) 76-81.

[64] Vaddi K, Luchi M. JAK inhibition for the treatment of rheumatoid arthritis: a new era in oral DMARD therapy. Expert Opin Investig Drugs 2012; 21(7) 961-973.

[65] Dymock BW, See CS. Inhibitors of JAK2 and JAK3: an update on the patent literature 2010-2012. Expert Opin Ther Pat 2013; 23(4) 449-501.

[66] Kaur K, Kalra S, Kaushal S. Systematic review of tofacitinib: a new drug for the management of rheumatoid arthritis. Clin Ther 2014; 36(7) 1074-1086.

[67] Kawalec P, Mikrut A, Wiśniewska N, Pilic A. The effectiveness of tofacitinib: a novel Janus kinase inhibitor, in the treatment of rheumatoid arthritis: a systematic review and meta-analysis. Clin Rheumatol 2013; 32(10) 1415-1424.

[68] Lee FB, Fleischmann R, Hall S, Wilkinson B, Bradley JD, Gruben D et al. Tofacitinib versus methotrexate in rheumatoid arthritis. N Engl J Med 2014; 370(25) 2377-2386.

[69] Meyer DM, Jesson MI, Li X, Elrick MM, Funckes-Shippy CL, Warner JD et al. Anti-inflammatory activity and neutrophil reductions mediated by the JAK1/JAK3 inhibitor, CP690,550 in rat adjuvant-induced arthritis. J Inflamm (London) 2010; 7 41.

[70] Yamaoka K, Tanaka Y. Targeting the Janus kinases in rheumatoid arthritis: focus on tofacitinib. Expert Opin Pharmacother 2014; 15(1) 103-113.

[71] Vyas D, O'Dell KM, Bandy JL, Boyce EG. Tofacitinib: the First Janus kinase (JAK) inhibitor for the treatment of rheumatoid arthritis. Ann Pharmacother 2013; 47(11) 1524-1531.

[72] Gaujoux-Viala C, Nam J, Ramiro S, Landewé B, Buch MH, Smolen JS et al. Efficacy of conventional synthetic disease-modifying antirheumatic drugs, glucocorticoids and tofacitinib: a systematic literature review informing the 2013 update of the EULAR recommendations for management of rheumatoid arthritis. Ann Rheum Dis 2014; 73(3) 510-515.

[73] http://pubchem.ncbi.nlm.nih.gov/summary/summary.cgi?cid=44205240 (Accessed 10/17/14)

[74] van Vollenhoven RF. Small molecular compounds in development for rheumatoid arthritis. Curr Opin Rheumatol 2013; 25(3) 391-397.

[75] Shi JG, Chen X, Lee F, Emm T, Scherle PA, Lo Y et al. The pharmacokinetics, pharmacodynamics and safety of baricitinib, an oral JAK1/2 inhibitor, in healthy volunteers. J Clin Pharmacol 2014 ; 54(12) 1354-1361.

[76] http://newdrugapprovals.org/2014/07/21/decernotinib-jak-inhibitor-for the treatment of autoimmune and inflammatory disease/ Accessed 8/20/14

[77] https://b-com.mci-group.com/AbstractList/EULAR2014.aspx Lack of differentiation of Janus kinase inhibitors in rheumatoid arthritis based on Janus kinase pharmacology and clinically meaningful concentrations. Accessed 8/20/14

[78] EULAR Meeting-Van Vollenhoven R et al. Ann Rheum Dis 2014; 73 Suppl 2 Accessed 8/20/14

[79] Malemud CJ. Suppression of autoimmune arthritis by small molecule inhibitors of the JAK/STAT pathway. Pharmaceuticals 2010; 3 1446-1455.

[80] Norman P. Selective JAK 1 inhibitor and selective Tyk2 inhibitor patents. Expert Opin Ther Pat 2012; 22(10) 1233-1249.

[81] Malerich JP, Lam JS, Hart B, Fine RM, Klebansky B, Tanga MJ et al. Diamino-1,2,4-triazole derivatives are selective inhibitors of TYK2 and JAK1 over JAK2 and JAK3. Bioorg Med Chem Lett 2010; 20(24) 7454-7457.

[82] Dalila AS, Mohd Said MS, Shaharir SS, Asrul AW, Low SF, Shamsul AS et al. Interleukin-23 and its correlation with disease activity, joint damage, and functional disability in rheumatoid arthritis. Kaohsiung J Med Sci 2014; 30(7) 337-342.

[83] Boniface K, Blom B, Liu YJ, de Waal Malefyt R. From interleukin-23 to T-helper 17 cells: human T helper cell differentiation revisited. Immunol Rev 2008; 226 132-146.

[84] Hayakawa N, Noguchi M, Takeshita S, Eviryanti A, Seki Y, Nishio H et al. Structure-activity relationship study, target identification, and pharmacological characterization of a small molecular IL-12/IL-23 inhibitor, APY0201. Bioorg Med Chem 2014; 22(11) 3021-3029.

[85] Tang C, Chen S, Qian H, Huang W. Interleukin-23: as a drug target for autoimmune inflammatory diseases. Immunology 2012; 135(2) 112-124.

[86] Liang Y, Zhu Y, Xia Y, Peng H, Yang XK, Liu YY et al. Therapeutic potential of tyrosine kinase 2 in autoimmunity. Expert Opin Ther Targets 2014; 18(5) 571-580.

[87] Qi Z, Shen L, Zhou H, Jiang Y, Lan L, Luo L et al. Phosphorylation of heat shock protein 27 antagonizes TNF-$\alpha$ induced HeLa cell apoptosis via regulating TAK1 ubiquitination and activation of p38 and ERK signaling. Cell Signal 2014; 26(7) 1616-1625.

[88] Malemud CJ, Haque A, Louis NA, Wang J: Immune response and apoptosis – Introduction. J Clin Cell Immunol 2012; S3: e001.

[89] Malemud CJ. Role of nonreceptor tyrosine and threonine kinase inhibitors. 2009; In. Gracia-Foncillas J. (Editor) Molecular Biology of Cancer: Toward New Therapies. Prous Science, Barcelona.

[90] Wong BR, Grossbard D, Payan G, Masuda ES. Targeting Syk as a treatment for allergic and autoimmune disorders. Expert Opin Investig Drugs 2004; 13(7) 743-762.

[91] Scott DL. Role of spleen tyrosine kinase inhibitors in the management of rheumatoid arthritis. Drugs 2011; 71(9) 1121-1132.

[92] Gomez-Puerta JA, Mócsai A. Tyrosine kinase inhibitors for the management of rheumatoid arthritis. Curr Top Med Chem 2013; 13(6) 760-773.

[93] Pine RR, Chang B, Schoettler N, Banquerigo ML, Wang S, Lau A et al. Inflammation and bone erosion are suppressed in models of rheumatoid arthritis following treatment with a novel SyK inhibitor. Clin Immunol 2007; 124(3) 244-257.

[94] http://pubchem.ncbi.nlm.nih.gov/summary/summary.cgi?cid=25008120 (accessed 10/17/14)

[95] Boström E, Ohrn F, Hanze E, Sandström M, Martin P, Wählby-Hamrén U. Exposure vs. response of blood pressure in patients with rheumatoid arthritis following treatment with fostamatinib. J Clin Pharmacol 2014 ; 54(12) 1337-1346 doi: 10.1002/jcph.341

[96] Baloum M, Grossbard EB, Mant T, Lau DT. Pharmacokinetics of fostamatinib, a spleen tyrosine kinase (SYK) inhibitor, in healthy human subjects following a single and multiple oral dosing in three phase I subjects. Br J Clin Pharmacol 2013; 76(1) 78-88.

[97] Platt AM, Benson RA, Mc Queenie R, Butcher JP, Braddock M, Brewer JM et al. The active metabolite of spleen tyrosine kinase inhibitor fostamatinib abrogates the CD4+T cell-priming capacity of dendritic cells. Rheumatology (Oxford) 2014 Jul 26 pii.keu273 [Epub ahead of print]

[98] Taylor PC, Genovese MC, Greenwood M, Ho M, Nasonov E, Oemar B et al. OSKIRA-4: a phase IIb randomised, placebo-controlled study of the efficacy and safety of fostamatinib monotherapy. Ann Rheum Dis 2014 Jul 29 pii:annrheumdis-2014205361. doi: 10.1136/annrheumdis-2014-205361 [Epub ahead of print]

[99] Scott IC, Scott DL. Spleen tyrosine kinase inhibitors for rheumatoid arthritis: where are we now? Drugs 2014; 74(4) 415-422.

[100] Thoma G, Drückes P, Zerwes G. Selective inhibitors of the Janus kinase Jak3-Are they effective? Bioorg Med Chem Lett 2014; 24(19) 4617-4621 pii:S9060-894X(14)00890-7. doi: 10.1016/j.bmcl.2014.08.046

[101] Chrencik JE, Patny A, Leung IK, Korniski B, Emmons TL, Hall T et al. Structural and thermodynamic characterization of the TYK2 and JAK3 kinase domains in complex with CP690550 and CMP-6. J Mol Biol 2010; 400(3) 413-433.

# 3

# Edible and Medicinal Mushrooms as Promising Agents in Cancer

Ken Yasukawa

## 1. Introduction

Conquering cancer is one of the major challenges facing mankind in the 21st century. The advancement of diagnostic techniques has made discovering miniscule tumors feasible, and early treatment of many types of cancers has consequently become a reality. However, while the development of anticancer drugs progresses, the number of people diagnosed with cancer continues to rise. The drug, tamoxifen, has been approved in the US to prevent breast cancer relapse. In addition, cancer prevention has become an important part of conquering cancer, with both primary and secondary prevention strategies. The former entails the prevention of cancer itself, while the latter involves the prevention of death once an individual has already developed cancer.

Edible mushrooms such as *Lentinula edodes* (shiitake) and *Grifola frondosa* (maitake) have been known from ancient folklore to possess properties that enhance biological defense responses (immune functions), and have been used in people with decreased immune function such as those with cancer, allergies and other disorders, and in elderly people. Many of these mushrooms contain compounds called β-glucans, which are high molecular weight polysaccharides of glucose linked together by glycosidic bonds. β-glucans are contained in mushrooms, yeast, fungi, and higher plants. In Japan, several mushroom-derived pharmaceutical products have been developed, and include schizophyllan from *Schizophyllum commune*, krestin from *Trametes versicolor*, and lentinan from *L. edodes* an anticancer polysaccharide from shiitake. In South Korea, meshima, a mycelia culture of *Phellinus linteus*, was developed as an anticancer drug. Antitumor activities of polysaccharides and peptide polysaccharides in these mushrooms have been reported. In addition to polysaccharides, unique substances such as sterols and triterpenes are reportedly present in mushrooms. Some of these compounds are promising anticancer agents. Please refer to a review published elsewhere for a description on herbal medicine extracts that have been anticipated for their cancer prevention effects [1]. In this chapter, we will introduce the anticancer activities of polysaccharides as well as the cancer prevention activities of sterols and triterpenes.

## 2. Mushroom-derived anticancer polysaccharides

Research on mushroom-derived β-glucans began when Chihara, Hamuro, and others at the National Cancer Center Research Institute in Japan isolated and purified lentinan, a β-1,3-glucan with branched chains formed by β-1,6-glycosidic bonds, from *L. edodes* in 1968 [2, 3]. Subsequently, many efficacy studies on lentinan, primarily concerning its antitumor activities, have been reported [4-6]. Ikekawa *et al.* intraperitoneally administered aqueous extracts of six types of edible mushrooms, and demonstrated their antitumor effects on cancer cell line sarcoma S-180 [7].

Upon such discoveries, polysaccharides lentinan and schizophyllan, glycoprotein krestin, and *P. linteus* mycelia extract meshima have been utilized as anticancer drugs.

Lentinan (Figure 1) demonstrated an effect to prolong the survival of patients with inoperable and relapsed stomach cancer in combination with a chemotherapeutic agent in a human double-blind controlled clinical trial. It has been revealed that its oral consumption, however, does not exhibit efficacy. In 1985, this compound was approved as an anti-malignant tumor agent (injectable solution), and has been prescribed to cancer patients as a pharmaceutical product. Subsequently, the antitumor effects of various mushroom extracts that contain β-glucan were reported in animal experiments [8]. However, most of these studies administered mushroom extracts that contain β-glucan to animals via injection, and there are very few reports that showed its effect via oral consumption. There is, however, one such rare report; an epidemiological study that suggests mushroom intake via oral consumption may be effective [9]. Intraperitoneal administration of lentinan suppressed 3-methylcolanthrene-induced tumor expression [5]. In *Lentinula edodes*, α-(1,4)-glucan binds with TLR-4, thereby inducing monocyte differentiation and exhibiting cytotoxic effects in A549 human lung carcinoma cells [10].

Schizophyllan derived from *Schizophyllum commune* (Figure 2) is typically structured with β1 → 3 linkage and on rare occasions with β1 → 6 linkage between D-glucose monomers [11]. Due to such structure, a rigid triple-helical structure is formed. In addition, this compound is used in anticancer drugs since it possesses antitumor activities [12]. However, it is administered via intramuscular injection, and its effects via oral route in the manner of food consumption have not been elucidated. Although the mechanism of the antitumor activities of β-glucans including schizophyllan is not completely understood, it is thought that they activate macrophages and natural killer (NK) cells through respective β-glucan receptors, induce a helper T1 cell-dominant immune response state, and consequently exhibit antitumor activities [13, 14].

Krestin, an anti-malignant tumor agent, is a protein-bound polysaccharide derived from the mycelia of *Trametes versicolor* CM-101 strain. Since this drug does not cause serious side effects

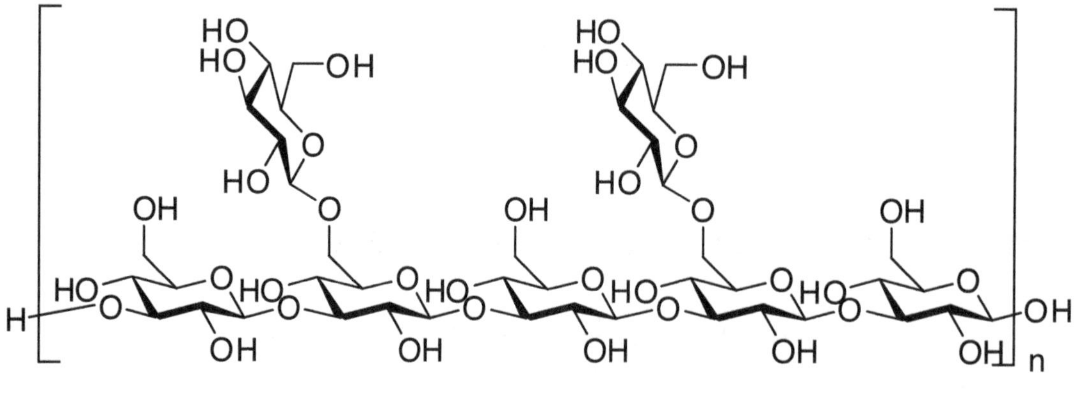

Figure 1. Structure of lentinan

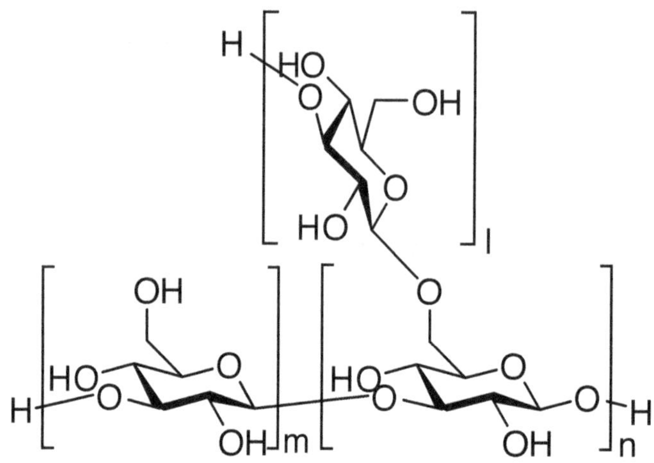

Figure 2. Structure of schizophyllan

with oral administration, there was a period of time in which it was used alone after its release in 1977. However, it is now evident that it has no effect by itself, and is now used in conjunction with other drugs. Krestin is thought to exhibit its antitumor actions by acting on the immune response mechanism that has decreased due to a cancer-bearing state. Krestin has a mean molecular weight of $9.4 \times 10^4$, and its sugar chain moiety consists of glucose (74.6%), galactose (2.7%), mannose (15.5%), xylose (4.8%), and fucose (2.4%), but mostly glucose in the form of β-glucans. The glucans have main chain β1 → 4 bond, and side chain β1 → 3 and 1 → 6 bond structures, and it has been suggested that branching occurs per number of sugar residues. Proteins and sugar chain moeities in Krestin are linked with each other by either *O*- or *N*-glycosidic bond [15]. In addition, coriolan, another antitumor polysaccharide derived from *Trametes versicolor*, was reported in 1971 [16].

*P. linteus* belongs to *Hymenochaetaceae* family, and is called *souou* in traditional Japanese medicine, and has been highly valued since ancient times. It has been referred to as the "mythical" mushroom since it grows extremely slowly in nature and artificial cultivation is also difficult. Research in South Korea succeeded in the mass cultivation of *P. linteus* Yoo (HKSY-PL2) strain, which has been shown to be more effective than most other strains. *P.*

*linteus* has properties to enhance the natural healing capability of the body, and was developed as a pharmaceutical product called meshima. Mycelia culture of *P. linteus* activated dendritic cells and macrophages through increased secretions of interleukin 12 (IL-12), interferon gamma (IFN-$\gamma$), tumor necrosis factor alpha (TNF-$\alpha$) by T-cells, and enhanced the antitumor effects of NK cells [17]. A proteoglycan generated by *P. linteus* acted as an immunostimulant and disrupted the Reg IV/EGFR/Akt signaling pathway, thereby exhibiting tumor-inhibitory effects [18]. In addition, polysaccharides from *P. linteus* activated the P27kip1-cyclinD1/E-CDK2 pathway and induced S-phase cell cycle arrest in HT-29 cells, resulting in cellular damage [19].

Through their immunostimulatory properties, mushroom-derived polysaccharides and glycoproteins augment anticancer drugs, alleviate side effects, and contribute greatly to quality of life (QOL) improvement.

## 3. Chemical carcinogenesis and two-stage carcinogenesis theory

It has been acknowledged that many types of cancers are caused by environmental carcinogenic agents. In 1915, Yamagiwa and Ichikawa succeeded in inducing cancer by rubbing coal tar on rabbit ears [20]. The significance from this study was the skin cancer had metastasized to the rabbit lung. In 1941, Berenblum *et al.* applied carcinogenic agent benz[*a*]pyrene (B[*a*]A) and croton oil (seed oil of *Croton tiglium*) on mouse skin, and proposed a two-stage carcinogenesis theory that tumorigenesis occurs similarly to when B[*a*]A is applied continually [21, 22]. Specifically, changes due to a carcinogenic agent were termed initiation, and changes due to croton oil were termed promotion. Later, Hecker reported the cancer-promoting ingredient of croton oil as 12-*O*-tetradecanoylphorbol-13-acetate (TPA). Many of these experiments are conducted using initiators 7,12-dimethylbenz[*a*]anthracene (DMBA) and TPA [23,24]. Fujiki *et al.* later reported on many mouse skin tumor promoters such as teleocidin [25]. Cancer begins when cells transform into latent cancer cells after undergoing initiation by receiving initiators or radiation. Subsequently, these cells become cancer cells after a long period of promotion process by promoters. Finally, after modifications through a process termed progression, the cells acquire the ability to divide infinitely, thereby clinically morphing to cancer. These steps occur in a continuous manner, and cannot be strictly distinguished from each other. When considering primary prevention, it is realistic to suppress the promotion process, which requires a long period of time and is known to be reversible to some degree. In addition, it has also become evident that cancer develops via similar mechanisms in many organs. Furthermore, TPA is known to activate Epstein-Barr virus (EBV). Although the prevalence of EBV is extremely high in Africa, the incidence of Burkitt's lymphoma greatly differs depending on the village [26]. It has been revealed that villages with greater incidence regularly utilized *Euphorbia tirucalli* and phorbol-esters, which are constituents of *Euphorbia tirucalli* and closely related to TPA. It is suggested these phorbol-esters are involved in the onset of Burkitt's lymphoma [27, 28].

## 4. Screening for cancer preventative substances

We are conducting a screening for an antitumor substance using a method in which the suppressive effect against tumor promoter-induced inflammation is examined as a positive outcome index [29]. This method was utilized by Hecker *et al.* when they isolated and identified TPA and this method has been confirmed to be advantageous with high correlation as it employs a carcinogenesis experiment and skin from inbred (syngeneic) mice. Specifically, when TPA is applied on the auricle of female ICR mice, maximum swelling was observed 6-10 hours later. The mushroom extracts suppressed the TPA effects, as seen by swelling inhibition, and were confirmed by two-stage carcinogenesis experiments on mouse skin. We induced inflammation with TPA in mice and investigated methanol extracts of 27 edible mushrooms, 8 mushroom supplements, and 3 medicinal mushrooms, discovering the presence of promising mushrooms as shown in Table 1. Specifically, inhibitory effects were observed in: *Russula delica, Lactarius deliciosus, Hypsizigus marmoreus* (*H. marmoreus*), *Mycoleptodonoides aitchisonii* (*M. aitchisonii*), *Naematoloma sublateritium* for edible mushroom; *Inonotus obliquus* (chaga), meshima, *Ganoderma lucidum* (reishi), deer horn shape *Ganoderma amboinense* (rokkaku reishi), *Pleurotus cornucopiae* (golden oyster mushroom) for mushroom supplements; and *Poria cocos* (poria) and polyporus as medicinal mushrooms [30]. Of these mushrooms, the application of methanol extracts of *H. marmoreus* [31], *M. aitchisonii* [30], poria [32], chaga [33], and meshima [34] suppressed the promotion process. These results indicated that edible and medicinal mushrooms are effective cancer preventing foods. In addition, there is a method in which the suppressive effect against the EBV activation that is involved in the onset of Burkitt's lymphoma is examined as a positive outcome index [35]. Substances that were confirmed to have inhibitory effects through this method are thought to contribute to cancer prevention in those infected with EBV.

| **Scientific name** | **IR (%)** |
|---|---|
| *Polyporus confluens* | 35** |
| *Russula delica* | 65** |
| *R. cyanoxantha* | 38** |
| *R. pseudodelica* | 41** |
| *R. sanguinea* | 41** |
| *Lactarius deliciosus* | 61** |
| *L. volemus* | 17 |
| *Armillariella mellea* | 12 |
| *Flammulina velutipes* | 30** |
| *Hypsizigus marmoreus* | 58** |
| *Lyophyllum decastes* | 54** |
| *L. connatum* | 53** |
| *L. shimeji* | 40** |
| *Pleurocybella porrigens* | 50** |

| Scientific name | IR (%) |
|---|---|
| *Tricholoma japonicum* | 49** |
| *T. matsutake* | 39** |
| *T. portentosum* | 41** |
| *Lycoperdon perlatum* | 20* |
| *Agaricus bisporus* | 36** |
| *Macrolepiota procera* | 11 |
| *Phaeolepiota aurea* | 15 |
| *Sarcodon aspratus* | 22* |
| *Mycoleptodonoides aitchisonii* | 62** |
| *Rhodophyllus crassipes* | 23* |
| *Naematoloma sublateritium* | 55** |
| *Pholiota squarrosa* | 33** |
| *Hygrophorus russula* | 36* |
| *Ganoderma lucidum* | 82** |
| *Ganoderma amboinense* | 79** |
| *Polyporus mylittae* | 33** |
| *Phellinus linteus* | 73** |
| *Inonotus obliquus* | 84** |
| *Pleurotus cornucopiae* var. *citrinopileatus* | 52** |
| *Hericium erinaceum* | 19 |
| *Sparassis crispa* | 49** |

IR: Inhibitory ratio at 1 mg/ear. * $p < 0.05$, $p < 0.01$ vs control group by Student's t test.

**Table 1.** Inhibitory effect of edible and medicinal mushrooms on TPA-induced inflammation in mice.

## 5. Cancer preventative effects of edible mushroom

Figure 3 illustrates the inhibitory effects of *M. aitchisonii* in mouse skin, two-stage carcinogenesis experiments. Specifically, Figure 3-A indicates the tumor incidence, where the vehicle control group showed the first tumor appearance in week 5 and tumor development in 93% of the mice in week 20. In contrast, mice that were given *M. aitchisonii* (*M. aitchisonii* group) showed the first tumor appearance in week 5 and tumor development in 53% of the mice in week 20. Figure 3-B shows the mean number of tumors at 20 weeks, where *M. aitchisonii* group presented 1.6 tumors in contrast to the vehicle control group that exhibited 11.2 tumors, confirming a 63% inhibitory effect [30]. Methanol extracts of *H. marmoreus* similarly suppressed the tumor promotion process [31].

A screening for suppressive ingredients was, therefore, conducted; using inhibitory effects against TPA-induced inflammation as an index, active ingredients were isolated and their

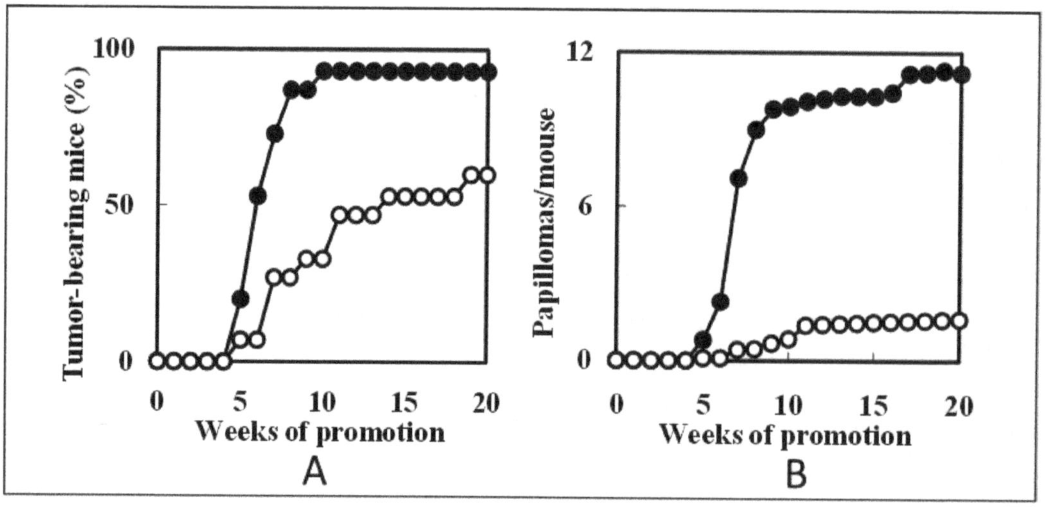


Data are expressed as percentage of mice bearing papillomas per mouse (A), and as average number of papillomas per mouse (B). ●, TPA + with vehicle alone;°, TPA with methanol extract of *M. aitchisonii*.

**Figure 3.** Inhibitory effect of the methanol extract from *Mycoleptodonoides aitchisonii* on the promotion of skin papillomas by TPA in DMBA-initiated mice [30].

chemical structures were elucidated. The active ingredients were ergosterol (**1**) and ergosterol peroxide (**2**) (Figure 4), which are normal ingredients of mushrooms, and these were stronger than non-steroidal anti-inflammatory drug indomethacin as shown by their 50% inhibitory effects ($ID_{50}$: 756 and 467 nM/ear, respectively vs. 908 nM/ear). These two sterols have been demonstrated to suppress the promotion process in mouse skin two-stage carcinogenesis experiments [31, 36]. Other sterols (**6-10**) have been reported to inhibit the TPA-induced EBV activation (Table 2.) [37].

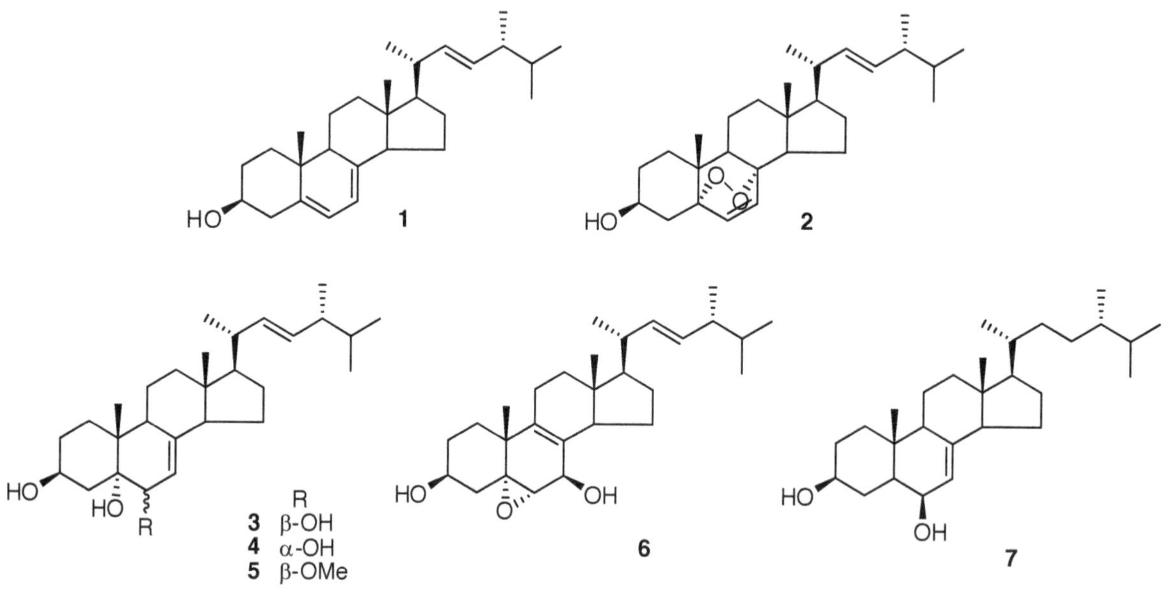


**Figure 4.** Structures of sterols from *Hypsizigus marmoreus*.

| Compound | $IC_{50}$ |
|---|---|
| Ergosterol (**1**) | 520 |
| Ergosterol peroxide (**2**) | 525 |
| Cerevisterol (**3**) | 518 |
| 6-Epicerevisterol (**4**) | 512 |
| 22,23-Dihydrocerevisterol (**5**) | 515 |
| 6-O-Methylcerevisterol (**6**) | 298 |
| (22E,23R)-5α,6α-Epoxyergosta-8,22-diene-3β,7β-diol (**7**) | 192 |
| β-Carotene | 397 |

$IC_{50}$: Mol ratio/32 pmol TPA.

**Table 2.** Inhibitory effects of sterols from *Hypsizigus marmoreus* on induction of the Epstein-Barr virus early antigen.

## 6. Cancer preventative effects of mushroom supplements

Mushroom supplements, such as meshima, chaga, and almond mushroom, are all believed to be beneficial for cancer, and utilized based on the wishes of cancer patients and their families. As shown in Table 1, supplements including reishi, rokkaku reishi, meshima, and chaga strongly suppressed TPA-induced inflammation [30]. Methanol extracts of Meshima and chaga strongly suppressed the promotion process in experiments involving DMBA and TPA carcinogens [33, 34]. Furthermore, chaga and meshima suppressed the promotion process through oral administration [38, 39].

Lanostane-type triterpenes depicted in Figure 5 were isolated and identified from chaga, and these triterpenes are known to show inhibitory effects in TPA-induced EBV activation (Table 3) [40, 41]. Eight types of lanostane-type triterpenes were isolated as active ingredients, and using the inhibitory effects against TPA-induced inflammation as an index, their 50% inhibitory effects ($ID_{50}$: 125-458 nM/ear) indicated that they are stronger than non-steroidal anti-inflammatory drug indomethacin (908 nM/ear) (Tasble 4) [33]. Of these triterpenes, inotodiol (**13**) and 3β-Hydroxylanosta-8,24-dien-24-al (**15**) suppressed the tumor promotion process [40, 41].

| Compound | $IC_{50}$ |
|---|---|
| Uvariol (**10**) | 392 |
| 3β-Hydroxylanosta-8,24-dien-21-al (**12**) | 232 |
| Lanosta-8,23*E*-diene-3β,22*R*,25-triol (**14**) | 231 |
| Lanosta-7:9(11),23*E*-triene-3β,22*R*,25-triol (**15**) | 228 |
| Oleanolic acid | 389 |

$IC_{50}$: Mol ratio/32 pmol/TPA.

**Table 3.** Inhibitory effects of lanostane-type triterpenes from *Inonotus obliquus* on induction of the Epstein-Barr virus early antigen.

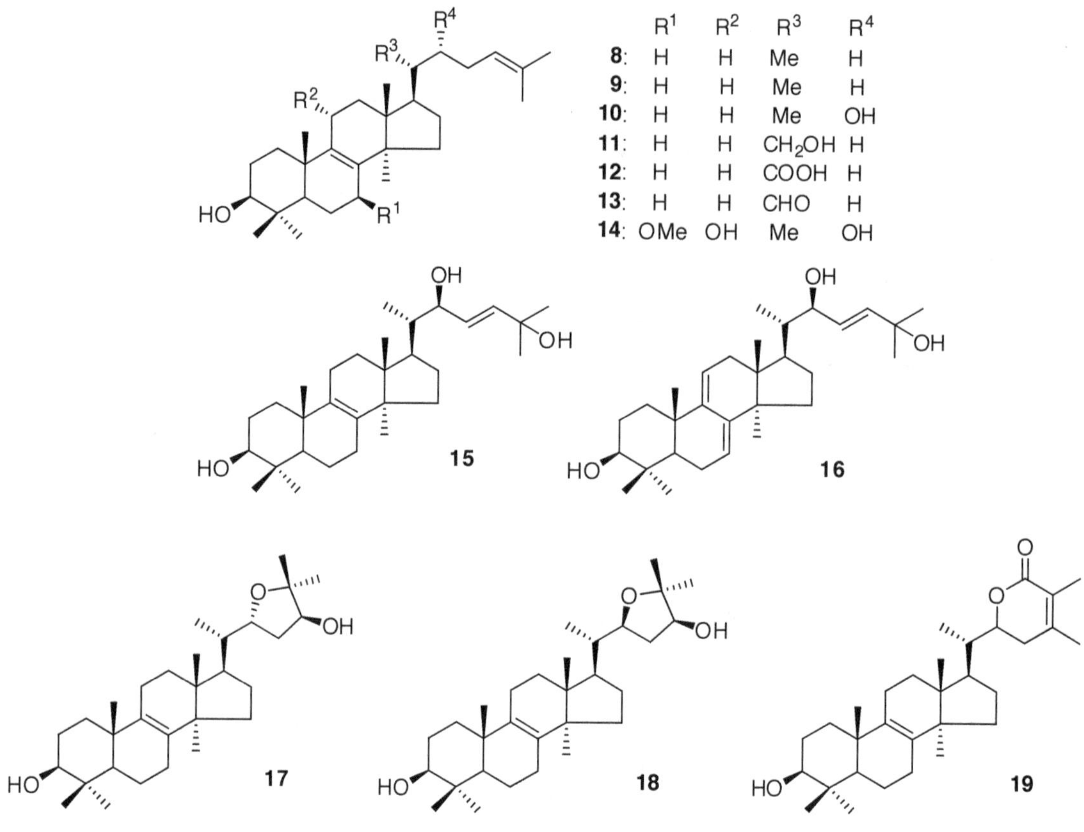


**Figure 5.** Structures of lanostane-type triterpenes from *Inonotus obliquus*.

| Compound | $ID_{50}$ (nM/ear) |
|---|---|
| Lanosterol (**8**) | 458 |
| Inotodiol (**9**) | 125 |
| Uvariol (**10**) | 134 |
| 3β-Hydroxylanosta-8,24-dien-21-al (**12**) | 389 |
| Methoxyinonotsutriol (**14**) | 272 |
| 3β,22-Dihydroxylanosta-7,9(11),24-triene (**16**) | 335 |
| Inotolacton B (**19**) | 265 |
| Indomethacin | 908 |

$ID_{50}$: 50% Inhibitory dose.

**Table 4.** Inhibitory effects of lanostane-type triterpenes from *Inonotus obliquus* on TPA-induced inflammation in mice.

Reishi belongs to the *Ganodermataceae* family, and is cut into appropriate sizes to be brewed in hot water and consumed as an extract since the fruiting body is woody and not suitable for direct consumption, or is consumed as medicinal alcohol. It has been described in *Shennong Ben Cao Jing* (or *The Classic of Herbal Medicine*) compiled in the Eastern Han Dynasty (25-220), as a life-prolonging miracle drug that nourishes life, and since then, it has been used for various medicinal purposes in China. Akihisa *et al.* isolated multiple lanostane-type triterpene acids from its fruiting body, and reported that they suppress EBV activation as shown in Table 5 [42-44]. Of these compounds 20-Hydroxylucidenic acid N (**21**) suppressed the promotion process in mouse skin two-stage carcinogenesis [42]. With regards to triterpenes from reishi, ganoderic acid T (**49**) exhibited anticancer activities by inducing apoptosis in metastatic lung cancer cells mediated through mitochondria dysfunction and p53 expression [45]. In addition, ganoderic acid T (**49**) suppressed the nuclear translocation of NF-κB and expression of MMP-9 and iNOS, thereby inhibiting invasion by cancer cells [46]. Ganoderic acid DM (**46**) displayed anticancer activities by inducing G1-phase cell cycle arrest and apoptosis in MCF-7 cancer cells [47]. Ganoderic acid A (**44**) and ganoderic acid H (**42**) suppressed breast cancer cell invasion by inhibiting AP-1 and NF-κB and consequently down-regulating Cdk4 expression [48]. Ganoderic acid Me (**48**) inhibited tumor invasion by suppressing MMP2/9 expressions [49]. Lucidenic acid B (**26**) exhibited anti-invasive activity through suppressing TPA-induced NF-κB and AP-1 DNA-binding activities thereby downregulating MMP-9 expression in HepG(2) cells [50]. Lucidenic acid B (**26**) induced apoptosis through mitochondrial cytochrome release and the activations of caspase-9 and caspase-3 [51].

| **Compound** | **$IC_{50}$** |
|---|---|
| Lucidenic acid F (**20**) | 352 |
| Methyl lucidenate F (**21**) | 285 |
| Lucidenic acid $D_2$ (**22**) | 287 |
| Methyl l ucidenic acid $D_2$ (**23**) | 290 |
| Lucidenic acid A (**24**) | 280 |
| Methyl l ucidenate A (**25**) | 287 |
| Lucidenic acid B (**26**) | 354 |
| Methyl lucidenate Q (**27**) | 283 |
| Methyl lucidenate L (**28**) | 275 |
| Lucidenic acid $E_2$ (**29**) | 280 |
| Methyl l ucidenate $E_2$ (**30**) | 288 |
| Lucidenic acid N (**31**) | 332 |
| Methyl l ucidenate C (**32**) | 331 |
| Lucidenic acid P (**33**) | 286 |
| Methyl l ucidenate P (**34**) | 293 |
| 20-Hydroxy lucidenic acid F (**35**) | 339 |
| 20-Hydroxy lucidenic acid $D_2$ (**36**) | 350 |
| 20-Hydroxy lucidenic acid $E_2$ (**37**) | 290 |
| 20-Hydroxy lucidenic acid N (**38**) | 288 |
| 20-Hydroxy lucidenic acid P (**39**) | 288 |
| 20(21)-Dehydrolucidenic acid A (**40**) | 350 |
| Methyl 20(21)-dehydrolucidenate A (**41**) | 357 |
| Ganoderic acid F (**42**) | 293 |
| Ganoderic acid $C_1$ (**43**) | 336 |

| Compound | $IC_{50}$ |
|---|---|
| Ganoderic acid A (**44**) | 291 |
| Ganoderic acid $C_2$ (**45**) | 290 |
| Ganoderic acid DM (**46**) | 352 |
| Ganoderic acid T-Q (**47**) | 281 |
| Ganodermanondiol (**50**) | 348 |
| Ganolactone (**51**) | 415 |
| Ganoderic acid E (**52**) | 281 |
| Methyl ganoderate F (**53**) | 289 |

$IC_{50}$: Mol ratio/32 pmol TPA.

**Table 5.** Inhibitory effects of lanostane-type triterpene acids from *Ganoderma lucidum* on induction of the Epstein-Barr virus early antigen.

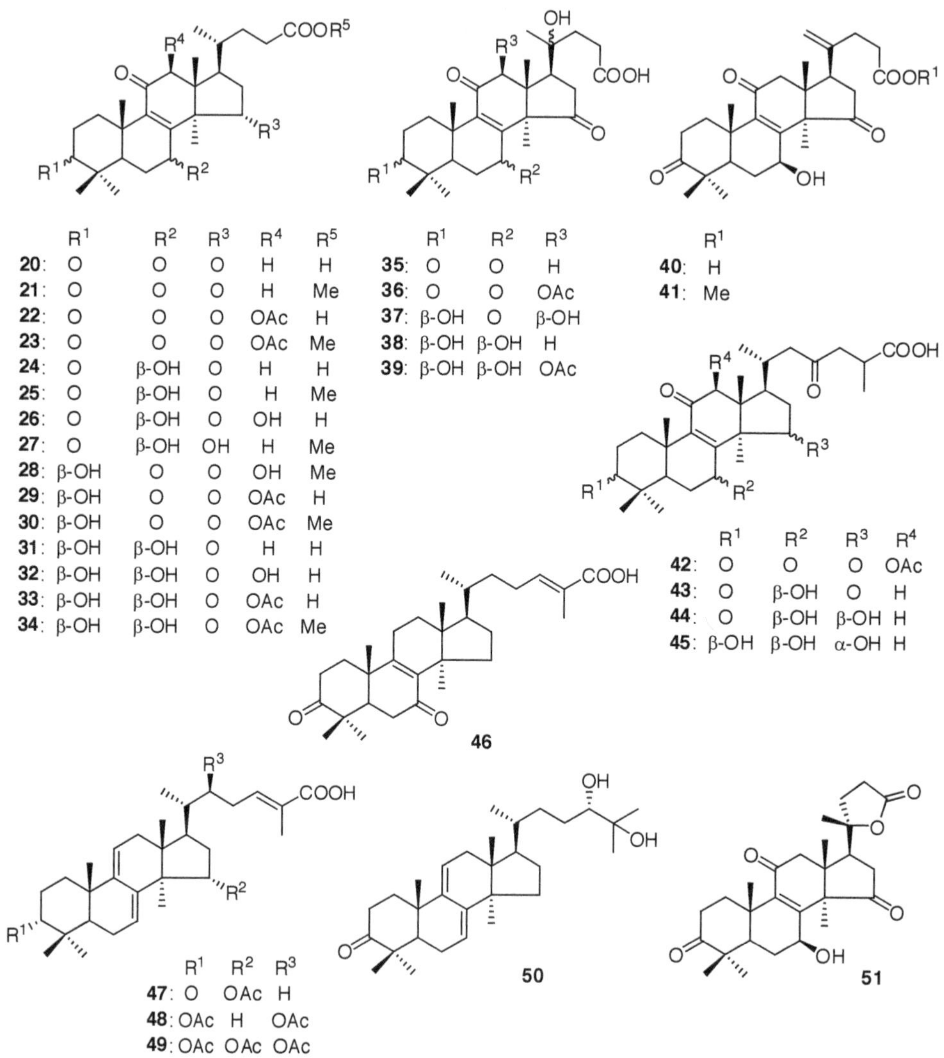


**Figure 6.** Structures of lanostane-type triterpene acids from *Ganoderma lucidum*.

*Piptoporus betulinus* is a fungus in the *Polyporaceae* family and the surface of its fruiting body had been used as a strop for razor blades. It is known that the Iceman, as evidenced by a mummy from 5,000 years ago found in the Tyrol region glacier, carried around this mushroom to prevent wound suppuration [52, 53]. Lanostane-type triterpenes (Figure 7) isolated from this mushroom suppressed TPA-induced inflammation [54].

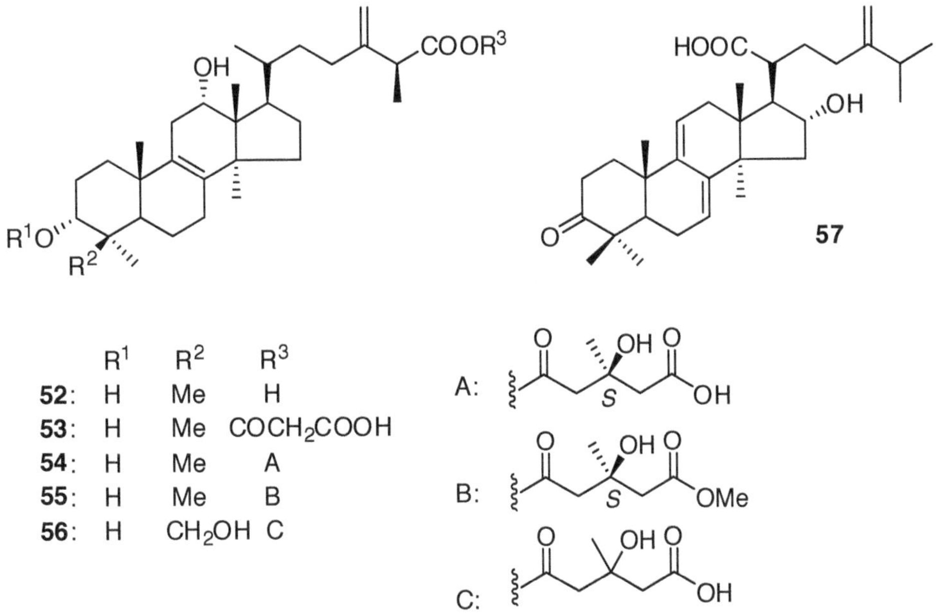


**Figure 7.** Structures of lanostane-type triterpenes from *Piptoporus betulinus*.

## 7. Cancer preventative effects and active ingredients of medicinal mushrooms

Of the medicinal mushrooms, polyporus (*Polyporus umbellatus; Polyporaceae* family) is an herbal medicine that possesses diuretic effects, but is also known to suppress TPA-induced inflammation. Screening for the active ingredients of this mushroom resulted in the isolation of insect metamorphosis hormone sterols, and the structures of eight compounds including new compounds polyporoid A (**58**), polyporoid B (**59**), and polyporoid C (**60**) were elucidated (Figure 8.) As shown in Table 6, the effects of these compounds in inhibiting TPA-induced inflammation ($ID_{50}$) were 117-682 nM/ear, which were greater than that of indomethacin [55].

The sclerotia of *Poria cocos* (*Polyporaceae* family) are referred to as poria, and due to their diuretic properties, and they are formulated in traditional Japanese medicine prescriptions. Additionally, they are also commonly formulated in traditional Japanese medicine prescriptions that are used as adjuvants. The oral administration of Juzentaiho-to and Rikkunshi-to, Japanese Kampo medicines, suppressed cancer promotion in mouse skin two-stage carcinogenesis experiments [56, 57]. It has been shown that, for an effect to appear, the immune response that

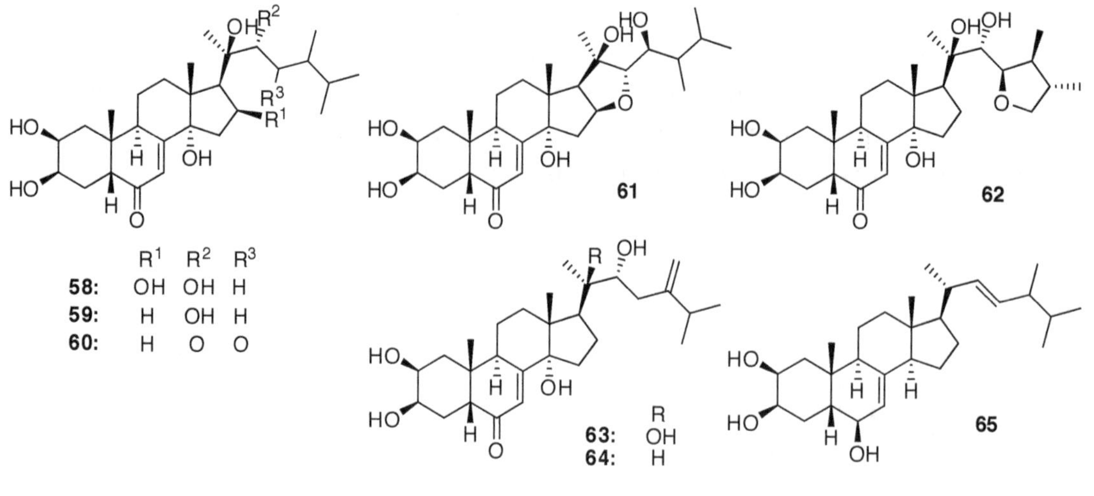


**Figure 8.** Structures of ecdysteroids from *Polyporus umbellatus.*

| Compound | $ID_{50}$ (nM/ear) |
|---|---|
| Polyporoid A (**58**) | 531 |
| Polyporoid B (**59**) | 682 |
| Polyporoid C (**60**) | 184 |
| Polyporusterone A (**61**) | 141 |
| Polyporusterone C (**62**) | 289 |
| Polyporusterone B (**63**) | 117 |
| Polyporusterone G (**64**) | 207 |
| Ergosta-7,22-diene-3β,5α,6β-triol (**65**) | 666 |
| Indomethacin | 838 |

$ID_{50}$: 50% Inhibitory dose.

**Table 6.** Inhibitory effect of ecdysterolids from *Polyporus umbellatus* on TPA-induced inflammation in mice.

is decreased during carcinogenic process be activated [57]. Of the formulated ingredients in these prescriptions, hoelen showed the strongest effect in suppressing TPA-induced inflammation [58]. A screening for the active ingredients of hoelen was therefore conducted, and multiple lanostane-type triterpene acids were isolated and identified (Figure 9) [32]. Of the poria-derived triterpenes, pachymic acid (**71**), 3-*O*-acetyl-16α-hydroxytrametenolic acid (**70**), dehydropachymic acid (**79**), 3β-hydroxylanosta-7,9(11),24-trien-21-oic acid (**75**), dehydroebuliconic acid (**81**), and poricoic acids A (**97**) and B (**94**) had inhibitory effects against TPA-induced inflammation ($ID_{50}$: 31-83 nM/ear), that were greater than that of indomethacin but similar to that of hydrocortisone ($ID_{50}$: 69 nM/ear). With regards to pachymic acid (**71**), 3-*O*-acetyl-16αhydroxytrametenolic acid (**70**), and poricoic acid B (**94**), all of which showed strong inhibitory effects, a mouse skin two-stage carcinogenesis experiment using DMBA and TPA demonstrated that they exhibited suppressive effects that were similar to that of the aforementioned ergosterol (**1**), ergosterol peroxide (**2**) and other triterpenes, even when 10% of the dosage of the latter compounds were administered [59]. These compounds have a carboxyl group (COOH) at the carbon 21 position (on side chain), and their suppressive effects decreased 90% when the COOH-group was methylated. It was discovered that COOH at the carbon 21 position plays an important role for activation [32]. Akihisa *et al.* isolated many new lanostane-type triterpene acids from poria, and reported their suppressive effects in TPA-induced EBV activation (Table 8) [60-62]. Moreover, they confirmed that 16-deoxyporicoic acid B (**93**), poricoic acid C (**95**), and 25-methoxyporicoic acid A (**102**) suppress the promotion process [60, 61]. Of these compounds, poricotriol A was revealed to induce apoptosis and possess antitumor effects [63]. Pachymic acid and dehydrotumulosic acid strongly suppress PL-$A_2$, which is related to inflammation [64].

| **Compound** | **$ID_{50}$ (nM/ear)** |
|---|---|
| 24-Dihydrolanosterol (**66**) | 501 |
| Lanosterol (**67**) | 469 |
| Tumulosic acid (**69**) | 440 |
| 3-*O*-Acetyl-16α-hydroxytrametenoic acid (**70**) | 31.1 |
| Pachymic acid (**71**) | 83.2 |
| 3β-Hydroxylanosta-7,9(11),24-trien-21-oic acid (**75**) | 59.4 |
| Dehydropachymic acid (**79**) | 38.0 |
| Dehydroeburiconic acid (**81**) | 57.9 |
| Polyporenic acid C (**82**) | 201 |
| 3-Epidehydrotumulosic acid (**84**) | 188 |
| Poricoic acid B (**94**) | 35.1 |
| Poricoic acid A (**97**) | 56.1 |
| Poricoic acid AM (**98**) | 148 |
| Poricoic acid D (**100**) | 243 |
| Indomethacin | 908 |
| Hydrocortisone | 68.9 |

$ID_{50}$: 50% Inhibitory dose.

**Table 7.** Inhibitory effect of lanostane-type triterpene acids from *Poria cocos* on TPA-induced inflammation in mice.

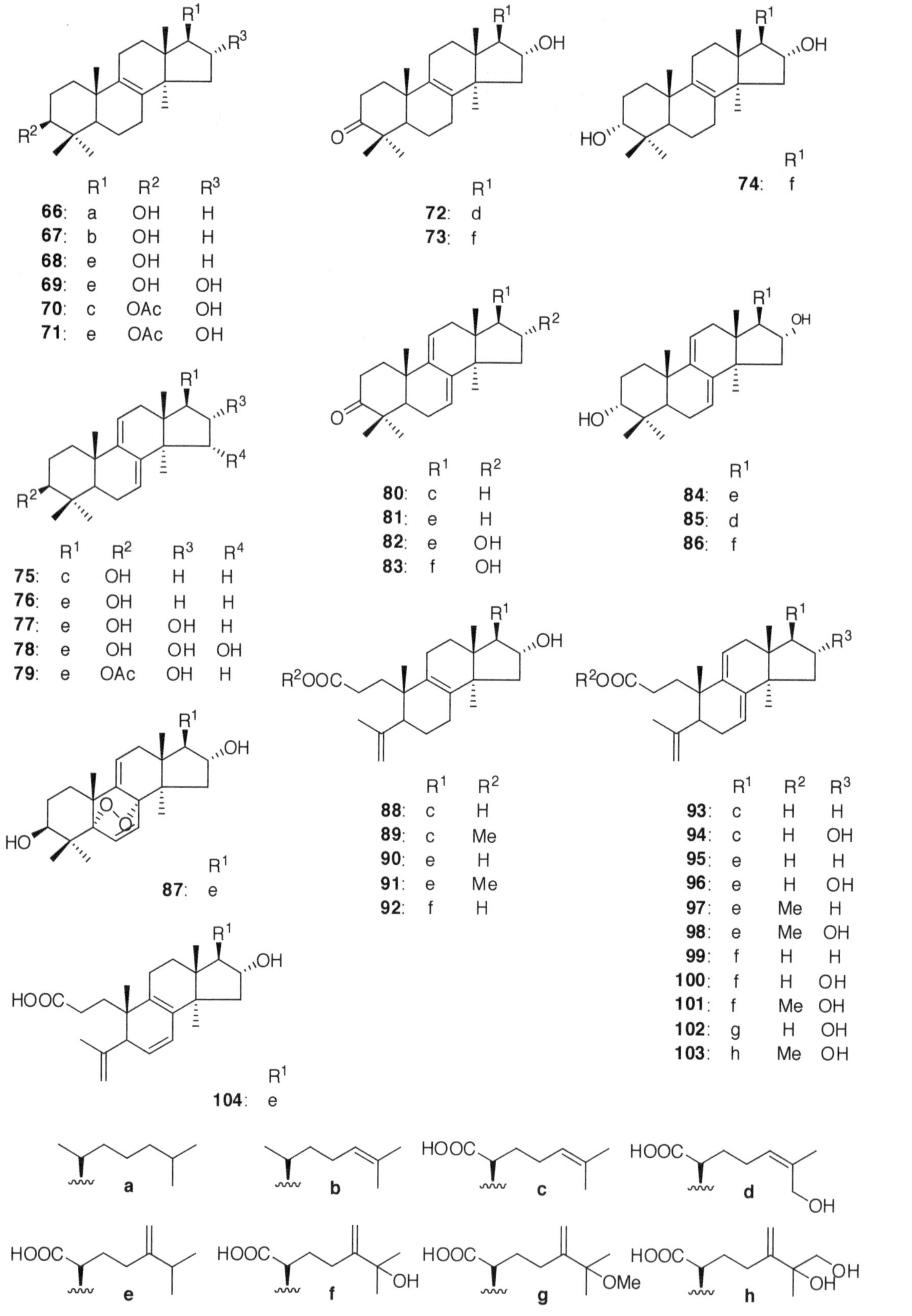


**Figure 9.** Structures of lanostane-type triterpene acids from *Poria cocos*.

| Compound | $IC_{50}$ |
|---|---|
| Eburicoic acid (**68**) | 465 |
| Pachymic acid (**71**) | 286 |
| 16α-Hydroxyeburiconic acid (**72**) | 348 |
| 16α,25-Dihydroxyeburiconic acid (**73**) | 299 |
| 25-Hydroxy-3-epitumulosic acid (**74**) | 238 |
| 3-Epidehydrotrametnolic acid (**75**) | 464 |
| Dehydroebricoic acid (**76**) | 460 |
| 15α-Hydroxydehydrotumulosic acid (**78**) | 268 |
| Dehydropachymic acid (**79**) | 284 |
| Dehydrotrametenonic acid (**80**) | 310 |
| Dehydroebriconic acid (**81**) | 405 |
| 16α,25-Dihydroxydehydroeburiconic acid (**83**) | 340 |
| 16α,27-Dihydroxydehydrotrametenoic acid (**85**) | 269 |
| 5α,8α-Peroxydehydrotumulosic acid (**87**) | 202 |
| Poricoic acid HM (**91**) | 219 |
| 25-Hydroxyporicoic acid H (**92**) | 202 |
| 16-Deoxyporicoic acid B (**93**) | 262 |
| Poricoic acid C (**95**) | 273 |
| Poricoic acid CM (**96**) | 332 |
| Poricoic acid AM (**98**) | 195 |
| 25-Hydroxyporicoic acid C (**99**) | 201 |
| Poricoic acid D (**100**) | 198 |
| Poricoic acid DM (**101**) | 207 |
| 25-Methoxyporicoic acid A (**102**) | 268 |
| 26-Hydroxyporicoic acid DM (**103**) | 187 |
| 6,7-Dehydroporicoic acid H (**104**) | 193 |
| β-Carotene | 397 |

$IC_{50}$: Mol ratio/32 pmol TPA.

**Table 8.** Inhibitory effects of lanostane-type triterpene acids from *Poria cocos* on induction of the Epstein-Barr virus early antigen.

## 8. Conclusion

Mushroom polysaccharides and glycoproteins have antitumor mechanisms such as activating various immunocompetent cells and reinforcing the tumor aggressiveness of the host. Many mushroom-derived polysaccharides have very weak effects when administered orally.

However, with the advancement in food technology, the development of these polysaccharides as food products is progressing and their development as oral pharmaceutical products is also anticipated.

Poria and reishi are listed in the first treatise of Shennong Ben Cao Jing, and viewed as herbal medicines that help maintain health. Although some mushroom triterpenoids show strong suppressive effects similar to that of hydrocortisone, most result in a moderate antitumour promotor effect. It is expected that these triterpenoids, such as pachymic acid, may inhibit phospholipase $A_2$. Nonetheless, since these mushrooms are edible and are used as supplements and herbal medicines, they are considered to have extremely low or no toxicity. Therefore, these triterpenoids from poria and reishi are a promising group of compounds. In particular, pachymic acid, ganoderic acid T, and lucidenic acid B, are leads in the search for cancer prevention drugs; the development of cancer prevention drugs with properties akin to tamoxifen is desired. When developing a preventative drug, the safety of the substance must first and foremost be considered.

There are many other challenges, such as further elucidating the mechanism, ascertaining the appropriate intake level, and supplying large amounts of the compound. The cooperation and collaboration of researchers from various fields will be necessary to address these issues.

## Acknowledgements

Dr. Michio Takido, my mentor and professor emeritus at School of Pharmacy, Nihon University, passed away on August 25, 2014. My research and attitude towards this research were greatly influenced by his guidance. This article is dedicated to Dr Takido with profound gratitude.

## Author details

Ken Yasukawa

Address all correspondence to: yasukawa.ken@nihon-u.ac.jp, yasukawa.ken@nihon-.ne.jp

School of Pharmacy, Nihon University, Funabashi, Chiba, Japan

## References

[1] Yasukawa K. Medicinal and edible plants as cancer preventive agents. In: Vallisuta O, Olimat SM (eds) Drug Discovery Research in Pharmacognosy. Rijeka: InTech; 2012. p181–208.

[2] Chihara G, Maeda Y, Hamuro J, Sasaki T, Fukuoka F. Inhibition of mouse sarcoma 180 by polysaccharides from Lentinus edodes (Berk.) sing. Nature 1969;222(5194) 687–688.

[3] Chihara G, Hamuro J, Maeda Y, Arai Y, Fukuoka F. Fractionation and purification of the polysaccharides with marked antitumor activity, especially lentinan, from *Lentinus edodes* (Berk.) Sing. (an edible mushroom). Cancer Research 1970;30(11) 2776–2781.

[4] Zákány J, Chihara G, Fachet J. Effect of lentinan on tumor growth in murine allogeneic and syngeneic hosts. International Journal of Cancer 1980;25(3) 371–376.

[5] Suga T, Shiio T, Maeda YY, Chihara G. Antitumor activity of lentinan in murine syngeneic and autochthonous hosts and its suppressive effect on 3-methylcholanthrene-induced carcinogenesis. Cancer Research 1984;44(11) 5132–5137.

[6] Hamuro J, Chihara G. Immunopotentiation by the antitumor polysaccharide lentinan, its immunopharmacology and physiology. In: The reticuloendoyhelial system. Vol. 8 (Hadden JW, Szentivanyl A, eds) Plenum Publ., New York, 1985, pp. 285–307.

[7] Ikekawa T, Uehara N, Maeda Y, Nakanishi M, Fukuoka F. Antitumor activity of aqueous extracts of edible mushrooms. Cancer Research 1969;29(3) 734–735.

[8] Ikekawa T. Beneficial effects of edible and medicinal mushrooms on health care. International Journal of Medicinal Mushroom 2001;3(4); 291–298.

[9] Hamuro J, Chihara G. Effect of antitumor polysaccharides on the higher structure of serum protein. Nature 1973;245(5419) 40–41.

[10] Lo TC-T, Hsu F-M, Chang CA, Cheng JC-H. Branched $\alpha$-(1,4) glucans from *Lentinula edodes* (L10) in combination with radiation enhance cytotoxic effect on human lung adenocarcinoma through the Toll-like receptor 4 mediated induction of THP-1 differentiation/activation. Journal of Agricultural and Food Chemistry 2011;59(22) 11997–12005.

[11] Komatsu N, Okubo S, Kikumoto S, Kimura K, Saito G, Sakai S. Host-mediated antitumor action of Schizophyllan, a glucan produced by *Schizophyllum commune*. Japanese Journal of Cancer Research (Gann) 1969;60(2) 137–144.

[12] Okamura K, Suzuki M, Chihara T, Fujiwara A, Fukuda T, Goto S, Ichinohe K, Jimi S, Kasamatsu T, Kawai N, Mizuguchi K, Mori S, Nakano H, Noda K, Sekiba K, Suzuki K, Suzuki T, Takahashi K, Takeuchi K, Takeuchi S, Yajima A, Ogawa N. Clinical evaluation of Schizophyllan combined with irradiation in patients with cervical cancer. Cancer 1986;58(4), 865–872.

[13] Ross GD, Vetvicka V. CR3 (CD11b, CD18): a phagocyte and NK cell membrane receptor with multiple ligand specificities and functions. Clinical and Experimental Immunology 1993;92(2) 181–184.

[14] Di Renzo L, Yefenof E, Klein E. The function of human NK cells is enhanced by β-glucan, a ligand of CR 3 (CD11b/CD18). European Journal of Immunology 1991;21(7) 1755–1758.

[15] Kobayashi H, Matsunaga K, Oguchi Y. Antimetastatic effects of PSK (Krestin), a protein-bound polysaccharide obtained from basidiomycetes: an overview. Cancer Epidemiol, Biomarkers & Prevention 1995;4(3) 275–281.

[16] Ito H, Hidaka H, Suigura M. Effects of coriolane, an antitumor polysaccharide, produced by *Coriolus versicolor* Iwade. Japanese Journal of Pharmacology 1979;29(6) 953–957.

[17] Huang H-Y, Chieh S-Y, Tso TK, Chien T-Y, Lin H-T, Tsai Y-C. Orally administered mycelia culture of *Phellinus linteus* exhibits antitumor effects in hepatoma cell-bearing mice. Journal of Ethnopharmacology 2011;133(2) 460–466.

[18] Li Y-G, Ji D-F, Zhong S, Zhu J-X, Chen S, Hu G-Y. Anti-tumor effects of proteoglycan from *Phellinus linteus* by immunomodulating and inhibiting Reg IV/EGFR/Akt signaling pathway in colorectal carcinoma. International Journal of Biological Macromolecules 2011;48(8) 511–517.

[19] Zhong S, Ji D-F, Li Y-G, Lin T-B, Lv Z-Q, Chen H-P. Activation of P27kip1-cyclin D1/E-CDK2 pathway by polysaccharide from *Phellinus linteus* leads to S-phase arrest in HT-29 cells. Chemico-Biological Interactions 2013;206(2) 222–229.

[20] Yamagiwa K, Ichikawa K. Experimental study of the pathogenesis of carcinoma. The Journal of Cancer Research 1918;3 (1) 1–29.

[21] Berenblum I. The cocarcinogenic action of croton resin. Cancer Research 1941;1(1) 44–48.

[22] Berenblum I. The mechanism of carcinogenesis. A study of the significance of cocarcinogenic action and related phenomena. Cancer Research 1941;1(10) 807–814.

[23] Hecker E. Phorbol esters from crotn oil, chemical nature and biological activities. Naturwissenschaften 1967;54(11) 282–284.

[24] van Duuren BL. Tumor-promoting agents in two-stage carcinogenesis. Progress in Expremental Tumor Research 1969;11(1) 31–68.

[25] Fujiki H, Suganuma M. Naturally-derived tumor promoters and inhibitors of carcinogenesis. Toxin Reviews 1996;15(2) 129–156.

[26] van den Bosch CA. Is endemic Burkitt's lymphoma an alliance between three infections and a tumour promoter? Lancet Oncology 2004;5(12) 738–746.

[27] Aya T, Kinoshita T, Imai S, Koizumi S, Mizuno F, Osato T, Satoh C, Oikawa T, Kuzumaki N, Ohigashi H, Koshimizu K. Chromosome translocation and *c-myc* activation by Epstein-Barr virus and *Euphorbia tirucalli* in B lymphocytes. Lancet 1991;337(8751) 1190.

[28] Imai S, Sugiura M, Mizuno F, Ohigashi H, Koshimizu K, Chiba S, Osato T. African Burkitt's lymphoma: A plant, *Euphorbia tirucalli*, reduces Epstein-Barr virus-specific cellular immunity. Anticancer Research 1994, 14(3A) 933–936.

[29] Yasukawa K, Takido M, Takeuchi M, Nakagawa S. Effect of chemical constituents from plants on 12-*O*-tetradecanoylphorbol-13-acetate-induced inflammation in mice. Chemical & Pharmaceutical Bulletin 1989;37(4) 1071–1073.

[30] Yasukawa K, Kanno H, Kaminaga T, Takido M, Kasahara Y, Kumaki K. Inhibitory effect of methanol extracts from edible mushroom on TPA-induced ear oedema and tumour promotion in mouse skin. Phytotherapy Research 1996;10(4) 367–369

[31] Yasukawa K, Aoki T, Takido M, Ikekawa T, Saito H, Matsuzawa T. Inhibitory effects of ergosterol isolated from the edible mushroom *Hypsizigus marmoreus* on TPA-induced inflammatory ear oedema and tumour promotion in mice. Phytotherapy Research 1994;8(1) 10–13.

[32] Kaminaga T, Yasukawa K, Takido M, Tai T, Nunoura Y. Inhibitory effect of *Poria cocos* on 12-*O*-tetradecanoylphorbol-13-acetate-induced ear oedema and tumour promotion in mouse skin. Phytotherapy Research 1996;10(7) 581–584.

[33] Akita A, Sun Y, Yasukawa K. Inhibitory effects of chaga (*Inonotus obliquus*) on tumor promotion in two-stage mouse skin carcinogenesis. Journal of Pharmacy and Nutrition Science 2015;5(1), 71-76.

[34] Yasukawa K, Kitanaka S, Takahashi H, Hirayama H, Shigemoto K. Inhibitory effect of natural fruit body of *Phellinus linteus* on tumor promotion in mice skin. The Japanese Journal of Pharmacognosy 2007;61(1), 14–17.

[35] Ohigashi H, Takamura H, Koshimizu K, Tokuda H, Ito Y. Search for possible antitumor promoters by inhibition of 12-*O*-tetradecanoylphorbol-13-acetate-induced Epstein-Barr virus activation; ursolic acid and oleanolic acid from anti-inflammatory Chinese medicinal plant, *Glechoma hederaceae* L. Cancer Letters 1986;30(2) 143–151.

[36] Yasukawa K, Akihisa T, Kanno H, Kaminaga T, Izumida M, Sakoh T, Tamura T, Takido M. Inhibitory effects of sterols isolated from *Chlorella vulgaris* on 12-*O*-tetradecanoyl- phorbol-13-acetate-induced inflammation and tumor promotion in mouse skin. Biological & Pharmaceutical Bulletin (Tokyo) 1996;19(4), 573–576.

[37] Akihisa T, Franzblau SG, Tokuda H, Tagata M, Ukiya M, Matsuzawa T, Metori K, Kimura Y, Suzuki T, Yasukawa K. Antitubercular activity and inhibitory effect on Epstein-Barr virus activation of sterols and polyisoprenepolyols from an edible mushroom, *Hypsizigus marmoreus*. Biological & Pharmaceutical Bulletin 2005;28(6) 1117–1119.

[38] Akita A, Yasukawa K. Inhibitory effect of chaga (*Inonotus obliquus*) on tumor promotion in two-stage mouse skin carcinogenesis, Japanese Journal of Complementary and Alternative Medicine 2011;8(1) 29–32.

[39] Yasukawa K, Takahashi H, Kitanaka S, Hirayama H, Shigemoto K. Inhibitory effect of an aqueous extract of *Phellinus linteus* on tumor promotion in mouse skin. Mushroom Science and Biotechnology 2007;15(2) 97–101.

[40] Nakata T, Yamada T, Taji S, Ohishi H, Wada S, Tokuda H, Sakuma K, Tanaka R. Structure determination of inonotsuoxides A and B in vivo anti-tumor promoting activity of inotodiol from the sclerotia of *Inonotus obliquus*. Bioorganic & Medicinal Chemistry 2007;15(1) 257–264.

[41] Taji S, Yamada T, Wada S, Tokuda H, Sakuma K, Tanaka R. Lanostane-type triterpenoids from the sclerotia of *Inonotus obliquus* possessing anti-tumor promoting activity. European Journal of Medicinal Chemistry 2008;43(11) 2373–2379.

[42] Akihisa T, Nakamura Y, Tagata M, Tokuda H, Yasukawa K, Uchiyama E, Suzuki T, Kimura Y. Anti-inflammatory and anti-tumor-promoting effects of triterpene acids and sterols from the fungus *Ganoderma lucidum*. Chemistry & Biodiversity 2007;4(2) 224–231.

[43] Akihisa T, Tagata M, Ukiya M, Tokuda H, Suzuki T, Kimura Y. Oxygenated lanostane-type triterpenoids from the fungus *Ganoderma lucidum*. Journal of Natural Products. 2005;68(4) 559–563.

[44] Iwatsuki K, Akihisa T, Tokuda H, Ukiya M, Oshikubo M, Kimura Y, Asano T, Nomura A, Nishino H. Lucidenic acids P and Q, methyl lucidenate P, and other triterpenoids from the fungus *Ganoderma lucidum* and their inhibitory effects on Epstein-Barr virus activation. Journal of Natural Products 2003;66(12) 1582–1585.

[45] Tang W, Liu J-W, Zhao W-M, Wei D-Z, Zhong J-J. Ganoderic acid T from *Ganoderma lucidum* mycelia induces mitochondria mediated apoptosis in lung cancer cells. Life Sciences 2006;80(3) 205–211.

[46] Chen N-H, Liu J-W, Zhong J-J. Ganoderic acid T inhibits tumor invasion in vitro and in vivo through inhibition of MMP expression. Pharmacological Reports 2010;62(1) 150–163.

[47] Wu GS, Lu JJ, Guo JJ, Li YB, Tan W, Dang YY, Zhong ZF, Xu ZT, Chen XP, Wang YT. Ganoderic acid DM, a natural triterpenoid, induces DNA damage, G1 cell cycle arrest and apoptosis in human breast cancer cells. Fitoterapia 2012;83(2) 408–414.

[48] Jiang J, Grieb B, Thyagarajan A, Sliva D. Ganoderic acids suppress growth and invasive behavior of breast cancer cells by modulating AP-1 and NF-κB signaling. International Journal of Molecular Medicine 2008;21(5) 577–584.

[49] Chen N-H, Liu J-W, Zhong J-J. Ganoderic acid Me inhibits tumor invasion through down-regulating matrix metalloproteinases 2/9 gene expression. Journal of Pharmacological Sciences 2008;108(2) 212–216.

[50] Wang C-J, Chau C-F, Hsich Y-S, Yang S-F, Yen G-C. Lucidenic acid inhibits PMA-induced invasion of human hepatoma cells through inactivating MAPK/ERK signal

transduction pathway and reducing binding activities of NF-κB and AP-1. Carcinogenesis 2008;29(1) 147–156.

[51] Hsu C-L, Yu Y-S, Yen G-C. Lucidenic acid B induces apoptosis in human leukemia cells via a mitochondria-mediated pathway. Journal of Agricultural Chemistry 2008;56(11) 3973–3980.

[52] Capasso L. 5300 years ago, the Ice Man used natural laxatives and antibiotics. The Lancet 1998;352(9143) 1864.

[53] Schlegel B, Luhmann U, Härtl A, Gräfe U. Piptamine, a new antibiotic produced by *Piptoporus betulinus* Lu 9-1. The Journal of Antibiotics 2000;53(9) 973–974.

[54] Kamo T, Asanoma M, Shibata H, Hirota M. Anti-inflammatory lanostane-type triterpene acids from *Piptoporus betulinus*. Journal of Natural Products 2003;66(8) 1104–1106.

[55] Sun Y, Yasukawa K. New anti-inflammatory ergostane-type ecdysteroids from the sclerotium of *Polyporus umbellatus*. Bioorganic & Medicinal Chemistry Letters 2008;18(9) 3417–3420.

[56] Haranaka R, Kosoto H, Hirama N, Hanawa T, Hasegawa R, Hyun SJ, Nakagawa S, Haranaka K, Satomi N, Sakurai A, Yasukawa K, Takido M. Antitumor activities of Zyuzen-taiho-to and Cinnamomi Cortex. Journal Medical and Pharmaceutical Society for Wakan-Yaku 1987;4(1) 49–58.

[57] Yasukawa K, Yu S-Y, Takido M. Inhibitory effect of oral administration of Rikkunshi-to on tumor promotion in two-stage carcinogenesis in mouse skin. Journal of Traditional Medicines 1996;13(2) 180–184.

[58] Yasukawa K, Yu S-Y, Kakinuma S, Takido M. Inhibitory effect of of Rikkunshi-to, a traditional Chinese herbal prescription, on tumor promotion in two-stage carcinogenesis in mouse skin. Biological & Pharmaceutical Bulletin 1995;18(5) 730–733.

[59] Kaminaga T, Yasukawa K, Kanno H, Tai T, Nunoura Y, Takido M. Inhibitory effect of lanostane-type triterpene acids, the components of *Poria cocos*, on tumor promotion by 12-O-tetradecanoylphorbol-13-acetate in two-stage carcinogenesis in mouse skin. Oncology 1996;53(5) 382–385.

[60] Akihisa T, Nakamura Y, Tokuda H, Uchiyama E, Suzuki T, Kimura Y, Uchikura K, Nishino H. Triterpene acids from *Poria cocos* and their anti-tumor-promoting effects. Journal of Natural Products 2007;70(6) 948–953.

[61] Akihisa T, Uchiyama E, Kikuchi T, Tokuda H, Suzuki T, Kimura Y. Anti-tumor-promoting effects of 25-methoxyporicoic acid A and other triterpene acids from *Poria cocos*. Journal of Natural Products 2009;72(10) 1786–1792.

[62] Ukiya M, Akihisa T, Tokuda H, Hirano M, Oshikubo M, Nobukuni Y, Kimura Y, Tai T, Kondo S, Nishino H..Inhibition of tumor-promoting effects by poricoic acids G

and H and other lanostane-type triterpenes and cytotoxic activity of poricoic acids A and G from *Poria cocos*. Journal of Natural Products 2002;65(4) 462–465.

[63] Kikuchi T, Uchiyama E, Ukiya M, Tabata K, Kimura Y, Suzuki T, Akihisa T. Cytotoxic and apoptosis-inducing activities of triterpene acids from *Poria cocos*. Journal of Natural Products 2011;74(2) 137–144.

[64] Cuéllar MJ, Giner RM, Recio MC, Just MJ, Máñez S, Ríos JL. Two fungal lanostane derivatives as phospholipase $A_2$ inhibitors. Journal of Natural Products 1996;59(10) 977–979.

# 4

# The Evolving Role of Natural Products from the Tropical Rainforests as a Replenishable Source of New Drug Leads

Ibrahim Jantan, Syed Nasir Abbas Bukhari, Mohamed Ali Seyed Mohamed, Lam Kok Wai and Mohammed Ahmed Mesaik

## 1. Introduction

More than 80, 000 of the 250, 000 species of flowering plants have been reported to be used by human civilizations for medicinal purposes [1]. This figure could be higher as information on the native uses of plants as medicines was mainly passed on verbally from one generation to another and has mostly stayed unregistered. Some of the traditional knowledge might be lost as some practitioners were secretive and reluctant to reveal enough information. Information on the ancient uses of plant materials as medicines can be found in archeological finds, archives, ancient documents, history books and pharmacopoeias. Fossil records date human use of plants as medicines at least to the Middle Paleolithic age some 60, 000 years ago [2]. The World Health Organization (WHO) estimated that as much as 80 per cent of the world's population relies on traditional forms of medicine, chiefly plants [3]. The tropical rainforest plants are biologically and chemically diverse resource as they synthesize a wide spectrum of organic molecules as defense agents against diseases, pests and predators. They have been shown to be the source of chemicals of diverse structures with promising biological activities and perhaps the most valuable source of therapeutic agents due to their rich biodiversity [4]. Tropical rainforests have been called the 'world's largest pharmacy', because over one quarter of natural medicines have been discovered within them; additionally, about 70% of the drugs used today are models of natural products. Plants have always been a rich source of natural products and historically provided many major new drugs. Natural products or natural product-derived compounds signify great structural variety, which is not usually found in synthetic compounds. Of the 1184 new chemical entities reported through 1981 to 2006, 60% were derived from or based on natural products. Twenty-five percent of all prescription medications are made using the various types of secondary metabolites from living organisms, mainly plants [5-9].

One hundred twenty-one prescription drugs are made from higher plants. This does not include antibiotics from microorganisms. Among the world's 25 best-selling pharmaceutical agents, 12 are natural product-derived [10], and natural products are playing key role in drug discovery programs of the pharmaceutical industry and various research organizations [11-13]. Half of these plant-based medicines come from the tropics, and 74% of these came from native folklore. Seventy percent of the plants identified as having anti-cancer characteristics by the US National Cancer Institute are found only in the tropical rainforests. Quinine, the first known antimalarial, comes from a neotropical tree, and curare, used as a poison for arrow tips by indigenous peoples in the Neotropics, is also useful for heart conditions. As new medical discoveries are being made all the time obviously, the tropical rainforests and their resources such as natural products find place in every part of our life. Plants have evolved and adapted over millions of years to withstand bacteria, insects, fungi and weather to produce unique, structurally diverse secondary metabolites.Therefore, natural products play a leading role in the research of leads for the development of drugs for treating human diseases [14]. The investigation of biological and chemical properties of natural products for the past two centuries has not only produced drugs for the treatment of several diseases, but has instigated the development of synthetic organic chemistry, and the arrival of medicinal chemistry as a major route to discover efficacious and novel therapeutic agents. Structural alteration of natural compounds or synthesis of novel compounds, based on designs following a natural compound scaffolding, have offered us a lot of vital new drugs in the fields of medicine, agriculture, and food spheres [15-16].

## 2. History of drug discovery and development

Medicinal plants have been used by mankind since ancient times as the main source of medicines. Originally the choice of plants to treat various ailments was on an irrational basis as it was strongly influenced by ideologies of the primitive societies which were deeply rooted in mysticism and superstition. They believed, for example, a person became ill because evil spirits dwelled in his body. Plants with unpleasant odor and taste, accompanied by enchantments and ceremonial dances, were used to get rid of the demons and the person would then recover from his illness. However, the selection of plants for medicinal purposes became more rational when it was influenced and shaped by new philosophies and religions [17]. In the search for remedies from plants many different theories of disease were proposed and the choice of plants was based on these ideas. Although the ancient peoples were ignorance on the etiology of disease and the mechanism by which the medicinal agents made the disease disappear, they tried to establish a relationship between them. One of the earliest theory was the concept of plant signature which claimed that God provided visual sign (signature) in plants that permits us to recognize and utilize them to cure diseases [18]. Signature plants were probably first recognized in ancient China, where there was classification that associated plant features to human organs. 'Yang' was linked to strong acting plants: diseases of upper half of the body were treated with upper parts of plants, whereas 'Yin' was related with plants possessing modest action and those with sweet, salty, sour and bitter tastes; underground parts of the plant were used to treat the diseases of lower parts of the body [19]. Signature plants emerged for medicinal uses in western cultures during the Middle Ages. Paracelsus Doctrine of Signature, published in the 16th century, was a theory based on signature plants [17].

The signature plants provided a way of reducing the complexity of selecting plants to treat diseases. However, the traditional medicine practitioners of many cultures did not depend on the Doctrine of Signatures alone for knowledge of the proper use of a medicinal plant. A wide range of plants were experimented by trial and error to treat diseases and discovered that certain plants were effective against a number of diseases. The 'crude clinical trials' were actually a screening process but they could also possibly have produced many adverse effects, casualties and possibly thousands of deaths resulted from the toxicity of some of the plants. Several thousands of plants had been screened and based on their long-term use by human, one might expect that plants presently in use in traditional medicine produced some beneficial effects and have low human toxicity. If a plant showed acute toxic effects following its use to treat illness it would then not be used at all. However, if a plant had chronic toxic effects it would be less likely be noticed and it would continue to be used [20]. Moreover, there was lack of reporting system to document these effects as most information was passed on only by word of mouth. The information derived from the empirical knowledge and theories on the use of plants, although has been regarded with interested skepticism, had contributed towards the early development of medicinal agents from plants. The traditional knowledge and practices on the use of medicinal plants for treating diseases rely exclusively on practical experience and observation passed on verbally from one generation to the next with little documentation. It is necessary to understand the contemporary relevance of empirical knowledge and the interpretation of this knowledge using modern methods in the chemical and biological studies of substances [20].

During the course of history, natural products have offered a variety of compounds that have extensive applications in the fields of medicine, food and agriculture [21]. Higher plants in particular have been the basis of medicinal agents for centuries, and presently they play key roles in the primary health care of 80% of the world [22]. Medicinal agents and natural products therefore, are also a significant feature in the health care systems of the residual 20% of the population living in developed countries, with more than half of all the drugs in clinical use having sourced from natural products [23].The earliest history of the identification of novel bioactive compounds from natural sources can be traced back in 1804 when a young German pharmacist had successfully isolated morphine from the seed pods of the poppy, *Papaver somniferum* [24]. Since then, it marked the birth of the study on purification and the effects of drugs from natural products. This classical example represents most of the drug discovery process from natural products, where majority of new drugs have been discovered by direct isolation from natural sources and molecular modification of natural products. The phenotypic screening and single target or bullet-based approach have been the dominant paradigms to discover natural small organic molecules from natural resources as new leads or models for the development of synthetic molecules for the discovery of drug targets.

Plant-based traditional medicine systems have been in existence for centuries in countries like China [25], India [26], the Malay Archipelago, and medicinal plants are used widely in African traditional health systems [27-28]. Many phytomedicines are registered and extensively used in Europe, and more than 600 botanical items have been legitimately documented in various editions of the United States Pharmacopoeia[29], however existing rules forbid most from being marketed as drugs. According to the WHO, majority of population still rely on plant-based traditional medicines for primary health care [30] and 80% of 122 plant derived drugs were related to their original ethnopharmacological purposes [31]. The knowledge associated with traditional medicines has promoted further investigations of medicinal plants as potential medicines and has led to the isolation of many natural products that have become well known pharmaceuticals. Until the 1950s almost all drug research relied heavily on vascular plants as sources of medicines. Plant-based traditional knowledge has become a recognized tool in search for new sources of drugs [32]. Most of the early discoveries of plant-derived drugs were by examining the use of these plants in traditional medicine. The phytochemicals isolated directly from plants were used unmodified as drugs. Morphine, isolated from opium poppy (*Papaver somniferum*) was the first plant-derived drug. Other examples include reserpine, an antihypertensive drug, from the root of *Rauvolfia serpentina*. the cardiac glycosides digoxin and digitoxin from *Digitalis lanata*, and the anticancer agents, vincristine and vinblastine from *Catharanthus roseus* [33]. The anticancer area, in particular, has made great use of natural products such as vinblastine and vincristine (vinca alkaloids), etoposide and teniposide (podophylltoxin analogues), paclitaxel (taxol), and camptothecin–derived topotecan. In the past ten years, 62% of the new anticancer-agents have been natural products or based on natural products models [31].

## 3. Conventional approach of drug discovery from natural products

History had shown that serendipity played a major role in the finding of novel drugs. One classical example that warrant a repetition was the discovery of penicillin, an antibiotic produced by *Penicillium notatum*, by Alexander Fleming in 1928. Henry Harris once said that 'Without Fleming, no Chain; without Chain, no Florey; without Florey, no Heatley; without Heatley, no penicillin.' After several years, the main active component was finally determined to be benzylpencillin which lysis the staphylococcal colonies on an agar plate [34]. The impact of the aforementioned example was so great that more scientists at that time started to look into natural products as the main source of leads. Since then, more structured strategies in natural products drug discovery were implemented in choosing plants for biological screening such as the ethnobotanical approach, chemotaxonomic approach or the phylogenetic survey screening, phenotypic screening and the single target or bullet-based approach.

The selection of plants based on traditional knowledge serves as the initial biological screening in a drug discovery program. The selection of plant samples for biological screening is generally based on the indigenous uses of plants. The ethnobotanical approach is more targeted and the most successful of the plant-surveying methods. The indigenous uses of plants offer important clues or information on the biological activities of those plants which are based on accumulated past knowledge and experiments by ancient civilization. Undeniably, some of the effectiveness of these plant extracts have been refuted due to the placebo effect in the patients, it is still one of the best approach for identifying leads. For example, plants used traditionally against diseases possibly caused by viruses are collected for anti-HIV screening [33]. The ethnobotanical field searches have generated many lead compounds which have been identified as drug candidates for the development of many therapeutic agents such as antiviral, antifungal and anticancer drugs. There are many important discoveries that lead to the development of more effective and safer drugs. Prostratin, a powerful antiviral agent, was found in the aqueous extract of *Homalanthus nutans* which is used in Samoa to treat yellow fever. A novel compound that kills parasitic worms in the stomach was isolated form *Curcuma comosa* which is used in Thailand to ease stomach pains and other gastrointestinal disorders. The extracts of ipecacuanha root, found in the genus of the Rubiaceae family, was used in the Aztec and Mayan cultures to treat amoebiasis and emetine, the bioactive compound responsible for the activity had been isolated from the plant [35]. Due to the adverse side-effects, a synthetic compound dehydroemetine was synthesized. Codeine which is found in the opium poppy, *Papaver somniferum*, is widely used for the treatment of moderate pain. The use of codeine can be traced back hundreds of years far back in the Egyptians and the Ancient Chinese history. Another plant extract known as ma huang or 'Yellow Hemp' has been used by the Chinese to treat asthma and hay fever for thousands of years [36]. It was not until 1926, when the active ingredient, ephedrine was introduced into the Western medicine as an orally active bronchodilator to treat acute asthma. Another important example is the use of cinchona bark from the species *Cinchona succirubra* by the Quechua, South American Indians in the treatment of fevers. The active ingredient, quinine was the first effective treatment for malaria caused by *Plasmodium falciparum*. Other plant that possess antimalarial activity was reported by the Chinese herbalist known as *Artemisia annua* or sweet wormwood which had been described in a 4$^{th}$ century text. Studies have shown that the active compound responsible for the antimalarial properties was artemisinin [33, 37].

Phylogenetic survey or chemotaxonomic method is a plant-collecting method where researchers select relatives of plants identified to yield useful compounds. The ecological survey is a selection made on the basis of defensive features of the plants against predators, indicating that they produce chemicals capable to exert an effect on animals. The non-targeted method (haphazard collection of plant samples) is practiced by researchers particularly in areas involving biological diversity, nonetheless the success rate is poor [33]. Taxol, derived from *Taxus brevifolia*, is a notable example of anticancer drug discovered by a random screening program. In phenotypic screening, pure compounds or extracts from plants are screened through *in vitro* followed by *in vivo* or *vice versa* to monitor the desirable change in phenotype before an effort is made to determine the biological target. Meanwhile the single target approach requires a molecular structure (active site or receptor) that will undergo a specific interaction with the so called plant extracts or pure compounds when they are administered to treat a certain disease. While these two pharmacological approaches are still commonly practiced in most of the universities and research centers in developing countries, the chances of finding bioactive compounds from plants are highly serendipitous. To minimize the time consumption and tedious laboratory work, a directed screening is principally carried out on medical folkloric plants.

Methods adopted in the natural products isolation or bioassays screening have been rather straightforward. Crude extracts obtained from the dried or fresh plants are extracted with aqueous or organic solvents such as water, methanol, chloroform, hexane, and ethyl acetate. The practical of this isolation method can be found since the Mesopotamian and Egyptian civilizations where natural products extraction had been a common practice to produce perfumes or pharmaceutical products. Simple soxhlet extraction, maceration, hydro-distillation, and other solvent extractor techniques have been employed in the past and present, albeit large quantity of plant samples are generally required to obtain pure compounds. Conventional chromatography methods such as column and planar chromatography which rely on the differential partitioning between the mobile and stationary phases play important roles in drug discovery from natural products. Before new chromatographic methods were developed, isolation of minor compounds from plant extracts was relatively difficult. In recent time, the weaknesses using these conventional methods have been gradually solved by the replacement with more advanced instruments such as high-throughput gradient flash and medium or high pressure liquid chromatography (HPLC). In general, methods of isolation can be divided into a few categories including extraction, precipitation, and chromatography. Before the invention of sophisticated analytical spectroscopy techniques such as nuclear magnetic resonance (NMR), mass spectrometry (MS), infrared spectroscopy (IR), and X-ray crystallography, determination of molecular structure of pure compounds from natural products had been the major obstacle in drug development. People had been using different sets of chemical transformations and measurement of physical data such as melting point and molecular weight for the compounds structure determination. Issues regarding chirality have been an on-going debate among the scientists when deciding on the structure of the isolated natural compounds.

When Fischer and Daniel Koshland suggested the lock and key model and induced fit theory, the chirality of natural compounds had become an important issue that needs to be resolved before the real mechanism of action can be proposed. Since single target approach relies heavily on the interactions between the bioactive compound and protein target; possibly specific enzyme or receptor, the real identities of the natural compounds need to be accurately determined. Nowadays, it is obligatory to include the proper and accurate structural elucidation data of the pure compounds before the pharmacological activity can be published in any research journals. Such remarkable improvements in the spectrometry techniques have definitely amplified the speed of drug discovery process from natural products. A single plant extract may consist of a considerable pool of metabolites. Attempt to isolate the right bioactive compound out of the hundreds mixture of other compounds is quite tedious and time consuming; similar to finding a needle in a haystack. Two conventional approaches that deserved a mention here are the extract-library screening and bioassay-guided isolation. These two techniques, popularized in the 1980s, are commonly used for screening, hit identification, and hit-to-lead development from the natural products, however received a competitive disadvantage when compared to the approaches using the synthetic chemical libraries [38]. The screening of extract-library normally carried out on cell cultures to study the cellular responses under controlled conditions. The extract that shows certain activity will then be subjected to a series of isolations until the pure active compound is obtained. A more recent bioassay-guided isolation method requires a step-by-step separation of extracted components based on differences in their physicochemical properties and assessing the biological activity where the process continues until the right bioactive compound is successfully isolated. One best example is the use of TLC plate, in which spraying with reactive media that respond with the compounds from extract will produce a color implying the presence of an active compound and further isolation work is required to obtain the compound. While these two methods are in disadvantage position compared to the more well-defined high throughput screening on synthetic chemical libraries, lately it received a renewed interest from both the academic institutions and drug industries. The practicality of discovering new drugs by conventional methods has been constantly receiving negative perception from the funding agencies and private companies. Considering the number of people who actually have the access to high throughput screening chemical libraries or other high throughput bioassays, authors truly believe that the use of the aforementioned conventional methods are still highly relevant in our society. Without a doubt, these old practices have definitely set a good platform in natural products drug discovery program.

## 4. De-emphasize of natural products research in the 80's

The interests in finding bioactive natural products from the tropical rainforests at several major pharmaceutical companies had generally declined in the early 1980s when microorganisms and fungi which were easy to collect and culture provided alternative sources. Dwindling interests on plants as source of drugs were also due to low success rate in the discoveries of plant-derived drugs, and advances in synthetic organic chemistry and biotechnology that offered more opportunities to design new drugs in the laboratory [33, 39]. Many pharmaceutical firms had abandoned exploring traditional knowledge of plants in mid-1980s in their search for new drugs.. The reductionist approach in finding bioactive natural products from the tropical rainforests had declined due to the many major hurdles faced by them such as difficulties in obtaining sufficient supply of high quality natural products screening libraries, ownership issues and research in this field is lengthy, expensive, highly complex and ineffective with low success rate. On the other hand, the process of drug development is often a risky and costly endeavor. Drug discovery and development process requires between 10 to 20 years and was estimated to cost US$ 802 million per drug in 2004 [40]. Most recently it was estimated that the cost of inventing and developing a drug could exceed US$1 billion or more. The average drug developed by a major pharmaceutical company costs at least $4 billion, and it can be as much as US$11 billion [41]. Natural products drug discovery has been marginalized in favor of the rational design of synthetic compounds to target specific molecules after the advent of high throughput screening (HTS), combinatorial chemistry and advancement in the knowledge of molecular mechanisms, cell biology and genomics.

Historically numerous complications linked with natural products, particularly plant-derived products, added to decreasing attention in their development within the pharmaceutical industry. A few years ago, there were major problems with obtaining authentic plant materials. Difficulty in the access to genetic resources and traditional knowledge by the multinationals and pharmaceutical firms and the absence of a legal framework for a fair and equitable sharing of benefits, arising from the commercial and other utilization of genetic resources with the resource countries resulted in the departure of many drug companies from investing in natural products from tropical rainforest plants as a source of drug leads. It was convenient to collect plants and exhibit that their extracts possessed interesting biological potential. However, when investigators returned to approve the potential and ultimately to develop and commercialize the product, failure resulted often due to inadequate records and loss of the original collections of plant. There were also problems regarding the assessment of biological activities of natural products, which commonly are complex combinations of materials. The interactions among the components of the mixtures, either the antagonism by a material of another's activity or the combined effect/addition of activities, often delivered unclear results. Identification and purification of active components from intricate natural products encompassing lots of numerous chemical substances, regularly of almost similar physical and chemical properties, were slow and expensive. Once the active component was isolated and purified, its chemical structure still needed to be documented. Moreover, natural product materials are often poor pharmaceuticals; their chemical stability may be minimal; they might have poor solubility or bioavailability characteristics; they may not formulate properly, etc., therefore not ensuing Lipinski's Rule of Five [42]. All these difficulties have stood stern challenges. The most accountable problem for restricted importance in plant-based natural product materials for pharmaceutical discovery and development has been hesitation regarding the availability of amounts of pure chemical substances. Quantities are required initially to generate information to understand and assess real prospective of the material for pharmaceutical application. Ultimately, the most restrictive thought is the amount required to fulfill market demand should a pharmaceutical develop into an effective drug. The market demand can vary from a scale of hundreds to thousands of kilograms yearly. It is recognized that the complete synthesis will not provide the intricate natural product to satisfy this market demand [43].

Subsequent to the 'Golden Age of Antibiotics' and the worldwide reassurance to discover new antibiotics, several main pharmaceutical companies at the time initiated natural product discovery (NPD) programs which highlighted not only on antifungal and antibacterial targets but also on infectious illnesses. These platforms provided compounds for the treatment of hypercholesteremia, tissue rejection in organ transplantations, cancer and microbial infections [44, 45]. Though majority of the larger pharmaceutical industries removed their NPD programs during the 1980s and early 1990s, it was the advent of programmed high throughput screening (HTS) which enhanced the impetus of biological testing and combinatorial chemistry started to be endorsed as a better method to producing 'drug-like' materials for HTS. As a result, several pharmaceutical companies sold their gatherings of screening extracts [46, 47] as it was believed that orthodox extract-derived monitoring resulted in the constant rediscovery of previously isolated compounds and that the structural intricacy of natural products required whole synthesis and derivatization which is both synthetically and economically difficult.

Owing to supply difficulties, the time required to develop a natural product from an extract to a pharmaceutical was believed to be excessively lengthy; HTS machineries rely on combinatorial chemistry to yield huge compound libraries. During the past two decades 'customary natural product chemistry' has predominantly been substituted by molecular target-based drug discovery, using great combinatorial libraries to discover effective 'hits' [45]. However, developments in technology and sophisticated instrumentation for the rapid identification of novel natural products and structure explanation keep enhancing the natural product discovery [44]. Since 1980s, it was thought that combinatorial chemistry would be the upcoming basis of numerous new carbon skeletons and drug front runners or novel chemical entities (NCEs). This has unquestionably not been the case because there has only been one combinatorial NCE permitted by the U.S FDA in that time frame, the kinase inhibitor sorafendib (approved by the FDA, 2005) to treat renal carcinoma [48]. Combinatorial chemistry has definitely altered the progress of new chemical leads following in the synthesis of structural analogues [48]. At that instance, combinatorial libraries included hundreds to thousands of novel compounds; however through the late 1990s synthetic chemists came to know that these libraries needed the intricacy of the complex natural products produced by nature [48]. The idea of diversity-oriented synthesis (DOS) was applied in which synthetic chemists would synthesize compounds analogous to natural products or that are based on natural product topologies. These compounds are currently being verified in a large variety and number of biological screens to define their role (s) as leads to new drug entities [48]. The examination of the degree of NCEs authorizations shows that natural products still add to or are involved in ~50% of all small molecule testing from 2000–2006 [49]. This is endorsed by the statistical data where out of 7000 natural compounds, 20 drugs have been discovered with a hit rate of 0.3% whereas HTS of synthetic compound libraries only achieved below 0.001% hit rate. Nonetheless the pharmaceutical industries have used considerable resources to both combinatorial chemistry and HTS [49]. Of the 1184 NCEs covering all diseases/sources/countries, 30% were discovered to be synthetic. It is also noteworthy that 52% of these compounds are whichever a natural product, a chemical modification or a mimic of a previously existing natural product pharmacophore [49]. Notwithstanding recompenses and the past accomplishments, majority of large pharmaceutical companies have reduced the use of natural products in drug discovery screening. This has been due to the apparent shortcomings of natural products and the expectations related with the use of assortments of compounds prepared by combinatorial chemistry approaches.

## 5. Revival of natural products research in the 90's

However, there was a revival of traditional knowledge-driven drug development in the later part of the eighties and this was partly due to the advances in chromatographic and spectroscopic techniques which have had a tremendous impact on the isolation and structure elucidation of the constituents of medicinal plants and the development of series of bioassay methodologies which were fast, easy to perform, quantitative and could selectively detect biologically active molecules at very low levels [50]. The phytochemicals can also be used as starting materials for the partial synthesis of drugs, as lead structures for molecular modification or as models to synthesize new drugs with improved therapeutic effects. In order to conduct preclinical and clinical trials and further develop a promising lead into a marketed drug, sustainable supply is necessary. The continuous supply problem is the major challenge for plant natural product drug discovery and development. Nevertheless, contemporary methodologies are accessible to overwhelm the difficulties. Advancement in technologies like biotechnology, fermentation, total chemical synthesis, sampling strategies and nanoscale NMR for structure determination are all vital to the accomplishment of natural products as drug leads. The novelty in the field of natural products, will result in a new wave revival of novel drugs in the upcoming future [51]. The past few years, though, have seen a reintroduced attention in the use of natural compounds and, more significantly, their part as a basis for drug development. The contemporary apparatus of chemistry and biology particularly, the numerous '-omics' technologies now let researchers to detail the precise nature of the biological effects of natural compounds on the human body, in addition to discover probable interactions, which grasps much potential for the development of novel treatments against numerous devastating diseases, including cancer and dementia. The recent revival of interest in natural products research is mainly due to disappointing results of combinatorial chemistry and HTS in delivering potent chemical leads. There is a new hope for the discovery of drug leads from the tropical rainforests. One reason why natural products are advantageous is that they provide complex molecules not accessible through synthesis. For example, taxol and rapamycin could not be synthesized cost effectively by standard medicinal chemistry, even including combinatorial chemistry approaches. Combinatorial synthetic methods are unlikely to produce molecules of the complexity of rapamycin and taxol.

Natural products have pointed the way to the future. A number of noteworthy advances in science and industry have been inspired by the quest of capturing the value of natural products. In 1982, the US National Cancer Institute began again to look for new drugs from the rainforests. There are good reasons for such renewed interest because they have already provided tangible evidence of their potential with remedies for a range of medical problems ranging from childhood leukemia to toothaches. Some examples of rainforest plants responsible for 25 percent of the drugs used in the clinic are included in Table 1. Most developments in capability and technology are nurturing a revival in natural products research and are either directly or indirectly addressing the historical obstacles to development of natural products [52-56]. There are three foremost reasons for the revitalization of natural product research; i). The potential of combinatorial chemistry to fill drug development projects with de novo synthetic small-molecule drug candidates is unsatisfied. ii). The applied problems of natural products drug discovery are being overawed by advances in separation equipment and in the speed and sensitivity of structure explanation. iii). A convincing case is being made for the essential usefulness of natural products as foundations of drug leads.

Possibly the strongest motivation for development of new natural products is the improvement in bioassay technology over the last few years. We now have automatic, specific and selective bioassays in which materials, comprising natural products preparations, can be evaluated quickly and cost-effectively. In reality, although the bioassay technology development facilitates faster and accurate substances evaluation, the availability of those evaluating substances has become very limited. Once the biological activity has been confirmed by a suitable bioassay or primary screen, the current separation and structure elucidation technology allow us to isolate, purify and determine the chemical structure of the active constituents in few days, or at maximum, a few weeks. The development of separation methods are mainly linked with high performance chromatography techniques [52]. The biodiversity of the earth is quickly declining and we frequently come across many articles in newspapers and journals on the rate, consequences, cause, etc., of loss of biological diversity. This will lead to the loss of chemical diversity and loss of potential uses of those chemicals have for mankind. Besides medicines, foodstuffs, fibers for clothing, building materials, etc. are chemicals derived from nature. The loss of those important organisms and their respective chemical diversity is the driving force for the revival of natural products research [56]. Globalization of world's economy increases the interest in pharmaceutical development. Since the discovery and development of new pharmaceuticals help to uphold the competitiveness of the industry, natural products research has been revisited as a way to increase the effectiveness of discovery and development [55].

| No | Drug | Origin | Use |
|---|---|---|---|
| 1 | Quinine | Cinchona tree (S. America) | Treat malaria |
| 2 | Neostigmine | Calabar bean (Africa) | Used to treat glaucoma and provides a blueprint for synthetic insecticides |
| 3 | Novacaine, cocaine | Coca plant (South America) | local less addictive anesthetics |
| 4 | Turbocurarine | Curare liana (America) | Native people used to poison arrow tips. Used as relaxants to treat muscle disorders like Parkinson's and Multiple Sclerosis. |
| 5 | Vincristine, vinblastine | Rosy periwinkle (Madagascar) | Hodgkin's disease and Pediatric leukemia |
| 6 | Cortisone | Wild yams (Central America) | Active ingredient in birth control pills |
| 7<br>8 | Calanolide A<br>Michellamine B | *Calophyllumlanigerum* (Borneo)<br>*Ancistrocladuskorupensis* (southwestern Cameroon) | Reverse transcript inhibitor (Anti HIV)<br>Reverse transcript inhibitor (Anti HIV-1, and HIV-2) |

**Table 1.** Drugs derived from rainforest plants

Many new approaches have been employed in the isolation and purification of NP, using various advanced fractionation techniques which includes the counter-current chromatography [57, 58] and structure elucidation by spectroscopic techniques (1D, 2D NMR spectroscopy, FTIR, UV, mass spectrometry, etc.) [59, 60]. The arrival of more compatible high-throughput screening technique provided an opportunity to screen natural products mixture within the quick span of time. Singh and Barrett [59] reported that pure bioactive compounds can be isolated from fermentation broths in 2 weeks and that the structures of more than 90% of new compounds can be elucidated within 2 weeks. Advanced NMR techniques permit to solve complex structures using less than 1 mg compound. Quinn et al. [61] showed that it was possible to prepare a screening library for highly diverse compounds from plants from analysis of the Dictionary of Natural Products, where the compounds were pre-selected based on drug-like in their physicochemical properties. It will be interesting to see if such a collection proves to be enriched in bioactive molecules. Besides the above, many alternative methods are also being explored in efforts to increase the speed and efficiency of using natural products in drug discovery. Multifaceted approach integrating traditional and modern techniques, i.e. combining botanical, phytochemical, medicinal chemistry, HTS, organic and combinatorial chemistry synthesis producing natural products-like compounds, biological, computational, molecular, multi-target approach, metabolomics, proteomic and genomic techniques will continue reviving the interest in using natural products as leads for the discovery of new drugs.

## 6. Modern approaches in drug discovery from natural products

The arrival of novel technologies in mass spectrometry, NMR and other spectroscopic techniques, bimolecular target or cell-based screening, early hit characterization and the utilization of computational methods have improved the impact of natural products in the HTS based drug discovery. Natural product extracts frequently contain a large number of constituents comprising those, which are difficult to separate. The unambiguous structures of pure compounds can be determined by the combination of conventional techniques like ultraviolet absorption spectroscopy (UV), IR, MS and NMR. In rare cases, where there is a difficulty in determining the absolute configuration, the single crystal X ray analysis is employed. The conventional separation techniques are time consuming and tiresome. The direct hyphenation of a proficient separation technique with efficient spectroscopic techniques such as HPLC-FTIR can be used to support the dereplication process [62]. HPLC-FTIR has been used to detect functional groups in main constituents of mixtures but has not found extensive application owing to limitations in compatibility; i.e. obtaining optimum separation accompanied by adequate detection [62].

One of the new technologies in drug discovery from natural products is the use of capillary electrophoresis (CE) in screening program first developed by Cetek Corporation and Cubist. The assay is able to identify active natural product compounds/ extracts and by detecting any shift in the protein when a ligand binds to it due to the conformational and surface charge changes. The CE technique can distinguish between weak and strong binding compounds in extracts prior to determining their concentration [63]. This technology has been applied to Cetek's internal drug discovery program in finding novel natural product compounds that inhibit the cancer target, HSP90, a molecular chaperonin that is responsible for maintaining the correct folding and stability of proteins [64]. Another interesting example which was recently reported by Wang, et al.showed that a CE method in conjunction with liquid chromatography-tandem mass spectrometry (LC-MS/MS) has been successfully applied in the screening of plant extracts, successfully identified a natural compound called baicalin from *Radix scutellariae* as a new protein kinase an inhibitor [65]. In an another separate study, Zhao and Chen, developed a simple and effective neuraminidase-immobilized capillary microreactor facbricated by glutaraldehyde cross-linking technology for screening of the neuraminidase inhibitors from traditional Chinese medicines. Six out of eighteen natural products including bavachinin, bavachin, baicalein, baicalin, chrysin, and vitexin have been found as potent inhibitors from the screening[66]. Some important aspects of CE that deserve a recognition in this chapter is its ease of use, versatility and high resolution separation components, high separation efficiency, and its low amount of sample and reagent consumption.

Flow injection analysis-NMR (FIA-NMR) encompasses a sample, which is injected as a plug into a fluid stream and then swept into the NMR detector coil. In a FIA-NMR, the mobile phase is used as a hydraulic push solvent which transfers the injected sample from the injector port to the NMR flow cell. The scout scan that is used to determine the location of the solvent peaks is obtained by the spectrometer once the pump stops. Finally a signal is sent to the solvent pump so that the old sample from the NMR flow-cell can be flushed out [67]. HPLC-NMR-MS is a novel and most advanced spectrometric method that is used in the de-replication of natural product extracts [68]. Despite being the most effective method, the benefit of the above said hyphenated methodology is the matching of the MS data to the NMR spectrum. In addition, the information of the functional groups (e.g., hydroxyl and amino moieties) that are delivered by the HPLC-NMR is readily identified by MS techniques. The advent of higher field magnets and cryo probes had proven HPLC-NMR to be a strong and effective spectroscopic instrument and applied to the crude extracts (NMR and UV profile from PDA HPLC detection). There is a significant improvement in the profiling sensitivity and de-replication of natural products due to the utilization of higher field magnets and the recent developments of the micro coil HPLC-NMR and capillary NMR (CapNMR) which has allowed for smaller amounts of samples to be examined in the order of 40–120 μL [69-71]. The micro coil HPLC-NMR is best suited for online HPLC-NMR which uses the on flow, stop flow or time silencing experiments to separate components present in greater concentrations and analyses the same [71-74], whereas the Capillary NMR uses the non-deuterated solvents in an off-line HPLC separation thereby offering a wide range of solvents with a low cost. The isolated compounds are re-dissolved in deuterated solvents and then injected into the CapNMR flow probe using volumes of around 6 μL with $^{1}$H-NMR spectra acquired for sample quantities in the order of 2–30 μg, thereby increasing the sensitivity with a prospect to classify the novel low level secondary metabolites [75].

Besides the above, the information obtained from the 1D and 2D NMR spectra is sufficient to classify the compounds in addition to the provision of a 'high-fidelity' snapshot of the constituents in the extract, thus providing the information which paves way for rational decisions about the top method of fractionation or to proceed with isolation further. Many recent publications have been reported using this approach [71-73].The technique and utilization of HPLC-NMR in natural products identification/classification is well recognized in the literature but applications of its uses have mainly dealt only with the chemical profiling of plants [76-78]. Numerous modes of HPLC-NMR (mostly on-flow and stop-flow modes) combine the resolving power of chromatography, which is interfaced with the structural understanding provided by NMR. The reductionist approach has not been very successful in discovering effective drugs to treat complex diseases, such as cancer, metabolic, cardiovascular and neurological diseases. Single-target drugs may not always induce the desired effect to the entire biological system even if they successfully inhibit or activate a specific target.There are limitations in the use of reductionist or mono-target approach in drug discovery. The approach yields only a limited understanding of complicated pathogenesis and multi-target pathologies of systemic diseases such as cancers, cardiovascular diseases and neurodegenerative disorders. There is difficulty in identifying relevant interventions to target such complexities. Bullet-based or mono-target drug intervention cannot effectively combat the complex pathologies of systemic diseases as they are regulated by complex biological networks and depend on multiple steps of genetic and environmental challenges to progress. Recently there is a growing interest to use innovative approaches to drug discovery from natural products by network pharmacology which integrates systems biology and pharmacology [79]. The integrated multidisciplinary concept of multiple targets, multiple effects and complex diseases in network pharmacology have enriched our understanding of complicated pathogenesis and multi-target pathologies of systemic diseases and reduced difficulty in identifying relevant interventions to target such complexities. The '-omic' technologies in system biology have now been widely used to correlate and elucidate multiple targets and network of human diseases and drug actions [80]. The concept of network pharmacology is especially useful in accurately translating and interpreting the therapeutic effects of herbal medicines into modern biochemical and biological meanings. Herbal medicines may serve as valuable resources for network-based multi-target drug discovery. The concept of network pharmacology is especially useful in accurately translating and interpreting the therapeutic effects of herbal medicines into modern biochemical and biological meanings. The efficacy of the multi-target drugs from herbal extracts are developed followed by identification of their major bioactive components and redevelopment of a completely new multi-component formulations composed of the major bioactive components in order to reach a synergistic and optimal combination [81].

Combining natural product chemistry and metabolomics approaches in drug discovery is a new strategy to discover new drugs. There are few reports in the scientific literature, which discuss the unison of classical natural product chemistry approaches with metabolomics to identify novel bioactive natural products. These have generally focused on the study of plants [82]. The identification of bioactive natural products from plants remains a multifaceted task because of their high chemical diversity and complexity. By measuring the metabolome of different extracts or fractions of a plant and combining these data with its corresponding biological activity, signals related to the compounds related to the displayed activity can potentially be determined. Systems biology is a most promising field encompassing tools in the post-genomics revolution such as transcript omics, proteomics, glycomics and fluxomics with an intention to characterize all gene and cell products completely inclusive of mRNA, proteins, glycan structures and metabolites. Metabolomics aims at constructing balanced observations using highly reproducible tools followed by the analysis of data to locate the correlations between the available data. The profiling of all the low molecular weight metabolites of an organism is not possible and hence this emerging field of metabolomics combines analytical chemistry, biochemistry and computational biology permitting the analysis of thousands of metabolites in any biological system. The principal analytical platforms are the Mass spectrometry with gas chromatography (MS-GC), liquid chromatography (LC) or capillary electrophoresis (CE) and NMR spectroscopy. A balanced extraction procedure to efficiently extract all the primary and secondary metabolites from tissues and the body fluids is used to obtain them in the natural form prior to the analysis in the various solvents used. The metabolite extraction procedures are more complicated and complex due to the diversified nature of small molecules present and due to the unavailability of a single analytical technique and platform which helps in analysis of all the metabolites simultaneously. Several separation techniques and methodologies need to be applied to achieve complete analysis of the metabolites [83]. Simultaneous analysis of hundreds of compounds is achieved by various tools in informatics that extracts information from the data, removing the background noise, detection and integration of peaks throughout large data sets and normalizing and transforming the resulting data matrices prior to any statistical analysis [84]. Metabolomics has a restricted access to the ability of identifying the signals with respect to the chemical nature. About 60 to 80 % of all detected compounds are unknown [84-85] even today and the metabolic discipline has created a large mass of spectral NMR library to tackle this problem. These unknown secondary metabolite structures can be one among the undiscovered resources of the natural products, fingerprinting, foot printing, profiling or target analyses are common terms used in this field. Fingerprinting aims to take a 'snapshot' of the organism where the signals cannot necessarily be used to detect/identify specific metabolites and depends strongly on the technique used. The signals are assigned to a metabolite irrespective of its nature to be a known or a novel compound. The term target analysis aims to determine and quantify a specific metabolite of interest [81].

The microarray is a new technology recently developed that has empowered the scientific community to understand the fundamental aspects underlining the growth and development of life as well as to explore the genetic causes of anomalies occurring in the functioning of the human body.DNA microarray technology can analyze and compares changes in DNA or protein. A chromosomal change in an abnormal individual could be identified when DNA from this individual is compared with DNA (control) from a healthy individual. It is very precise and useful in that it is capable to detect much smaller changes compared to conventional karyotyping technique. This competent technique enabled us to understand the elemental aspects underlining the growth and development of life as well as to explore the genetic causes of anomalies occurring in the functioning of the human body. Microarray technology has been utilized extensively in pharmacogenomics where comparative analysis of the genes from an unhealthy and a normal cell will help the identification of the biochemical constitution of the proteins synthesized by the abnormal/unhealthy genes. The information obtained from the analysis then could be utilized for synthesis and design of drugs which fight the abnormal proteins and reduce their effect [86].Kwon and his colleagues have developed an *in vitro* approach utilizing a multi-enzyme containing microarray system for high-throughput synthesis of polypeptide derived product and their subsequent full polyketide-based library screening of the human tyrosine kinase (TK), on a single glass microarray. The TK inhibitors are expected to treat chronic myeloid leukemia, gastrointestinal stromal tumours and breast cancer [87, 88].

A drug discovery program aims to find novel bioactive natural products, which possess some form of potent biological activity. However the isolation of known and undesirable natural products with no pharmacological interest or chemical is inevitable. The term dereplication which is a process of identifying known compounds responsible for the activity of an extract prior to bioassay-guided isolation becomes popular among the natural products researchers [89, 90]. Dereplication strategies generally involve a combination of bioassay, separation science, spectroscopic methods, and database searching and can be regarded as chemical or biological screening processes. There are a number of ways in which natural product programs approach dereplication, which is based upon availability of screening methods/instrumentation, time and the cost to identify possible 'biological leads or novel compounds' from a crude extract. At present there are many advanced methodologies and protocols that distinguish novel entities from known natural compounds at an early stage of a drug discovery program or in a natural product isolation strategy [90]. The dereplication process can be easily done by screening the compounds through the commercially available databases, reducing the time taken for structure elucidation of known compounds. One example is the Chapman and Hall Dictionary of Natural Products [91]; The Dictionary of Marine Natural Products (on-line) (subset of the Dictionary of Natural Products) containing over 30, 000 compounds [92]; MarinLit- The Marine Natural Products Database containing up to date bibliographic data on marine organisms with the number of references from 1, 200 journals/books and data for ~21, 000 compounds [93]; AntiMarin is a more recent database, in which the number of methyl groups, the number of sp3-hybridised methylene or methine protons, alkene, acetal, ether and formyl groups can be searched [94, 95]. Besides, SciFinder Scholar and SCOPUS are important research discovery tools (Chemical Abstracts on-line) [96, 97] and NAPRALERTTM is a database of all natural products, including ethnomedical information, pharmacological/biochemical information of extracts of organisms *in vitro, in situ, in vivo,* in humans (case reports, non-clinical trials) and clinical studies [98]. The availability of these scientific databases such as the ones mentioned to the research and academic institutions, is a fundamental and crucial step in a well-governed natural product program. With the rise in the number of novel drug targets, computational methods such as high throughput virtual screening, ligand docking tools, ADME (absorption, distribution, metabolism and excretion) profiling and other modern computational tools and softwares have been applied to accelerate the drug discovery process. Some of the common natural products libraries and databases as listed below allow the prompt screening of large number of natural compounds to be done in short period of time against a variety of drug targets. Dictionary Of Natural Products (*http://dnp.chemnetbase.com/intro/index.jsp*); UCSD Marine Natural Products Database (*http://naturalprod.ucsd.edu/*); Natural Products Alert (*http://napralert.org/*) ; ZINC (*http://zinc.docking.org/browse/catalogs/natural-products*) ; InterBioScreen (*http://www.ibscreen.com/products.shtml*); AnalytiCon Discovery (*http://www.ac-discovery.com/*); Molecular Diversity Preservation International (*http://www.mdpi.org/*). Computer-generated models of proteins including novel enzyme and receptor targets apart from the protein crystal structures that are deposited in Protein Data Bank (*http://www.pdb.org/*) can be easily generated by homology modeling subsequently followed by simple molecular docking to examine the interactions between the natural compounds and the protein targets. Bioassays can then be conducted selectively on the natural hits or leads retrieved without the neccesities of wasting the precious amount of the compounds and avoid expensive and time consuming experimental methods. Examples of molecular docking softwares currently available are AutoDock, AutoDockVina, FlexX, FRED, GOLD, eHiTS, and Lead finders. Some examples using high throughput virtual screening including the work of Wang et al. where ten natural compounds have been successfully identified as flacipain-2 (FP-2) inhibitors [99] and Liu et al. who have identified a natural product-like STAT3 dimerization inhibitor by structure-based virtual screening [100].

Other bioinformatics tools such as ligand and structure-based pharmacophore screening have also been reported to be successful in assisting the process of drug discovery from natural products. Chen et al. have proposed a three-dimentional quantitative structure-activity relationship pharmacophore model based on known mTOR inhibitors. Virtual screening using the best pharmacophore model successfully retrieved 20 natural products as potential mTOR inhibitors scaffolds[101]. It is also important to mention here that from the previous study by Doman showed that out of 365 molecules suggested by docking, 127 (34.8%) of them inhibited the activity of enzyme protein tyrosine phosphatase-1B (PTP1B) while only 85 (0.021%) out of approximately 400, 000 molecules were retrieved from high-throughput experimental assay. That is around 1700-fold enrichment of hit rate from structure-based docking over random screening [102].On the other hand, incorporation of chemoinformatic tools in drug discovery from natural products allow the compounds to be screened for their ADMET (absorption, distribution, metabolism, excretion, and toxicity) properties before they are enrolled in any drug development programs. Screening of natural compounds using the Pfizer 'Rule of 5' allows the researchers to remove any molecules that do not obey the rules. Since these rules were derived from a set of experimental observations of thousands of known drugs and drug-like molecules, a trained medicinal chemist/biochemist can easily use the *in silico* data as a guide in determining the potential drug-like natural compounds followed by the synthesis of further analogues so that they would have a favorable drug-like properties. A good drug-like molecule in general obey the following rules (i) molecular weight ≤ 500, (ii) calculated logP ≤ 5, (iii) number of hydrogen bond donors ≤ 5, and (iv) number of hydrogen bond acceptors ≤ 10. The introduction of *in silico* screening and natural products facilities for high-throughput screening in academic labs as well as in drug companies reduce the cost from random screening of very large collections of compounds. *In silico* or virtual screening helps to filter down the number of compounds used in real screens [103]. On the other hand, bioinformatic tool such as the Dictionary of Natural Products gives structural information on 150, 000 different compounds that could be used in virtual screening, even though the compounds would still have to be physically available for any predicted activity to be confirmed through testing in a relevant assay. Finally, clustering of chemically related scaffolds can be very useful in guiding the synthesis of new compounds, but obviously there is a delay and expense in the synthesis.

An academic collaboration has established the Drug Discovery Portal (see http://www.ddp.strath.ac.uk/) in an attempt to combine the techniques of virtual screening of chemically diverse natural products and their synthetic analogues with the rapid availability of physical samples for testing, This allows a wide variety of compounds from academic laboratories in many different institutions in a database that can be used for virtual screening. Academic biology groups also propose new and novel protein structures as targets for virtual screening with the Portal's database (and with conventional commercially available databases). When hits are predicted from the *in silico* screening, the compounds can be obtained from the originating chemist for confirmatory tests. Often, there is an immediate link to expertise for the preparation of analogues to help start a lead optimization program. Nevertheless, access to the Portal is freely available for the academic group. The continued expansion of the chemical database means that there is a valuable and growing coverage of chemical space of many novel chemical compounds. Although the compounds in the Portal's database will generally have already been disclosed in a thesis or in a chemistry journal, very few of them have been previously tested for biological activity. This is a common feature of known natural products: of the 150, 000 structures in the CRC Dictionary of Natural Products only 1% of them have been investigated. The introduction of metabolomics technologies in natural product discovery processes will be beneficial on multiple levels. By increasing the number of identifications in our metabolomics data, compounds with novel structures can be easily obtained and tested for any disease under investigation. Furthermore, multi-parallel analysis using metabolomics technologies will also enhance the throughput of chemical characterization processes of many different species from natural resources. Since natural product chemists have collected a lifetime of compound libraries of active and also inactive pure compounds, these data can be used to construct the mass spectral and NMR spectral libraries, undoubtedly help the biological interpretations of metabolomics data to be done with less difficulty. The advancements in analytical instrumentation and sophisticated hyphenation of separation techniques with high sensitive detectors have allowed for greater detection of small molecule compounds measurable in biological systems (i.e., primary and secondary metabolites). These technologies can be used to advance the discovery of natural product chemistry to identify potential novel drugs candidates which will assist in sustaining health and the fight against disease and illness. In the case of NMR of crude extracts, patterns can be easily visualized and interpreted using the multivariate data analysis. This can be carried out in a comparative manner distinguishing differences between relatively similar extracts or it can be linked with a specific (generally *in vitro*) biological activity. Ultimately this enables the construction of a complex database of the metabolome [104-106].

## 7. Scientific interests and recent advances in natural products research from the tropical rainforests

Plant derived natural compounds have continuously captivated scientists globally on grounds of being biocompatible, and are considered as potentially safe and effective therapeutic agents. Table 2 shows examples of natural products derived from plants that have become well known pharmaceuticals [107-116].

| No. | Drug/Chemical | Action/Clinical Use | Plant Source |
|---|---|---|---|
| 1 | Betulinic acid | Anticancerous | *Betula alba* |
| 2 | Bromelain | Anti-inflammatory, proteolytic | *Ananascomosus* |
| 3 | Camptothecin | Anticancerous | *Camptothecaacuminata* |
| 4 | (+)-Catechin | Haemostatic | *Potentillafragarioides* |
| 5 | Cissampeline | Skeletal muscle relaxant | *Cissampelospareira* |
| 6 | Codeine | Analgesic, antitussive | *Papaver somniferum* |
| 7 | Colchicine | Antitumor agent, anti-gout | *Colchicum autumnale* |
| 8 | Curcumin | Choleretic, Antitumor agent | *Curcuma longa* |
| 9 | Demecolcine | Antitumor agent | *Colchicum autumnale* |
| 10 | Deserpidine | Antihypertensive, tranquillizer | *Rauvolfiacanescens* |
| 11 | L-Dopa | Anti-parkinsonism | *Mucunasp* |
| 12 | Digoxin | Cardiotonic | *Digitalis purpurea* |
| 13 | Etoposide | Antitumor agent | *Podophyllumpeltatum* |
| 14 | Glasiovine | Antidepressant | *Octeaglaziovii* |
| 15 | Irinotecan | Anticancer, antitumor agent | *Camptothecaacuminata* |
| 16 | Kheltin | Bronchodilator | *Ammivisnaga* |
| 17 | Monocrotaline | Antitumor agent (topical) | *Crotalaria sessiliflora* |
| 18 | Neoandrographolide | Dysentery | *Andrographispaniculata* |
| 19 | Podophyllotoxin | Antitumor anticancer agent | *Podophyllumpeltatum* |
| 20 | Quinine | Antimalarial, antipyretic | *Cinchona ledgeriana* |
| 21 | Qulsqualic acid | Anthelmintic | *Quisqualisindica* |
| 22 | Sanguinarine | Dental plaque inhibitor | *Sanguinariacanadensis* |
| 23 | Scopolamine | Sedative | *Datura species* |
| 24 | Sparteine | Oxytocic | *Cytisusscoparius* |
| 25 | Taxol | Antitumor agent | *Taxusbrevifolia* |
| 26 | Teniposide | Antitumor agent | *Podophyllumpeltatum* |
| 27 | Tetrandrine | Antihypertensive | *Stephaniatetrandra* |
| 28 | Theophylline | Diuretic, brochodilator | *Theobroma cacao and others* |
| 29 | Topotecan | Antitumor, anticancer agent | *Camptothecaacuminata* |
| 30 | Trichosanthin | Abortifacient | *Trichosantheskirilowii* |
| 31 | Vinblastine | Antitumor, Antileukemic agent | *Catharanthusroseus* |
| 32 | Vincristine | Antitumor, Antileukemic agent | *Catharanthusroseus* |
| 33 | Scopolamine | Sedative | *Datura species* |
| 34 | Taxol | Antitumor agent | *Taxusbrevifolia* |

**Table 2.** Natural products derived from plants [107-116]

## 7.1. Anti-inflammatory agents

Natural products (and conventional medicines) offer great anticipation in the identification of bioactive compounds and their development into drugs for the treatment of inflammatory diseases. Plants have been the source of several conventional medicine systems through the world for centuries and continue to deliver mankind with new medicines to treat anti-inflammatory conditions. Previously, the plant-derived medicines were dispensed in the form of crude drugs like tinctures, teas, powders, poultices, and other herbal preparations. This eventually serves as the basis of the current modern drug discovery [117]. Numerous records can be found in conventional medicine concentrating on the relief from pain and inflammation. People who are suffering from inflammation in the ancient times were treated with phyto-chemicals eventually lead to the discovery of the first anti-inflammatory, analgesic drug aspirin. The discovery of aspirin was based on the previously known analgesic and antipyretic features of the bark of willow-tree since 400 BC by the Greeks and Romans. In 1899, aspirin or also known as acetylsalicylic acid was introduced as the first potent drug for the treatment of rheumatic disease [118]. Hippocrates said 'let your food be your medicine'. Another very well studied natural anti-inflammatory agent is curcumin which is derived from the turmeric root. Turmeric is a yellow spice intrinsic to Asia, commonly relished as both a food and a dye. Turmeric appears as yellow in curry powder, and is a viscous compound found in turmeric rhizomes. Many scientific reports have shown that curcumin exhibits strong anti-inflammatory powers and extremely effective at relieving pain, and most important of all it is nontoxic. Like the NSAID's, curcumin inhibits the pro-inflammatory mediator cyclo-oxygenase-2 (COX-2) although it is not selective to a single isoform. Besides, curcumin also affects the activity of other important factors in inflammation such as NF-kappa β, PPAR Gamma transcription factors, and 5-LOX [119]. By inhibiting the activity of all these features of inflammation, curcumin delivers much superior anti-inflammatory and pain-relieving activity than most drugs.

Ginger root which is a common spice found in food, also comprises a number of scientifically confirmed pain relieving mediators. Ginger consists a protein-digesting enzyme called zingibain, which seems to relieve arthritis pain by reducing inflammation. In reality, the anti-inflammatory activity of ginger relates positively with aspirin. Ginger root also contains two groups of compounds called as the shagaols and gingerols. These compounds are strongly antioxidants, therefore serving to stop cells from untimely destruction because of exposure to environmental toxins and by-products of metabolism. Still more, these compounds are strong anti-inflammatory agents, and are recognized to relieve inflammation throughout the body [120]. Provided that oxidation and inflammation are part and parcel of all chronic degenerative diseases, ginger can play an important role in disease risk reduction. On the other hand, plants such the Amazon bark cats' claw and the common spice rosemary are also found to exhibit potent anti-inflammatory and pain-relieving characteristics. In toxicity studies, these plants were proven to be highly nontoxic. Besides, plants such as hops also contain well known anti-inflammatory mediators. This herb is commonly found in beer brewing, comprises a group of compounds called the humulones which were shown to inhibit phorbol ester-induced COX-2 expression in mouse skin by blocking activation of NF-kappaB and AP-1: IkappaB kinase and c-Jun-N-terminal kinase as respective potential upstream targets [121].

Propolis has been used in folk medicine for thousands of years and gain wide recognition for its possible therapeutic uses, because of the wide range of the biological and pharmacological activities. Among the well-known and one of the major properties the anti-inflammatory effect.

Though there are good numbers of studies focused on the biological activities of propolis together with its botanical sources, studies on Chinese propolis are insufficient. The anti-inflammatory effects of the ethanol extracts from Chinese propolis (EECP) and poplar buds (EEPB) from *Populus canadensis* were investigated *in vitro* for their modulating effects on the RAW 264.7 cells and the inflammatory cytokines production and by measuring nuclear factor (NF)-κB activation in TNF-α or IL-1β stimulation HEK 293 cells using reporter gene assays. Their possible modulatory effects on LPS-induced endotoxemia and acute pulmonary damage as acute inflammatory signs were also tested in mice. Both *Populus Canadensis* EECP and EEPB displayed a strong free-radical scavenging action and significant *in vitro* anti-inflammatory effects by modulating key inflammatory mediators of mRNA transcription, inhibiting the production of specific inflammatory cytokines, and blocking the activation of nuclear factor (NF)-κB [125]. A group of scientists investigated the antioxidant capacities and anti-inflammatory activities of ethanol extracts of leaves of *Cassia alata, Eleusine indica, Carica papaya, Eremomastax speciosa* and the stem bark of *Polyscias fulva,* collected in Cameroon. The ethanolic extracts displayed robust antioxidant activities against both hydrogen peroxide and superoxide anion reactive oxygen species. The highest antioxidant activities was observed with the *Cassia alata*. The effect of plant extracts on γδ T cells and in DC was evidenced by the dose dependent reduction in TNF-α production in the presence of *Cassia alata, Carica papaya, Eremomastax speciosa Eleusine indica,* and *Polyscias fulva*. γδ T cells proliferation was affected to the greatest extent by *Polyscias fulva* [126].*Celastrus paniculatus* Willd., an important medicinal plant widely used in Ayurveda, is enriched with remarkable nervine, cognition enhancing, and other therapeutic properties. Antioxidant and anti-inflammatory activities of the aqueous, methanol, and chloroform extracts of *C. paniculatus* seeds were evaluated using DPPH radical scavenging assay, Trolox equivalent antioxidant capacity (TEAC), Ferric reducing antioxidant power assay (FRAP), and lipoxygenase inhibition assay, respectively. Total phenolic content was also determined. Almost all the assays suggested chloroform extract to have the strongest antioxidant property and the highest phenolic content. However, aqueous extract showed maximum anti-inflammatory activity [127].

### 7.2. Anticancer agents

Plants have a long history of use in the treatment of cancer. The medicinal herbs that are traditionally used for anti-cancer treatment and that are anti-angiogenic through multiple interdependent processes (including effects on gene expression, signal processing, and enzyme activities) include *Goniothalamus species (*Custard-apple family*), Artemisia annua* (Chinese worm wood), *Viscum album* (European mistletoe), *Curcuma longa* (curcumin), *Scutellaria baicalensis* (Chinese skullcap), resveratrol and proanthocyanidin (grape seed extract), *Magnolia officinalis* (Chinese magnolia tree), *Camellia sinensis* (green tea), *Ginkgo biloba,* quercetin, *Poriacocos, Zingiber officinalis* (ginger), Panax ginseng, *Rabdosia rubescens* hora (Rabdosia), and Chinese destagnation herbs [128]. The exploration of anticancer agents from plant sources has started since the 1950s. More than 3000 plants species have been reported to be involved in the development of anticancer drugs [129]. Numerous compounds from tropical rainforest medicinal plant species with potential anticancer activity have been identified.

Positively, most of the new plant secondary metabolites and their derivatives have been utilized in clinical cancer trials [130-132]. Of all available anticancer drugs between 1940 and 2002, nearly half were natural products or their derivatives with another 8% considered natural product mimics [131]. The anticancer agents from plant origin which are currently in clinical use can be classified mainly to four classes: the first class is the vinca alkaloids e.g. vincristine, vinblastine, vindesine, vinorelbine; second class the podophyllotoxin and its derivatives which includes etoposide, teniposide; the fourth is taxanes under which come the paclitaxel, docetaxel and the fifth class is the camptothecin and its derivatives (e.g. topothecan, irinothecan). Other groups include anthracyclines (doxorubicin, daunorubicin, epirubicin, idarubicin). As a matter of fact, half of the anti-cancer drugs which are globally accepted and in use today were either natural products or their derivatives and were developed based on of knowledge gathered from naturally existing small or macromolecules [133, 134]. In addition to this there is numerous active biomolecules identified in fruits and vegetables and can used in anticancer treatment. These agents include the curcumin which is mainly isolated from turmeric, resveratrol found in red grapes, peanuts and berries, the genistein exist in the soybeans, the diallyl sulfide and S-allyl cysteine in allium, the allicin of garlic, the lycopene in tomato, the capsaicin in red chilies, beside the diosgenin in fenugreek, 6-gingerol in ginger, ellagic acid in pomegranate, ursolic acid naturally found in apple, pears, and prunes. Similarly the catechins in green tea, eugenol in cloves, indole-3-carbinol in cruciferous vegetables, and beta carotene in carrots [128, 135].

Vinblastine and vincristine were isolated from *Catharanthus roseus* (L.) G. Don (Apocynaceae) (formerly *Vincarosea* L.) and have been used clinically for over 40 years[136]. The vinca alkaloids and several of their semi-synthetic derivatives block mitosis with metaphase arrest by binding specifically to tubulin resulting in its depolymerization [137]. Podophyllotoxin was isolated from the resin of *Podophyllum peltatum* L. (Berberidaceae) but was found to be too toxic in mice so derivatives were made with the first clinically approved drug being etoposide [138]. The epipodophyllotoxins bind tubulin, causing DNA strand breaks during the G2 phase of the cell cycle by irreversibly inhibiting DNA topoisomerase II [138]. Paclitaxel was originally isolated from *Taxus brevifolia* Nutt. (Taxaceae) and was clinically introduced to the U.S. market in the early 1990s [139, 140]. The taxanes, including paclitaxel and derivatives, act by binding tubulin without allowing depolymerization or interfering with tubulin assembly [141, 142]. Camptothecin was isolated from *Camptotheca acuminata* Decne. (Nyssaceae) but originally showed unacceptable myelosuppression [139, 143]. Interest in camptothecin was revived when it was found to act by selective inhibition of topoisomerase I, involved in cleavage and reassembly of DNA [143]. The taxanes and the camptothecins together account for approximately 30% of the worldwide accepted and marketed anticancer drugs in 2002, costing over US$ 2.75 billion [143]. Besides these, irinotecan was isolated from the same *Camptotheca acuminata* tree in China for metastatic colorectal cancer and 9AC for ovarian, stomach cancer, and T-cell lymphoma. Like camptothecin, this drug is also currently in clinical trials and have already been approved by the FDA [144]. Numerous derivatives of all four compound classes have been synthesized, some of which are currently in clinical use. All of these natural products have led to significant biological discoveries related to their unique mechanisms of action.

### 7.3. Immunomodulatory agents

Immunomodulators are used to enhance or suppress host defense responses in the treatment of those diseases in which defective immune responses play an important role in determining disease outcomes. These include primary and secondary immunodeficiencies that accompany long-standing infections, as well as debilitating diseases like cancer, rheumatoid arthritis, systemic lupus erythematosus and long-standing infections, leading to acquired immune deficiencies. Immunosuppressive drugs are commonly used in the treatment of inflammation and allergic disorders and rejection of transplanted organs, while immunostimulant drugs are highly desirable for the treatment of immunodeficiency and infectious diseases [145]. Many therapeutic effects of plant extracts have been recognized and recommended based on their impact on human immunity [146]. A good numbers of herbal preparations such as *Phyllanthus debelis, Tinospora cordifolia, Trogonella foenumgraecum, Pouteria cambodiana, Centella asiatica, Panax ginseng* and *Picrorhiza scrophulariiflora* have been found to display a wide range of immunomodulatory effects [147-150]. The idea of modulation of the immune response to relieve the diseases has existed in early system of medicine together with Ayurveda and Unani. Additionally, plants have been widely used as a source of medicine in these systems to support health and to uphold body's resistance against infections [151]. Phytochemicals such as polysaccharides, lactones, alkaloids, diterpenoids and glycosides, isolated from several plants have been reported to contain potential immunomodulatory agents [151, 152]. Several types of immunomodulators have also been identified from isolates and extracts of bacteria and fungi, mammalian proteins such as interferons, interleukins and cytokines and some synthetic chemicals [153]. Several types of immunomodulators have been identified, including isolates and extracts of bacteria and fungi, mammalian proteins such as interferons, interleukins and cytokines and some synthetic chemicals [153]. Natural products and their derivatives represent a new class of novel immunomodulating agents. However, only little information is available about the immunological effects exerted by medicinal plants from the tropical rainforests which have been used traditionally for treatment of various ailments.

Plants belonging to family Meliaceae, such as, *Azadirachta indica, Mumronia pumila, Melia azedarch, Cedrela lilloi* and *Trichilia elegans* etc. show strong anti-inflammatory and anti-rheumatic properties [154] *C. lilloi* and *T. elegans* constrained the phagocytic capability and oxidative metabolism by opsonized zymosan as stimulus in peritoneal macrophages [155]. Lima et al. [156] reported that *Pisumsativum* agglutinin (PSA) prompts immunomodulatory effects by activating spleen lymphocytes *in vivo*. Our previous study on the screening of 20 medicinal plants for their phagocytic properties have indicated that the methanol extracts of some plants including *Phyllanthus amarus* exhibited strong immunomodulatory effects on polymorphonuclear neutrophils and macrophage cells [157]. The standardized methanol extracts of *P. amarus* and *P. urinaria* and their biochemical markers phyllanthin and hypophyllanthin, were able to modulate the innate immune response of phagocytes especially on the chemotactic migration of phagocytes, phagocytic ability and on the release of reactive oxygen species (ROS) [158]. The withanoloid, coagulin-H from *Withania coagulans* was found to have extremely potent IL-2 inhibitory activity. A complete suppression of PHA-activated T-cell was observed at 2.5 μg/mL concentrations and this suppression activity was similar to that of prednisolone. Similarly the IL-2 production was inhibited ($IC_{50}$ = 0.35 mg/mL). Molecular docking technique revealed the better interaction of coagullin-H at amino acids at the receptor binding site of the IL-2 protein compared with prednisolone [159]. The natural compound cheiradone, from a *Euphorbia* species was identified to interfere with angiogenesis process, inhibiting the *in vivo* and *in vitro* vascular endothelial growth factor (VEGF) in stimulated angiogenesis process. All stages of VEGF-induced angiogenesis were inhibited with an $IC_{50}$ values that range between 5.20 and 7.50 μM. In addition to this activity it inhibited VEGF binding to VEGF receptor-1 and 2 with $IC_{50}$ values of 2.9 and 0.61 μM respectively. However, cheiradone had no effect on fibroblast growth factor (FGF)-2 or epidermal growth factor (EGF) activity. [160]. Recently, a study using a transgenic mouse model of melanoma exhibited that the anticancer effects of popular kampo medicine were mediated by an improved antigen-specific antitumor cytotoxic T-lymphocyte response [151, 161].

## 8. Conclusions

Despite the scientific interests and advances in the past few decades of natural products research, to date efforts to discover new bioactive agents from the flora for use as chemical leads in the development of new drugs have not experienced the expected progress. There is a need to strategize research approach which should be based on the integration of human and technology resources available and the establishment of smart partnerships between academic and research institutions, industries and multinational drug coorporations. We need to learn from the past successful research experiences to increase the chances of discovering new drugs from the tropical rainforests. The right research strategy has to be used but it will take more than a few decades for countries of the tropical rainforests to establish their research and drug design capacity and be a serious competitor in the pharmaceutical markets. We have to be up-to-date with the newly emerging technologies which are already playing highly significant roles in natural product research such as the advances in high-throughput screening methodologies, the development of molecular biology and biotechnology and the use of virtual technology in rational drug design. The role of combinatorial chemistry in drug discovery and the future impact of genomics, proteomics and metabolomics in medicinal plant research should also be given due consideration. The potential of rainforests natural products to become new drugs is still on the horizon. The recent adoption of the Nagoya Protocol of the Convention on Biological Diversity on 29 October 2010 in Nagoya, Aichi Province, Japan, on access to genetic resources and the fair and equitable sharing of benefits arising from their utilization should encourage more pharmaceutical firms to venture into natural research to discover new drug leads [162]. The protocol provides a transparent legal framework for the effective implementation of a fair and equitable sharing of benefits between participating parties arising out of the utilization of genetic resources. However, the number of plants that have been studied extensively to search for new drugs is very few. A very small fraction, which is less than 5% of tropical forest plant species have been scanned for their chemical composition and medicinal values [163]. The figures are not unusual as systematic drug discovery programmes from plants are largely carried out by multinational drug corporations or research groups of the industrialized countries which possess the technology resources and well-equipped research facilities but have little access to the tropical plant genetic resources. In tropical countries rather most tropical countries there is little and minor concern for systematic research effort, to screen plants for new drugs, and the reason is the capacity to investigate these resources to their full potential and other aspects is very limited in these countries. Neverthless instead of this, several commercial activities such as clearing of forests for agricultural purposes and timber extraction predominate and are rapidly destructing the plant genetic resources.

Chemical prospecting in the tropical rainforests for potential drugs is still progressing. The prospective for drug discovery from plants and other natural sources is huge, but little time remains to discover this speedily diminishing resource. Given the quick devastation of tropical habitats, particularly the rainforests, and the degradation of marine ecologies, this deficiency of information is alarming. The wealth of potential drugs has two potential sources: either from the rainforest or from the laboratory. We need to stress here that the future of drug discovery lies in neither of these options alone, rather it embodies both the rainforest and the laboratory. Combinatorial laboratory technique, which is a relatively newly emerging technique, is growing in proficiency with support from pharmaceutical companies. And as new combinatorial libraries emerge, the ability and chance to quickly synthesize and derivative a biologically active compound increases. But even with this technology, there cannot be a substitution for the biodiversity that can be found within the boundaries of the rainforests.

## Author details

Ibrahim Jantan[1*], Syed Nasir Abbas Bukhari[1], Mohamed Ali Seyed Mohamed[1,2], Lam Kok Wai[1] and Mohammed Ahmed Mesaik[1]

*Address all correspondence to: profibj@gmail.com

1 Drug and Herbal Research Center, Faculty of Pharmacy, UniversitiKebangsaan Malaysia, Jalan Raja Muda Abdul Aziz, Kuala Lumpur, Malaysia

2 School of Life Science, B.S. Abdur Rahman University, Seethakathi Estate, Vandalur, Chennai, India

## References

[1] Duke JA. Database of biologically active phytochemicals and their activities. Boca Raton, FL: CRC Press; 1992.

[2] Solecki R. Shanidar IV, a Neanderthal Flower Burial in Northern Iraq. Science 1975;190:880-81.

[3] Farnsworth NR, Akerele O, Bingel AS, Soejarto DD, Guo Z. edicinal plants in therapy. Bulletin of the World Health Organization 1985;63:965-981.

[4] Jantan I. Medicinal Plant Research in Malaysia: Scientific Interests and Advances. Malaysia Journal of Health Science 2004;2:27-46.

[5] Mishra BB, Tiwari VK. Natural products: An evolving role in future drug discovery. European Journal of Medicinal Chemistry 2011;46:4769–4807.

[6] Rey-Ladino J, Ross AG, Cripps AW, McManus DP, Quinn R. Natural products and the search for novel vaccine adjuvants. Vaccine 2011;29:6464–6471.

[7] Cragg GM, Newman DJ. Biodiversity: A continuing source of novel drug leads. Pure and Applied Chemistry 2005;77:7-24.

[8] Haefner B. Drugs from the deep: Marine natural products as drug candidates. Drug Discovery Today 2003;8:536–544.

[9] Butler MS. The role of natural product in chemistry in drug discovery. Journal of Natural Products 2004;67:2141-2153.

[10] O'Neill M, Lewis JA. Human Medicinal Agents from Plants. In: Kinghorn AD, Balandrin MF.(eds). ACS Symposium Series 534; Washington, DC1993. p. 48.

[11] Kinghorn AD, Balandrin MF. Human Medicinal Agents from Plants. In: Kinghorn AD, Balandrin MF.(eds). ACS Symposium Series 534; Washington, DC1993.

[12] Josef M, John AG, Steven MG. Marine Natural Products Chemistry. Chemical Reviews 1993; 93:173-194.

[13] Berdy JH. Progress in Industrial Microbiology. In: Bushell ME, Grafe U.(eds.). Amsterdam: Elsevier; 1989. p. 27.

[14] Newman DJ, Cragg GM. Natural products as sources of new drugs over the last 25 years. Journal of Natural Products 2007;70:461-477.

[15] Guo ZR. Modification of natural products for drug discovery. ActaPharmaceutica-Sinica 2012;47:144–157.

[16] Valli M, Pivatto M, Danuello A, Castro-Gamboa I, Silva DHS, Cavalheiro AJ, et al. Tropical biodiversity: Has it been a potential source of secondary metabolites useful for medicinal chemistry? Quimica Nova 2012;35: 2278–2287.

[17] Shellard EJ. Medicines from plants with special reference to herbal products in Great Britain. Planta Medica 1987;53:121-123.

[18] Bernards CM. Sophistry in medicine: Lessons from the epidural space. Anesthesia and Pain Medicine 2005;30:55-66.

[19] Foster GM, . Hippocrates' Latin American Legacy. Humoral Medicine in the New World. Longhorne (USA): Gordon and Breach Science Publisher; 1994.

[20] Jantan I. The Scientific Values of Malaysian Herbal Products. MalaysianJournal of Health Science 2006;4:59-70.

[21] Dias DA, Urban S, Roessner U. A historical overview of natural products in drug discovery. Metabolites 2012. p. 303–336.

[22] Farnsworth NR, Akerele O, Bingel AS, Soejarto DD, Guo Z. Medicinal plants in therapy. Bulletin of the World Health Organization 1985;63:965-981.

[23] Balandrin MF, Kinghorn AD, Farnsworth NR. Human Medicinal Agents from Plants. In: Kinghorn AD, Balandrin MF.(eds). ACS Symposium Series 534; Washington, DC1993. p. 2.

[24] Dias DA, Urban S, Roessner U. A historical overview of natural products in drug discovery. Metabolites 2012. p. 303–336.

[25] Hson-Mou C, Paul P-H, But. Pharmacology and Applications of Chinese Materia-Medica. In. Singapore: World Scientific Publishing Company; 1986.

[26] Kapoor LD. CRC Handbook of Ayurvedic Medicinal Plants. Boca Raton, FL: CRC Press; 1990.

[27] Iwu M. Handbook of African Medicinal Plants. In. Boca Raton, FL: CRC Press; 1993.

[28] Watt M, Breyer-Brandwijk MG. Medicinal and Poisonous Plants of Southern and Eastern Africa. In. Edinburgh: E. and S. Livingstone Ltd; 1962.

[29] Tyler VE. Human Medicinal Agents from Plants. In: Kinghorn AD, Balandrin MF. (eds). ACS Symposium Series 534; Washington, DC1993. p. 25.

[30] Farnsworth NR, Akerele O, Bingel AS, Soejarto DD, Guo Z. Medicinal plants in therapy. Bulletin of the World Health Organization 1985;63:965-981.

[31] Fabricant DS, Farnsworth NR. The value of plants used in traditional medicine for drug discovery. Environmental Health Perspectives 2001;109:69-75.

[32] Sharma PP, Mujundar AM. Traditional knowledge on plants from Toranmal Plateau of Maharastra. Indian Journal of Traditional Knowledge 2003;2:292-296.

[33] Cox PA, Balick MJ. The ethnobotanical approach to drug discovery. Scientific American 1994:82-87.

[34] Hare R. New light on the history of penicillin. Med Hist 1982;26:1-24.

[35] Sinha BM. *Emetine in amoebiasis*. Antiseptic 1946;43:776-778.

[36] Abourashed EA, El-Alfy AT, Khan IA, Walker L. Ephedra in perspective--a current review. Phytotherapy Research 2003;17:703-712.

[37] Miller LH, Su X. Artemisinin: discovery from the Chinese herbal garden. Cell 2011;146:855-859.

[38] Gray AI, Igoli J, O, Edrada-Ebel R. Natural products isolation in modern drug discovery programs. Methods in Molecular Biology 2012;864:515-534.

[39] Rollinger JM, Langer T, Stuppner H. Strategies for efficient lead structure discovery from natural products. Current Medicinal Chemistry 2006;13:1491-1507.

[40] Michael D, Jean PG. Key factors in the rising cost of new drug discovery and development. Nature Reviews Drug Discovery 2004;3:417-429.

[41] Matthew H. The Truly Staggering Cost Of Inventing New Drugs Phrama & Health 2012. Available from: http://www.forbes.com/sites/matthewherper/2012/02/10/the-truly-staggering-cost-of-inventing-new-drugs/.

[42] Lipinski CA, Lombardo F, Dominy BW, Feeney PJ. Experiments and computational approaches to estimate solubility and permeability in drug discovery and development settings. Advanced Drug Delivery Reviews 1997;23:3-25.

[43] McChesney JD, Venkataraman SK, Henri JT. Plant natural products: back to the future or into extinction? Phytochemistry 2007;68 2015-2022.

[44] Baker DD, Chu M, Oza U, Rajgarhia V. The value of natural products to future pharmaceutical discovery. Natural Product Reports 2007;24:1125-1244.

[45] Ojima I. Modern natural products chemistry and drug discovery. Journal of Medicinal Chemistry 2008;51:2587–2588.

[46] Nussbaum FV, Brands M, Hinzen B, Weigand S, Habich D. Antibacterial natural products in medicinal chemistry - exodus or revival?. Angewandte Chemie 2006;45: 5072-29.

[47] Luzhetskyy A, Pelzer S, Bechthold A. The future of natural products as a source of new antibiotics. Current opinion in investigational drugs 2007;8:608-613.

[48] Newman DJ. Natural products as leads to potential drugs: An old process or the new hope for drug discovery? Journal of Medicinal Chemistry 2008;51:2589–2599.

[49] Newman DJ, Cragg GM. Natural products as sources of new drugs over the last 25 years. Journal of Natural Products 2007;70:461-477.

[50] Koehn FE. The evolving role of natural products in drug discovery. Nature 2005;4:206-220.

[51] Butler MS. The role of natural product in chemistry in drug discovery. Journal of Natural Products 2004;67:2141-2153.

[52] Brown EC, Newman DJ. The US National Cancer Institute's natural products repository; origins and utility. Journal of Environmental Monitoring 2006;8:800–805.

[53] Fullbeck M, Michalsky E, Dunkel M, Preissner R. Natural products: sources and databases. Natural Product Reports 2006;23:347–356.

[54] Gomord V, Chamberlain P, Jefferis R, Faye L. Biopharmaceutical production in plants: problems, solutions and opportunities. Trends in Biotechnology 2005;23:559–565.

[55] Jung HG. Chemical genomics with natural products. Journal of Microbiology and Biotechnology 2006;16:651-660.

[56] Koehn FE. The evolving role of natural products in drug discovery. Nature 2005;4:206-220.

[57] Vuorela P. Natural products in the process of finding new drug candidates. Current Medicinal Chemistry 2004;11:1375-1389.

[58] Wu S, Yang L, Gao Y. Multi-channel counter-current chromatography for high throughput fractionation of natural products for drug discovery. Journal of Chromatography A 2007;1180:99-107.

[59] Singh SB, Barrett JF. Empirical antibacterial drug discovery–foundation in natural products. Biochemical Pharmacology 2006;71:1006-1015.

[60] Harvey AL. Natural products as a screening resource. Current Opinion in Chemical Biology 2007;11:480-484.

[61] Quinn RJ, Carroll AR, Pham NB, Baron P, Palframan ME, Suraweera L, et al. Developing a drug-like natural product library. Journal of Natural Products 2008;71:464-468.

[62] Urban S, Separovic F. Developments in hyphenated spectroscopic methods in natural product profiling. Frontiers in Drug Design & Discovery 2005;1:113-166.

[63] Pierceall WE, Zhang L, Hughes DE. Affinity capillary electrophoresis analyses of protein–protein interactions in target-directed drug discovery. Methods in Molecular Biology 2004;261:187-198.

[64] Belenky A, Hughes D, Korneev A, Dunayevskiy Y. Capillary electrophoretic approach to screen for enzyme inhibitors in natural extracts. Journal of chromatography A. 2004;1053(1-2):247-251.

[65] Wang T, Zhang Q, Zhang Y, Kang J. Screening of protein kinase inhibitors in natural extracts by capillary electrophoresis combined with liquid chromatography-tandem mass spectrometry. Journal of Chromatography A 2014;1337:188-193.

[66] Zhao H, Chen Z. Screening of neuraminidase inhibitors from traditional Chinese medicines by integrating capillary electrophoresis with immobilized enzyme microreactor. Journal of Chromatography A 2014;1340:139-45.

[67] Wolfender J-L, Ndjoko K, Hostettman K. Liquid chromatography with ultraviolet absorbance-mass spectrometric detection and with nuclear magnetic resonance spectroscopy: A powerful combination for the on-line structural investigation of plant metabolites. Journal of Chromatography A 2003;1000:437-55.

[68] Wolfender J-L, Queiroz EF, Hostettman K. The importance of hyphenated techniques in the discovery of new lead compounds from nature. Expert Opinion in Drug Discovery 2006;1:237-260.

[69] Schroeder FC, Gronquist M. Extending the scope of NMR spectroscopy with micro-coil probes. Angewandte Chemie 2006;45:7122–7131.

[70] Lewis RJ, Bernstein MA, Duncan SJ, Sleigh CJ. A comparison of capillary-scale LC-NMR with alternative techniques: Spectroscopic and practical considerations. Magnetic Resonance in Chemistry 2005;43:783-789.

[71] Dias D, Urban S. Phytochemical analysis of the southern australian marine alga, Plocamium mertensiiusing HPLC-NMR. Phytochemical Analysis 2008;19:453–470, .

[72] Dias DA, Urban S. Application of HPLC-NMR for the rapid chemical profiling of a Southern Australian Sponge, Dactylospongia sp. Journal of Separation Science 2009;32:542-548.

[73] Lin Y, Schiavo S, Orjala J, Vouros P, Kautz R. Microscale LC-MS-NMR platform applied to the identification of active cyanobacterial metabolites. Analytical Chemistry 2008;80: 8045–8054.

[74] Sun Lin J, Mahyudin NA, Chamyuang S, Blunt JW, Cole T, Lang G, et al. Less is more: Dereplication and discovery using CapNMR techniques. 12th International Symposium of Marine Natural Products; 2007 4–9 Feb; Queenstown, New Zealand.

[75] Dias DA, White JM, Urban S. Laurenciafiliformis: Phytochemical profiling by conventional and HPLC-NMR approaches. Natural Product Communications 2009;4:157-172.

[76] Clarkson C, Stærk D, Hansen SH, Smith PJ, Jaroszewski JW. Discovering new natural products directly from crude extracts by HPLC-SPE-NMR: Chinane diterpenes Harpagophytum procumbens. Journal of Natural Products 2006;69:527-530.

[77] Cogne A-L, Queiroz EF, Marston A, Wolfender JL, Mavi S, Hostettmann K. On-line identification of unstable iridoids from Jamesbrittenia fodina by HPLC-MS and HPLC-NMR. Phytochemical Analysis 2005;16:429-439.

[78] Zschocke S, Klaiber I, Bauer R, Vogler B. HPLC-coupled spectroscopic techniques (UV, MS, NMR) for the structure elucidation of phthalides in Ligusticum chuanxiong. Molecular Diversity 2005;9:33-39.

[79] Harrold JM, Ramanathan M, Mager DE. Network-based approaches in drug discovery and early development. Clinical Pharmacology and Therapeutics.2013;94(6): 651-658.

[80] Emig D, Ivliev A, Pustovalova O, Lancashire L, Bureeva S, Nikolsky Y, Bessarabova M. Drug target prediction and repositioning using an integrated network-based approach. PLoS One. 2013 Apr 4;8(4):e60618. doi: 10.1371/journal.pone.0060618.

[81] Gui-biao Zhang, Qing-ya Li, Qi-long Chen, and Shi-bing Su. Network Pharmacology: A New Approach for Chinese Herbal Medicine Research Evidence-Based Complementary and Alternative Medicine Vol 2013 (2013), Article ID 621423, 9 pageshttp://dx.doi.org/10.1155/2013/621423

[82] Rochfort S. Metabolomics reviewed: A new "Omics" platform technology for systems biology and implications for natural products research. Journal of Natural Products 2005;68:1813-1820.

[83] Roessner U, Beckles DM. Metabolite measurements. In: Junker B, Schwender J, editors. Plant Metabolic Networks. Heidelberg, Germany: Springer; 2009.

[84] Roessner U, Nahid A, Hunter A, Bellgard M, editors. Metabolomics—The combination of analytical chemistry, biology and informatics. 2nd ed. Heidelberg, Germany: Springer; 2011.

[85] Beckles DM, Roessner U. Plant Metabolomics—Applications and opportunities for agricultural biotechnology. Altmann A, P.M. H.(eds.). Boston, MA, USA: Elsevier/Academic Press; 2011.

[86] Ferrer-Alcón M, Arteta D, Guerrero MJ, Fernandez-Orth D, Simón L, Martinez A. The use of gene array technology and proteomics in the search of new targets of diseases for therapeutics. Toxicology Letters 2009;186:45-51.

[87] Kwon SJ, Lee MY, Ku B, Sherman DH, Dordick JS. High-throughput, microarray-based synthesis of natural product analogues via in vitro metabolic pathway construction. ACS Chemical Biology 2007;2:419-425.

[88] Chan CY, Huang PH, Guo F, Ding X, Kapur V, Mai JD, et al. Accelerating drug discovery via organs-on-chips. Lab Chip 2013;3:4697-4710.

[89] Colegate SM, Molyneux RJ. Bioactive Natural Products: Detection, Isolation and Structure Determination. Boca Raton, FL, USA: Boca Raton, FL; 2008. p. 421- 437.

[90] Sarker SD, Latif Z, Gray A. Methods in Biotechnology: Natural Product Isolation. D S, editor. Totowa, NJ, USA: Human Press; 2006. p. 528.

[91] Blunt JW, Munro MHG (2009). Dictionary of Marine Natural Products. [(accessed on 21 July 2009)]. http://dmnp.chemnetbase.com/

[92] Buckingham J. The Dictionary of Natural Products 2001 [cited 2011 22 August]. Available from: http://dmnp.chemnetbase.com/.

[93] MarinLit. 2011 [updated 23 June cited 2011 23 June]. Available from: http://www.chem.canterbury.ac.nz/marinlit/marinlit.shtml.

[94] Blunt JW, Munro MHG, Laatsch H. AntiMarin Database 2012 [cited 2012 10 April]. Available from: http://www.chem.canterbury.ac.nz/marinlit/marinlit.shtml.

[95] Lang G, Mayhudin NA, Mitova MI, Sun L, S vdS, Blunt JW, et al. Evolving trends in the dereplication of natural product extracts: New methodology for rapid, small-

scale investigation of natural product extracts. Journal of Natural Products 2008;19:1595-1599.

[96] SciFinder Scholar [cited 2011 2 July]. Available from: http://www.cas.org/SCIFINDER/SCHOLAR/.

[97] SCOPUS. [cited 2011 25 August]. Available from: http://www.scopus.com/home.url.

[98] Napraler. [cited 2011 3 May]. Available from: http://www.napralert.org/.

[99] Liyan W, Shoude Z, Junsheng Z, Lili Z, Xiaofeng L, Lei S, et al. Identification of diverse natural products as falcipain-2 inhibitors through structure-based virtual screening. Bioorganic & Medicinal Chemistry Letters 2014;24:1261-1264.

[100] Liu LJ, Leung KH, Chan DS, Wang YT, Ma DL, Leung CH. Identification of a natural product-like STAT3 dimerization inhibitor by structure-based virtual screening. Cell Death and Disease 2014;5:1293.

[101] Chen L, Wang L, Qiong G, Jun X. An in silico protocol for identifying mTOR inhibitors from natural products. Molecular Diversity 2014.

[102] Doman TN, McGovern SL, Witherbee BJ, Kasten TP, Kurumbail R, Stallings WC, et al. Molecular docking and high-throughput screening for novel inhibitors of protein tyrosine phosphatase-1B. Journal of Medicinal Chemistry 2002;45:2213-2220.

[103] Fabricant DS, Farnsworth NR. The value of plants used in traditional medicine for drug discovery. Environmental Health Perspectives 2001;109:69-75.

[104] Politi M, Peschel W, Wilson N, Zloh M, Prieto JM, Heinrich M. Cannabis water extracts and tinctures analysed by NMR spectroscopy; different strategies to reduce the content of D9-THC. Phytochemistry 2008;69:652-670.

[105] Verpoorte R, Choi YH, Kim HK. Ethnopharmacology and systems biology: A perfect holistic match. Journal of Ethnopharmacology 2005;100:53-56.

[106] Wang M, Lamers RJAN, Korthout HA, Van Nesselrooij JHJ, Witkamp RF, Van der Heijden R. Metabolomics in the context of systems biology: Bridging traditional Chinese medicine and molecular pharmacology. Phytotherapy Research 2005;3:173-182.

[107] Om P, Amit K, Pawan K, Ajeet. Potential of Plants and Natural Products: A Review. American Journal of Pharmacological Sciences 2013;1:104-115.

[108] Madhuri L, Pandey G. Some anticancer medicinal plants offoreign Origin. Current Science 2009;96:779-783.

[109] Desai AG, Qazi GN, Ganju RK, El-Tamer M, Singh J, Saxena AK, et al. Medicinal plants and cancer chemoprevention. Current Drug Metabolism 2008;9:581-591.

[110] Mohammad S. Anticancer agents from medicinal plants. Bangladesh Journal of Pharmacology 2006;1:35.

[111] Monteiro LS, Bastos KX, Barbosa-Filho JM, de Athayde-Filho PF, Diniz M, F, Sobral MV. Medicinal Plants and Other Living Organisms with Antitumor Potential against Lung Cancer. Evidence-Based Complementary and Alternative Medicine 2014;2014:604152.

[112] Hotwani K, Baliga S, Sharma K. Phytodentistry: use of medicinal plants. Journal of Complementary and Integrative Medicine 2014.

[113] en T, Samanta SK. Medicinal Plants, Human Health and Biodiversity: A Broad Review. Advances in Biochemical Engineering / Biotechnology 2014.

[114] Sultana S, Asif HM, Nazar HM, Akhtar N, Rehman JU, Rehman RU. Medicinal plants combating against cancer--a green anticancer approach. Asian Pacific Journal of Cancer Prevention 2014;15:4385-4394.

[115] Pan SY, Litscher G, Gao S, H, SF Z, Yu Z, Chen H, et al. Historical perspective of traditional indigenous medical practices: the current renaissance and conservation of herbal resources. Evidence-Based Complementary and Alternative Medicine 2014.

[116] Ling X, Bochu W. A review of phytotherapy of gout: perspective of new pharmacological treatments. Pharmazie 2014;69:243-456.

[117] Newman DJ, Cragg GM, Snader KM. The influence of natural products upon drug discovery. Natural Product Reports 2000;17:215–234.

[118] van Der Heijden R, Jacobs DI, Snoeijer W, Hallard D, Verpoorte R. The Catharanthus alkaloids: pharmacognosy and biotechnology. Current Medicinal Chemistry 2003;11:607-628.

[119] Menon VP[1], Sudheer AR. Antioxidant and anti-inflammatory properties of curcumin. Exp Med Biol. 2007;595:105-125.

[120] Dugasani, S.; Pichika M.R.; Nadarajah, V.D.; Balijepalli, M.K.; Tandra, S.; Korlakunta, J.N. Comparative antioxidant and anti-inflammatory effects of [6]-gingerol, [8]-gingerol, [10]-gingerol and [6]-shogaol. Journal of Ethnopharmacology. 2010; 127: 515–520.

[121] Lee JC, Kundu JK, Hwang DM, Na HK, Surh YJHumulone inhibits phorbol ester-induced COX-2 expression in mouse skin by blocking activation of NF-kappaB and AP-1: IkappaB kinase and c-Jun-N-terminal kinase as respective potential upstream targets. Carcinogenesis. 2007 Jul;28(7):1491-1498.

[122] Viladomiu M, Hontecillas-Magarzo R, Kingston D, Eaton A, Zhang X, Philipson C, et al. Immune modulatory mechanisms of Oncostemum bojerianum extracts during Clostridium difficile infection in mice (MUC4P.845). The Journal of Immunology. 2014;192(1 Supplement):133.21.

[123] Lin J-T, Liu C-W, Chen Y-C, Hu C-C, Juang L-D, Shiesh C-C, et al. Chemical composition, antioxidant and anti-inflammatory properties for ethanolic extracts from Pleu-

rotus eryngii fruiting bodies harvested at different time. LWT - Food Science and Technology. 2014;55(1):374-382.

[124] Toffoli-Kadri MC, Carollo CA, Lourenço LD, Felipe JL, Brandini Néspoli JH, Wollf LGC, et al. In vivo and in vitro anti-inflammatory properties of Achyrocline alata (Kunth) DC. Journal of Ethnopharmacology. 2014;153(2):461-468.

[125] Wang K, Zhang J, Ping S, Ma Q, Chen X, Xuan H, et al. Anti-inflammatory effects of ethanol extracts of Chinese propolis and buds from poplar (Populus×canadensis). Journal of Ethnopharmacology. 2014;155(1):300-311.

[126] Sagnia B, Fedeli D, Casetti R, Montesano C, Falcioni G, Colizzi V. Antioxidant and Anti-Inflammatory Activities of Extracts from <italic>Cassia alata, Eleusine indica, Eremomastax speciosa, Carica papaya</italic> and <italic>Polyscias fulva</italic> Medicinal Plants Collected in Cameroon. PLoS ONE. 2014;9(8):e103999.

[127] Arora N, Pandey-Rai S. GC–MS analysis of the essential oil of Celastrus paniculatus Willd. seeds and antioxidant, anti-inflammatory study of its various solvent extracts. Industrial Crops and Products. 2014;61(0):345-351.

[128] Wang SJ, Zheng CJ, Peng C, Zhang H, Jiang YP, Han T, Qin LP (2013). Plants and cervical cancer: an overview. Expert Opin Investig Drugs 22(9):1133-1156

[129] Shoeb M.. Anticancer agents from medicinal plants. Bangladesh Journal of Pharmacology 2006; 1:35-41.

[130] Newman DJ, Cragg GM, Snader KM. The influence of natural products upon drug discovery.Natural Product Reports. 2000; 17: 215–234.

[131] Newman DJ, Cragg GM, Snader KM.Natural products as sources of new drugs over the period 1981–2002. Journal of Natural Products. 2003; 66: 1022–1037.

[132] Butler MS.The role of natural product chemistry in drug discovery. Journal of Natural Products. 2004; 67: 2141–2153.

[133] Cragg GM, Newman DJ, Weiss RB. Coral reefs, forests, and thermal vents: the world-wide exploration of nature for novel antitumor agents. Semin Oncol 1997;24:156-163.

[134] Newman DJ, Cragg GM. Natural products as sources of new drugs over the last 25 years. Journal Natural Products2007;70: 461–477.

[135] Bhanot A, Sharma R, Noolvi MN. Natural sources as potential anti-cancer agents: A review. International Journal of Phytomedicine 2011:3; 9-26

[136] van Der Heijden R, Jacobs DI, Snoeijer W, Hallard D, Verpoorte R. The Catharanthus alkaloids: pharmacognosy and biotechnology. Current Medicinal Chemistry 2003;11:607-628.

[137] Okouneva T, Hill BT, Wilson L, Jordan MA.The effects of vinflunine, vinorelbine, and vinblastine on centromere dynamics. Molecular Cancer Therapeutics 2003; 2:427–436.

[138] Gordaliza M, Garcia PA, del Corral JM, Castro MA, Gomez-Zurita MA. Podophyllotoxin: distribution, sources, applications and new cytotoxic derivatives. Toxicon 2004;44:441-459.

[139] Wall ME, Wani MC. Camptothecin and taxol: from discovery to clinic Journal of Ethnopharmacology 1996; 51: 239–253.

[140] Oberlies NH, Kroll DJ. Camptothecin and taxol: historic achievements in natural products research. Journal of Natural Products 2004;67:139-135.

[141] Schiff PB, Fant J, Horwitz SB. Promotion of microtubule assembly in vitro by taxol Nature 1979;277:665-667.

[142] Horwitz SB. Personal recollections on the early development of taxol. Journal of Natural Products 2004;67:136-138.

[143] Cragg GM, Newman DJ. A tale of two tumor targets: topoisomerase I and tubulin. The Wall and Wani contribution to cancer chemotherapy. Journal of Natural Products 2004;67:232-244.

[144] Taylor L. "Plant based drugs and medicines." Raintree Nutrition 2013 [cited 2003 12 Mar]. Available from: http://www.rain-tree.com/plantdrugs.htm.

[145] Patil, U.S., Jaydeokar, A.V., Bandawane, D.D. (2012), Immunomodulators: A Pharmacological Review. International Journal of Pharmacy and Pharmacology Science, 4(L) 30-36.

[146] J. M. Van der Nat, J.P.A.M. Klerx, and K.T.D. De Silva, and R. P. Labadie, "Immunomodulatory activity of an aqueous extract of *Azadirachta indica* stem bark, " Journal of Ethnopharmacology 1987; 19: 125–13, 1987.

[147] S. Diwanay, D. Chitre, and B. Patwardhan, "Immunoprotection botanical drugs in cancer chemotherapy, " Journal of Ethnopharmacology 2004; 90: 49–55.

[148] M. Gautam, S. Diwanay, S. Gairola, S. Shinde, P. Patki, and B. Patwardhan, "Immuno-adjuvant potential of Asparagus racemosusaqueous extract in experimental system. Journal of Ethnopharmacology 2004; 91:251–255.

[149] L. Yu, M. Zhao, B. Yang, and W. Bai, "Immunomodulatory and anti-cancer activities of phenolics from *Garcinia mangostana* fruit pericarp, " Food Chemistry, 1984;116: 969–973.

[150] M. G. Jayathirtha, and S. H. Mishra, "Preliminary immunomodulatory activities of methanol extracts of *Eclipta alba* and *Centella asiatica,* " Phytomedicine 2004; 11: 361–365.

[151] Winkler C, Wirleitner B, Schroecksnadel K, Schennach H, Mur E, Fuchs D. In vitro effects of two extracts and two pure alkaloid preparations of Uncaria tomentosa on peripheral blood mononuclear cells. Planta Med. 2004 Mar;70(3):205-10.

[152] Patwardhan and Gautam. Drug Discovery Today 2005;10(7): 495-502.

[153] Schepetkin I and Quinn, MT. Botanical Polysaccharides: Macrophage Immunomodulation and Therapeutic Potential. International Immunopharmacology 2006;6: 317-333.

[154] Sen P, Mediratta PK, Ray A. Effects of Azadirachta indica on some biochemical, immunological and visceral parameters in normal and stressed rats. Indian Journal of Experimental Biology 1990;30:1170-1175.

[155] Nores MM, Courreges MC, Benencia F, Coulombie FC. Immunomodulatory activities of Cedrela lilloi and Trichilia elegans aqueous leaf extracts. Joural of Medicinal Chemistry 1997;55:99-106.

[156] Lima JE, Sampaio ALF, Gracas MD, Henriques MO, Fidalgo CB. Lymphocyte activation and cytokine production by Pisum sativum agglutinin (PSA) in vivo and in vitro. Immunopharmacology 1999;41:147-155.

[157] Jantan, N. H. Harun, A. W. Septama, S. Murad, and M. A. Mesaik, "Inhibition of chemiluminescence and chemotactic activity of phagocytes in vitro by the extracts of selected medicinal plants, " Journal of Natural Medicine 2011; 65: 400–405.

[158] Yuandani, Ilangkovan M, Jantan I, Mohamad HF, Husain K, A. Razak AF.Inhibitory effects of standardized extracts of Phyllanthus amarus and Phyllanthus urinaria and their marker compounds on phagocytic activity of human neutrophils. Evidence-Based Complementary and Alternative Medicine 2013, Article ID 603634 pages, Doi./ 10.1155/2013/603634.

[159] Mesaik MA, Zaheer-Ul-Haq, Murad S, Ismail Z, Abdullah NR, Gill HK, Atta-Ur-Rahman, Yousaf M, Siddiqui RA, Ahmad A, Choudhary MI. Biological and molecular docking studies on coagulin-H: Human IL-2 novel natural inhibitor.Molecular Immunology. 2006;43 (11):1855-1863.

[160] Hussain S, Slevin M, Mesaik MA, Choudhary MI, Elosta AH, Matou S, Ahmed N, West D, Gaffney J. Cheiradone: a vascular endothelial cell growth factor receptor antagonist. BMC Cell Biology 2008;9:7) 1-10.

[161] Plaeger SF. Clinical immunology and traditional herbal medicines. Clinical and Diagnostic Laboratory Immunology 2003;10:337-338.

[162] Nagoya Protocol http://www.cbd.int/abs/about/

[163] Zakrzewski PA. Bioprospecting or biopiracy? The pharmaceutical industry's use of indigenous medicinal plants as a source of potential drug candidates. University of Toronto Medical Journal 2002;79:252-254.

5

# Lipids and Liposomes in the Enhancement of Health and Treatment of Disease

Simon A. Young and Terry K. Smith

## 1. Introduction

The discovery of liposomes initially came from studies by Bangham and Horne who observed by electron microscopy the self-association of the lipid phosphatidylcholine (mixed with or without cholesterol) in water formed 'spherulites' of varying sizes which had not a recognizable lamellar shell comprising a lipid bilayer [1]. The self-assembling 'spherulites', subsequently named liposomes from the greek *lipo* (fat) and *soma* (body), were recognised to be functionally analogous to studied biological membrane systems due to the similar rates of diffusion of ions [2]. However only when an ionophore, valinomycin, was utilised demonstrating selective diffusion of $K^+$ over $Na^+$ from liposomes containing equal concentrations of the ions, could liposomes be confirmed as entirely sealed membrane vesicles [3]. Furthermore Papahadjopoulos and Watkins showed the differential permeability to anions and cations could be significantly altered with liposomes of different phospholipid compositions [4]. Natural liposomes have bilayers composed of phospholipids and/or cholesterol and as such are poorly antigenic, typically non-toxic and physiologically inert. Liposomes can vary in size from 25 nm to 2.5 μm and are classified within three broad categories [5]: Multilamellar vesicles (MLV), which structurally resemble an onion with multiple concentric phospholipid bilayers separated by aqueous layers,large unilamellar vesicles (LUV) and small unilamellar vesicles (SUV) which have a single lipid bilayer surrounding the aqueous core. Typically multiple unilamellar vesicles of differing sizes can form inside of each other generating multilamellar structures.

The concept of liposomes as drug-carriers to aid in selectivity was explored in the early nineteen seventies predominantly through the work of drug-transport scientists such as Gregoriadis who initially looked at the fate of protein-containing liposomes delivered into animals [6]. The theory that liposomes stay intact and circulate in the bloodstream before accumulating in specific tissues where they release their molecules into cells was confirmed using radiolabelled proteins entrapped in liposomes. The radioactive signal from the proteins was barely detected in the bloodstream, but predominantly in the lysosomes of cells of the liver and spleen, showing the liposomes stayed intact prior to the radiolabelled proteins being taken up by the cells. This and related studies revealed the physiological behaviour of liposomes such as their integrity and long life span in the mammalian bloodstream. It was only through the use of cell culture it was confirmed that cargo carried by liposomes was directly delivered through endocytosis into the lysosomes and thus into the intracellular environment of cells [7]. These initial studies demonstrated the huge potential for liposomes as model systems, and a number of various applications were subsequently explored as listed here: The effect of surface charge on ion permeability [8]; their susceptibility to phospholipase hydrolysis [9]; the function of integral membrane ion transporters [10]; the delivery of active enzymes to functionally deficient cells [11]; their use as immunological adjuvants [12]; as stimulants of interferon production [13]; their interaction with polyene antibiotics [14]; their incorporation of local and general anaesthetics [15]; the inclusion and presentation of virus surface proteins [16]. Since those early experiments, there has been a continued interest in the use of liposomes and currently there are applications in a wide variety of scientific fields (Figure 1).

In this chapter we will focus on the use of lipids and liposomes in the enhancement of a number of health related areas and cover the development of new synthetic molecules, which have great potential in advancing improvements in health and the treatment of disease.

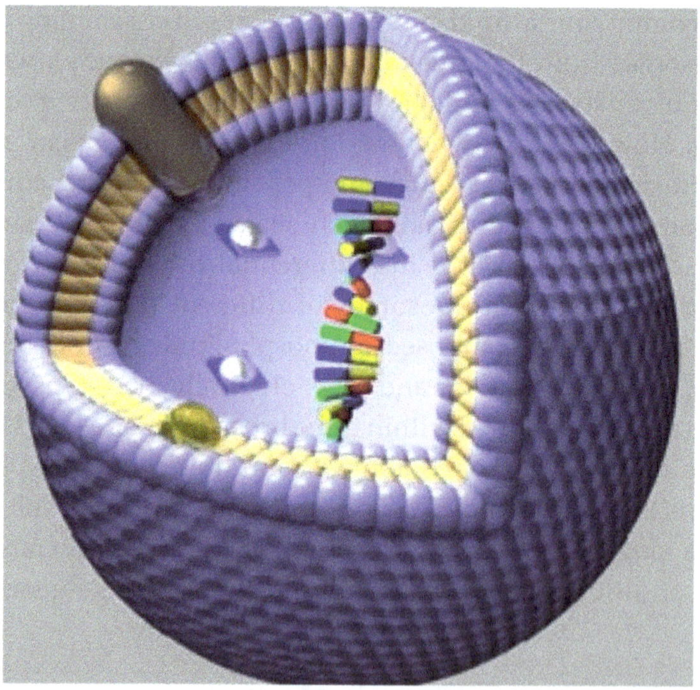

**Figure 1.** A schematic representation of a liposome. The liposome can facilitate the carrying of various cargo, water-soluble drugs, DNA or RNA, in the internal hydrophilic region, water-insoluble drugs within the hydrophobic region of the bilayer, or protein linked or incorporated into the phospholipid bilayer.

## 2. Current applications in treating disease

### 2.1. Non-communicable diseases

It is evident that with their physiological attributes, liposomes are an attractive means to deliver drugs to treat a variety of communicable and non-communicable diseases. Typically, drugs for the treatment of human diseases can often have a number of biochemical and pharmacological issues such as poor stability and solubility, rapid breakdown and lack of targeted delivery. As a result there are common problems in the use of such drugs, including the lack of a strong therapeutic cure and the necessity to consume high doses, which can result in unwanted side effects. If the disease is localised to a specific body tissue, the lack of selective targeting can result in poor bioavailability of the drug at the required site, potentially resulting in toxicity in other tissues, thus restricting the dose concentration. The use of natural phospholipid based liposome formulations having minimal toxicity, extended stability in the human body, tissue selectivity and a delayed release of the active compound at the site of action suggests clear benefits for drug development and treatment. In addition multiple compounds can be distributed by the same liposomes for added therapeutic impact. Equally, compounds of varying lipophilicities can transported, partitioning in the different hydrophobic and hydrophilic environments of the liposomes. Particle size is a critical factor both in the circulatory half-life of liposomes and also (along with the number of bilayers) dictates the amount of encapsulated drug [17]. In general, drug delivery systems are on the nanoscale, liposomes having diameters of 100 nm or less tend to have a good therapeutic index compared to conventional anticancer therapies. Typically liposomes for drug therapies approved for humans contain the neutrally charged phosphatidylcholine as the major membrane constituent, though occasionally cholesterol (up to a third of the total lipid content) is incorporated to reduce membrane instability due to serum protein binding. Thirty years ago, the application of liposomes to deliver an anti-cancer anthracycline drug doxorubicin trapped in negatively charged or neutral liposomes (called OLV-DOX) showed that it retained its antitumour activity in mice [18]. Importantly the use of the liposomal formulation reduced the accumulation of the drug in murine cardiac tissues, minimising toxicity and thus significantly improving their survival. When tested in humans however the OLV-DOX worked poorly, being rapidly cleared from the bloodstream with significant premature release of the drug, giving rise to potential cardiotoxicity [19]. These failings limited the application of liposomes in cancer treatment at that time, only resolved by the subsequent experimental trialling of polyethylene glycol (PEG) incorporation in phospholipid liposomes. The PEG was found to create a hydrophilic surface on the liposomes, reducing uptake by the reticuloendothelial system and thus increasing the circulation time of these so-called 'stealth' liposomes. This resulted in a revolution in liposome design and so in 1995 Doxil (PEGylated liposome-trapped doxorubicin) the first of the so-called 2$^{nd}$ generation was approved by the US Food and Drug Administration as the first liposome drug delivery system for human use [20]. Doxil was found to have extended stability in the bloodstream and reduced compound leakage resulting in increased accumulation in solid tumours (up to 22-fold) and reduced toxicity to non-target organs. Every year over 300,000 patients with ovarian cancer or Kaposi's sarcoma are now routinely intravenously treated with

Doxil [21] and it is occasionally utilised in cases of breast cancer and also in combination with bortezomib for multiple myeloma.

Alongside Doxil, to date five other liposomal formulations are approved for human cancer treatment (Table 1). Myocet, a related non-PEGylated liposome formulation of doxorubicin is used in combination with cyclophosphamide for breast cancer [22]. DaunoXome, a liposome formulation of daunorobicin is similarly used to treat Kaposi's sarcoma [23]. DepoCyt, a formulation of unusually large liposomes containing cytarabine is active against malignant lymphomatous meningitis [24], while Marqibo is a more typical nanoscale formulation of liposomes of vincristine utilised for acute lymphoblastic leukemia [25]. Recently, more success has come from the trial use of such liposome formulations in combination with standard anti-cancer drugs, one example being a Doxil and carboplatin composition which shows a better therapeutic index and less toxicity than the standard paclitaxel/carboplatin mixture used to treat ovarian cancer in the elderly [26]. Similarly in comparison to a standard treatment, a combination of Doxil, bortezomib and dexamethasone showed a strong therapeutic response and improved tolerability in patients with multiple myeloma [27].

| Market Product | Drug used | Target diseases | Company |
|---|---|---|---|
| Doxil or Caelyx | Doxorubicin | Kaposi's sarcoma | SEQUUS, USA |
| DaunoXome | Daunorubicin | Kaposi's sarcoma, breast & lung cancer | NeXstar, USA |
| Amphotec | Amphotericin-B | Fungal infections, Leishmaniasis | SEQUUS, USA |
| Ventus | Prostaglandin-E1 | Systemic inflammatory diseases | The liposome company, USA |
| Alec | Dry protein free powder of DPPC-PG | Expanding lung diseases in babies | Britannia Pharm, UK |
| Epaxal–Berna Vaccine | Inactivated hepatitis A virions | Hepatitis A | Swiss serum & vaccine institute, Switzerland |
| Avian retrovirus vaccine | Killed avian retrovirus | Chicken pox | Vineland lab, USA |
| Novasome | Smallpox vaccine | Smallpox | Novavax, USA |
| Depocyt | Cytarabine | Cancer therapy | Skye Pharm, USA |
| Topex-Br | Terbutaline sulphate | Asthma | Ozone, USA |

**Table 1.** Current products utilising liposomes

A major issue in cancer treatments is the failure of many forms of chemotherapy due to the phenomenon of multidrug resistance. As a result, the tactic of using drug combinations has become widely adopted due to the greater therapeutic index and efficacy in reversing the multidrug resistant phenotype [28]. In a combination treatment drugs can have one of three effects, synergistic, additive or antagonistic and this can be shaped by their specific molar ratios in the formulation [29]. Unfortunately in an *in vivo* setting, the combinatorial effect can be weakened due to disrupted pharmacokinetics of the drugs in the system, leading to incorrect dose ratios at the site of action [30]. Based on prior research, it was clear that the pharmacokinetic issues of combination therapies can be eliminated by the use of liposome formulations, resulting in delivery of the drugs to their site of action at the correct effective ratio [31]. Equally important in the enhancement of health is the use of liposomes in the treatment of cardiovascular disease, the leading cause of deaths worldwide. Again relatively early in liposome research, it was observed that liposomes carrying the MRI contrast agent 99mTc-DTPA accumulated in regions of the heart experimentally induced to undergo myocardial infarction (MI), a common cause of death [32]. In MI, during the ischemic phase, the exhaustion of nucleotide pyrophosphates causes extensive myocardial cell damage [33]. The obvious solution, the infusion of adenosine triphosphate (ATP) intravenously to increase myocardial cell energy levels is sub-optimal due to the molecule's short circulatory half-life and strong charge. The relatively unstable ATP could however be protected and successfully delivered using liposomes and clearly accumulated in canine myocardia damaged by ischemia [34]. Subsequently it was discovered that targeted ATP-containing liposomes can significantly protect against the subsequent effects of ischemia in an *ex vivo* rat heart model [35]. When translated into an animal model, ATP-loaded liposomes reduced the amount of irreversible myocardial damage by greater than 50% compared to control treated rabbits [36].

Another significant agent in the prevention and treatment of ischemic injury and indeed heart failure, coronary artery disease and hypertension in general, is Coenzyme Q10 (CoQ10) [37]. Evaluation of CoQ10 loaded liposomes again in the aforementioned rabbit model revealed that only 30% of the affected myocardia was at risk of irreversible damage compared to the control, indicative of significant protection and great potential in this approach [38]. In humans, the use of large-scale trials of adenosine on clinical patients with acute MI has shown some promise but again is a poor compound with a short half-life and hypotensive and brachicardic inducing properties [39]. These issues may be overcome based on an experimental study using PEGylated liposomes of adenosine which generated non-toxic and cardioprotective effects against MI in rats [40]. In treating another common cause of ischemic damage, thrombus formation, a range of thrombolytic drugs have been developed. Due to its need for constant infusion and potential to cause haemorrhage, one of the first thrombolytic drugs, heparin was quickly assessed in a liposomal formulation [41]. Liposomal heparin was much more effective in its thrombolytic effects, being retained in the plasma longer and generated a prolonged activity due to a gradual release of the agent. Ultimately an inhalable formulation successfully replaced the intravenous version in rat models of deep vein thrombosis and pulmonary embolism giving promise to future clinical trials [42].

### 2.2. Communicable diseases

As significant as the development of liposomes in the treatment of non-communicable human diseases has been, the field of anti-parasitic drug development generated the first liposomal formulation to be mass marketed. With no vaccines effective against any of the primary parasitic infections, anti-parasitic drug treatment remains the main approach. Many current anti-parasitic compounds were developed over 50 years ago and though effective, are hardly comparable to the modern view of the biochemical and clinical properties of an ideal drug. Due to the fact that many anti-parasitic drugs have solubility issues, low bioavailability and poor absorption by the gastrointestinal tract, it was an obvious choice to test the potential of liposomes for anti-parasitic drug delivery. AmBisome, a natural liposome configuration of the potent anti-leishmanial amphotericin B was the first liposome drug based formulation to be commercialised in 1990 (Table 2) [43]. A sterol biosynthesis inhibitor, amphotericin B is the standard second-line treatment for visceral leishmaniasis (caused by *Leishmania donovani*) and is essential in endemic disease areas in India due to the extensive development of resistance against the standard pentavalent antimonial compounds [44]. AmBisome is particularly effective against *Leishmania* (2 to 5-fold more potent than the free drug) due to the fact that the parasite infects the very macrophages which clear the liposomes from the bloodstream, increasing the therapeutic effect and additionally reducing the nephrotoxicity of amphotericin B. Initially liposomes containing antimonial compounds were tested in a hamster model of visceral leishmaniasis and were greater than 700 fold more active than the free drug version showing the significant potential of liposome use [45]. Interestingly antimonial encapsulated liposomes were also shown to be potent against cutaneous leishmaniasis where the parasites alternatively reside in peripheral tissues [46].

| Drug | Route of Administration | Targeted Diseases |
|---|---|---|
| Amphotericin-B | Oral | Mycotic infection, Leishmaniasis |
| Insulin | Oral, Ocular, Pulmonary and Transdermal | Diabetic mellitus |
| Ketoprofen | Ocular | Pain muscle condition |
| Pentoxifylline | Pulmonary | Asthma |
| Salbutamol | Pulmonary | Asthma |
| Tobramycin | Pulmonary | Pseudomonas infection, aeruginosa |
| Benzocain | Transdermal | Ulcer on mucous surface with pain |
| Ibuprofen | Oral | Rheumatoid arthritis |
| Adrenaline | Ocular | Glucoma, Conjectivitis |
| Penicillin G | Pulmonary | Meningococal, staphylococcal |
| Methotrexate | Transdermal | Cancer |

**Table 2.** Therapeutic applications utilising liposomes

While AmBisome remains the only liposomal antiparasitic agent on the market, other liposome formulations have been developed showing potency against *Leishmania spp*. Liposomes modified with sugars improved the targeting of antileishmanial pentamidine to infected macrophages with increased potency as a result [47]. Similarly, delivery of the alkylphospholipid miltefosine (hexadecylphosphocholine) in a liposomal form proved twice as active against *L. donovani* and actually even increased the susceptibility of a miltefosine-resistant parasite line [48]. Far less exploration has been done to assess the value of liposomal agents against the causative agents of Human African Trypanosomiasis (HAT) and Chagas' disease,

*Trypanosoma brucei* and *Trypanosoma cruzi* respectively. Both species of parasite have disseminating infections and localise to tissues of the body where there is limited interaction with liposomes. However a number of *in vitro* and *in vivo* studies using liposomes have evaluated potential anti-trypanosomal effects. Two related investigations demonstrated that phosphatidylcholine/stearylamine only liposomes at low concentrations (100 μM) non-toxic to erythrocytes, rapidly killed both *T. cruzi* [49] and *T. brucei* [50] through destabilization of their plasma membranes. Notably this effect was not seen with identical concentrations of the individual lipid components, suggesting the vesicle structure was important for activity. The surprising failure of liposomes containing benznidazole to improve on the potency of this classical anti-*T. cruzi* treatment was hypothesised to be due to a lack of drug delivery [51], though the anti-leishmanial AmBisome demonstrated some success in supressing *T. cruzi* infections *in vivo* [52].

With so many anti-malarial drugs commercially available and in development, the focus of liposome development in this field is on the protection of drugs from premature metabolism, to generate a slow release to improve the therapeutic index and reduce toxicity. To this end, liposomes of Artesunate, a semi-synthetic derivate of artemisinin, were found to release only 30% of the drug in 24 h in an *in vitro* test, giving promise to this method as a means to reduce the dosing frequency of antimalarial drugs [53]. In a rabbit model, Arteether directed for chloroquine resistant *Plasmodium falciparum*, when trapped in dipalmitoylphosphatidylcholine, dibehynoylphophatidylcholine, cholesterol liposomes persisted longer with greater bioavailabilty in the gastrointestinal tract when compared to the aqueous suspension [54]. Similarly, liposomes of chloroquine, the widely used 4-aminoquinoline antimalarial, modified with an antibody to selectively deliver to infected erythrocytes were found to cure the majority of chloroquine-resistant *Plasmodium berghei*-malarial infections in mice [55], proving that targeted liposomes can be very efficient in overcoming drug resistance. In the treatment of systemic mycoses such as aspergillosis, there are few antifungal agents available, but due to its broad spectrum of action amphotericin-B is potent against a wide range of fungi. In the form of AmBisome and other related formulations (e.g. Abelcet and Amphocil) they are even more effective in treatment of infections [56]. These formulations have also proved valuable in treating *Candida albicans* infections in immunocompromised patients, eradicating an efficient pathogen that is able to form fungal biofilms [57].

Understandably as the second most lethal infectious disease, many therapeutic cures for tuberculosis (TB) have been available for over 50 years, but there are often patient issues with the length of treatment and dose burden. As a result, treatment failures are common and can promote the development of multi-drug resistant strains. Due to their potential to overcome these problems, the development of drug carrying liposomes has become an important focus in anti-tubercular studies. A ground-breaking study demonstrated that gentamicin loaded liposomes had significantly greater antibacterial activity than the free drug, reducing the bacterial load in the spleen and liver in a mouse model of *Mycobacterium avium* [58]. As well as similar results utilising second-line antibiotics, lung-targeted liposomes were created comprised of a mixture of phosphatidylcholine, cholesterol, dicetylphosphate, O-steroyl amylopectin and monosialogangliosides, distearylphosphatidylethanolamine-poly(ethylene glycol) 2000 to deliver with less toxic effects, isoniazid and rifampicin for more efficient chemotherapy [59]. As the predominant site of infection for TB is the respiratory system, many efforts are now being made to develop aerosolised liposome formulations to successfully deliver anti-tubercular drugs to the lungs by inhalation [60].

The strength of liposomes in supporting in the treatment of disease goes beyond purely as drug delivery vehicles as they can be powerful tools to deliver vaccines, notably against viral infections (Table 1). Significantly, liposomes can be engineered to deliver a variety of immunogenic molecules, whether protein, nucleic acid or carbohydrate to stimulate a strong protective response. A notable commercially available preparation, Epaxal is a vaccine based on inactivated intact Hepatitis A virus adsorbed on to liposomes (thus named virosomes) which in a single dose are well tolerated and highly immunogenic giving good seroprotection [61]. Marketed nearly twenty years ago, Inflexal V, a vaccine preparation against Influenza virus consists of the viral heamagglutinin and neuraminidase surface proteins displayed in phosphatidylcholine based liposomes [62]. In particular, Inflexal V mimicking a natural influenza infection is a paradigm for liposome based vaccines with its safe but strong immunogenicity covering a wide range of ages and health conditions.

### 2.3. Other medical conditions

In addition to the treatment of disease, liposomes have the capability to aid in many other medical-related conditions (Table 2). Notable examples of their use include in analgesia, alleviation of macular degeneration, and as surfactants for pulmonary diseases. A variety of liposome preparations have been marketed for use in analgesia or post-surgical pain-relief. DepoDur and EXPAREL are liposome preparations of morphine and bupivacaine respectively and when intravenously injected, demonstrate stability and extended release properties to give prolonged anaesthesia or analgesia [63,64]. The typical therapy for neovascular age-related macular degeneration requires repeated intravitreal injections of an anti-vascular endothelial growth factor drug, effective in stabilising vision but an encumbrance for patients. The creation of Visudyne, a liposome based formulation of the photosensitiser Verteporfin which requires only intravenous injection has simplified patient treatment with relative success [65]. A common problem in pulmonary diseases such as respiratory distress syndrome is a lack of pulmonary surfactant, the phospholipid-protein complex needed to contribute a functional respiratory surface at the mammalian lungs. Curosurf, a modified natural surfactant isolated from pig lungs contains the essential phospholipid-associated surfactant proteins B and C, and is widely used successfully in clinical treatment [66].

## 3. New approaches utilising synthetic lipids and fatty acids

### 3.1. Non-natural lipids and fatty acids

While having many advantages, natural liposomes utilised for the treatment of disease have some drawbacks. Typically they are difficult to produce and are inherently unstable reducing the potential storage time. In recent years a new generation of liposomes have been developed with altered biochemical properties designed to improve stability, functionalization and drug release in addition to altered immunogenic and selective targeting properties. Construction of these liposomes was only possible due to the use of non-natural fatty acids and lipids in the particles. As an alternative to the standard inclusion of cholesterol in liposomes for increased stability, a series of sterol-modified phospholipids were constructed [67]. These involved the covalent attachment of cholesterol to the glycerol backbone of phosphatidylcholine, replacing a fatty acid chain and resulting in sterol modified liposomes (SML). Other hydrophobic molecules such as porphyrins and photosensitive agents can similarly replace a fatty acid chain, [68]. In generating synthetic lipids, there are also many simple changes to the lipid headgroup possible, vastly changing their chemical and biophysical properties [69]. Common modifications can include the addition of a polymer, nucleic acid, carbohydrate, amino acid or an assortment of functional chemical moieties for the downstream covalent attachment of ligands.

### 3.2. Advantages of using synthetic lipids in liposomes

As mentioned above, liposomes incorporating synthetic lipids can have three main advantages, extended stability of the liposome, directed cell targeting and controlled release of the cargo and examples of the modifications are discussed here:

Sterol modified liposomes carrying doxorubicin had similar therapeutic efficacy to the standard Doxil in a colon carcinoma model, but with greater overall stability in circulation, improved uptake into the liver and spleen [70]. This and other studies show the potential of SMLs as drug delivery systems that are easy to synthesise from commercially available molecules. Similarly the use of synthetic lipids incorporating porphyrins or photosensitive agents to generate liposomes known as porphysomes which have applications in photodynamic therapy and diagnostics. Importantly these porphysomes demonstrate good pharmacokinetics in mice, are safe at high doses, accumulate in tumours and can be imaged for diagnostic purposes [68]. The use of the synthetic polyethylene glycol (PEG-2000) modified 1,2-distearoyl-*sn*-glycero-3-phosphoethanolamine in liposomes greatly altered the surface hydrophilicity and by decreasing cell uptake, extended the circulatory half-life as mentioned previously for Doxil [20].

Utilising liposomes constructed with synthetic lipids can create a number of novel functions. In addition to the aforementioned polymer coating, modified headgroups are useful for the attachment of cargo or specific ligand targeting. Often these modifications result in improved targeting and biodistribution of liposomes by interacting with ligands present on specific cells or tissue types. One notable example is nucleic acid modified lipids, which can result in the physical interaction of the liposomes with single-stranded nucleic acids via base pairing. This has proved biologically important in the efficient targeting of the nucleic acid binding drug cisplatin to its site of action overcoming previous limitations in drug delivery and showing potency against a number of sensitive and resistant cancer cell lines [71]. Liposomes have also been generated using lipids synthesised with a range of functional groups to bind a number of ligands. Most common is a maleimide lipid, although others with ester, ether, avidin, thiol, hydrazine and carboxylic acid moieties in the headgroup have also been constructed [72]. The maleimide group can react with a free thiol and thus can allow liposomes to couple to any exposed cysteine on a protein such as a single chain antibody. This approach has proved useful in the modification of amyloid-β-targeting liposomes, made of sphingomyelin/cholesterol/phosphatidic acid and functionalised through a terminal maleimide group on PEG-phosphatidylethanolamine to display an anti-transferrin receptor antibody. This design gave the liposomes the ability to cross an *in vitro* blood brain barrier model of human brain capillary endothelial cells and thus hold huge potential for the successful delivery of therapeutics to the central nervous system targeting amyloid-β and other defective proteins in Alzheimer's disease [73].

In an ideal scenario in the liposomal drug delivery system, the liposomes should be stable in the circulation till they reach their destination and rapidly release their contents to have the desired effect. In optimising the release of cargo from liposomes, a number of methods are possible. Some such as altering the liposome formulation to destabilise the membrane or increasing the hydrophilicity of the cargo are applicable to natural liposomes. However, through the use of synthetic lipids, it is possible to control the release of liposome content with various environmental cues, either external such as heat, light or ultrasound; or internal e.g. pH or redox environment. This relies on the use of lipids to create liposomes that are sensitive to specific stimuli to trigger the delivery of material at the appropriate time and place. This is particularly useful in the delivery of small interfering RNAs (siRNA) where the use of pH responsive ionisable lipids containing amine headgroups means that liposomes release the nucleic acid only into the cytosol of the cell [74].

## 4. The use of lipids and liposomes as molecular tools

### 4.1. Molecules for imaging

The routine application of modified or synthetic lipids in liposomes and their subsequent biocompatibility *in vivo* or *ex vivo* demonstrated that such particles could also be visualised through the incorporation of fluorescently tagged lipids. This methodology effectively replaces the original inconsistent approach of using liposomes carrying fluorescein as cargo for imaging studies [75]. There are a number of commercially available synthetic lipid species which have a fluorophore replacing a lipid fatty acid chain or alternatively replacing or conjugated to a phospholipid headgroup. Common fluorophores attached to lipids include non-polar 4,4-difluoro-4-bora-3*α*,4*α*-diaza-*s*-indacene (BODIPY), polar nitrobenzo-2-oxa-1,3-diazole (NBD) and dansyl groups, hydrophobic pyrene and the highly fluorescent rhodamine dyes [76]. Importantly, in selecting a fluorophore to use in labelling lipids and liposomes, it is common to use dyes that emit light in the 650-1100nm far red/near infrared region to avoid the conflict with the UV responsive autofluorescence of most eukaryotic tissues. When fluorescent lipids are constructed into liposomes, the simple visualisation of the labelled particles has aided in the study of a number of areas of research such as drug delivery, disease diagnosis and membrane fusion events. A recent study using fluorescence microscopy specifically revealed that carbocyanine dye modified liposomes containing the antileishmanial agent meglumine antimoniate were taken up faster by *Leishmania major* infected macrophages compared with non-infected cells, most likely due to parasite-modified phagocytosis [77]. The attachment of the fluorescent curcumin molecule to 1,2-dipalmitoyl-3-(2-(1,7-bis(4-hydroxy-3-methoxyphenyl)-3,5-dioxohept-6-enylthio)ethyl phospho)-*sn*-glycerol (DPS) has a clinically relevant application for the diagnosis of Alzheimer's disease. As curcumin targets the Aβ peptide, injection of DPS-curcumin containing liposomes into the brains of mice revealed the nanoparticles could successfully target and stain the pathology causing Aβ deposits *in vivo* [78]. These types of imaging based studies may be further extended in a dual approach, for example in the efficient bimodal imaging of tumour angiogenesis through the use of rhodamine conjugated phosphatidylethanolamine and gadolinium-DTPA-bis(stearylamide) lipids for optical imaging and magnetic resonance imaging studies respectively [79]. These liposomes were additionally constructed with RGD cyclic peptide moieties conjugated to maleimide-PEG-DSPE, specifically to target the αvβ3 integrin highly expressed in angiogenesis. This and other studies [reviewed in 80] have strongly validated the use of these modified lipids in an effective streamlined approach for the *in vivo* visualisation and treatment of angiogenesis, a critical process in metastatic tumour biology.

### 4.2. Immune system modulators

Due to their biophysical properties, cell targeting and entering abilities, liposomes were candidate adjuvants to aid in the modulation of the human immune system. Initially it was observed that negatively charged liposomes of a certain composition of natural phospholipids carrying diphtheria toxin could induce an enhanced antibody response prior to release of the true antigen [81]. Subsequently this use was more deliberate, for example in the delivery of *Shigella flexneri* lipid A containing liposomes to stimulate an immune reaction [82]. To date, the wide use of liposomes containing monophosphoryl lipid A has proved highly effective in safely enhancing immune responses to candidate vaccines to HIV-1, malaria and a number of cancers [reviewed in 83]. Significantly, liposomes have been developed to act as primary adjuvants, incorporating lipids whose headgroup is covalently bound to antigens. Through the use of synthetic lipids like 1,2-dipalmitoyl-*sn*-glycero-3-phosphoethanolamine-N-[4-(*p*-maleimidophenyl)butyramide], a range of peptide, carbohydrate, lipid and even antibody-like molecules can be attached [84]. These modified liposomes can be administered via oral or nasal routes rather than injection and in addition to little or no toxicity have significant capability to be both prophylactic and therapeutic vaccines. One caveat however is that even early in liposome research it was clear that in certain circumstances any headgroup modified lipids could be adjuvants, and based on the evidence to date, it is likely that most synthetic lipids will induce some sort of immune response [69]. While the use of liposomes to stimulate the immune system to exert a seroprotective effect as discussed is desirable, there are situations where an immune suppressive effect may be desired. A directed suppression of the immune system is a desirable goal in the treatment of autoimmune disease, allergies and preventing the rejection of organ transplants. Administering liposomes coated in the bisphosphonate aldronate successfully caused an anti-inflammatory effect in a rabbit model through the systemic inactivation and depletion of macrophages and monocytes [85], similarly seen in models of tissue graft rejection [86] and arthritis [87]. These and other related liposomes based strategies have great potential to deliver therapeutic success in a safe manner for many immune-related conditions [88].

### 4.3. Nucleic acid carriers

It is clear liposomes have an enormous ability to transport an assortment of molecules to a variety of cells and tissue types and a rapidly expanding field is the delivery of nucleic acid into cells. In genetic modification, the delivery of genetic material to augment the existing genes or alternatively silence and/or remove genes has become essential. Some current approaches to deliver genetic material into cells and tissues include chemical-based and viral based methods and can be inefficient with membrane permeability issues and potentially cytotoxic effects. Particularly in exploring the concept of gene therapy, replacing a defective copy with a functional wild-type copy, the development of non-viral based vectors to deliver nucleic acid into cells has focused on liposomes due to their ability to carry large fragments of DNA and their low toxicity and immunogenicity. In the development of liposome based nucleic acid delivery systems, it was discovered that a cationic synthetic lipid N-[1-(2,3-dioleyloxy)propyl]-N,N,N-trimethylammonium chloride (DOTMA) would form liposomes that would readily interact with negatively charged DNA and stably hold it in the aqueous interior [89]. Typically cationic lipids have a positively charged polar amino head group on top of a lipid-like hydrophobic domain. In contrast, neutral or negatively charged lipid based liposomes can't form electrostatic interactions to bind and hold any negatively charged molecules. This ground-breaking research opened up the field of using cationic liposomes to deliver material and there are a now a wide range of synthetic phospholipid and cholesterol analogues that generally form positively charged liposomes [90]. Cationic liposomes have great promise as nucleic acid delivery agents as they are highly efficient, readily interacting with negatively charged membranes for uptake into cells to deliver their cargo. Since the initial discovery, many cationic liposomes have been used to deliver nucleic acids not just into cells in culture, but also animals and even in patients in phase I and II clinical trials though with some dose-dependent toxicity issues [90].

More recently, a revolution in the use of liposomes in nucleic acid delivery has come about through the discovery of small interfering RNAs (siRNA). These siRNA are molecules which are designed to bind the messenger RNA of a specific gene and thus silence its expression. This approach could potentially revolutionise the treatment of diseases such as cancer where suppression of gene expression is of paramount importance. However, the use of siRNA in a clinical setting has been restricted because the molecules have a short half-life, show poor uptake into cells and are rapidly cleared from the system. Again the application of liposome technology has resurrected this form of therapy with the potential of liposomes specifically targeting the siRNA to the appropriate tissue in high concentrations, preventing degradation of the molecule and therefore providing a safe non-toxic delivery system in humans and animals. Typically by using phosphatidylcholine based neutral liposomes, an efficient and stable targeted delivery of siRNAs into tumour tissues was observed in a variety of animal models, significantly with a concomitant inhibition of tumour growth [reviewed in 91].

### 4.4. Decoys for pathogens

Possibly the most unusual application for liposomes comes from the development of particles that when administered into an individual would impersonate the host cell type recognised by invading pathogens, trapping the infectious agent and thus reducing the potential for disease. A recent example is the use of liposomes bearing the glycan sialylneo-lacto-N-tetraose c (LSTc), an analogue of the influenza virus targeting sialic acid molecule found on the surface of respiratory tract cells. Decoy liposomes containing LSTc conjugated to 1,2-dioleoyl-*sn*-glycero-3-phosphoethanolamine successfully bind influenza virus particles in competition assays in culture and in a mouse model prevent virus spread and increase the survival time even under challenge of a lethal dose [92]. This is significantly better than using free sialic acid analogues, which have shown some success, but are not suitable due to toxicity and solubility issues. Importantly due to their mode of action, the decoy liposomes should have the ability to successfully target both newly emerging and established drug resistant influenza strains without discrimination. This approach has the possibility to become a key preventative treatment against a wide range of pathogens that target specific cell surface receptors.

## 5. Lipid analogues as cytotoxic molecules

### 5.1. Alkyllysophospholipids

Of all the lipid analogues that have be synthesised to date, the alkyllysophospholipids (ALPs) are probably the most studied for their toxicity to cells. This series of ether lipids was born out of the observation that the natural lipid lysophophatidylcholine (lysoPC) possessed potent immunomodulatory properties but was rapidly metabolised, reducing its effectiveness [93]. To increase the stability but retain the activity of this molecule, lysoPC analogues were synthesised that incidentally had inhibitory effects on tumour growth [94]. With a chemical structure containing a long alkyl chain, ALPs insert into the lipid bilayer of cell membranes and act similarly to a detergent at high concentrations causing cell lysis. At more physiologically relevant concentrations, ALPs have a number of biological effects relating to the disruption of cell membranes, including influencing membrane domains, phospholipid turnover and lipid associated signalling pathways [95]. The consequences of these diverse modes of action include growth inhibition, cell stress, cell cycle arrest and apoptosis. The most commonly studied ALPs are listed in table 3 showing the timeline of their development and primary publications. For their chemical structures see [95].

| Alkyllysophospholipid | Year | Targeted disease | Ref. |
|---|---|---|---|
| Edelfosine (ET-O-$CH_3$) | 1967 | Cancer, Leishmaniasis, Human African Trypanosomiasis | 96 |
| Miltefosine (HePC) | 1983 | Cancer, Leishmaniasis, Human African Trypanosomiasis | 97 |
| Ilmofosine | 1984 | Cancer, Leishmaniasis, Human African Trypanosomiasis | 98 |
| Erucylphosphocholine (ErPC) | 1992 | Cancer | 99 |
| Perifosine (D-21266) | 1997 | Cancer, Leishmaniasis | 100 |
| Erufosine (ErPC3) | 2002 | Cancer | 101 |

**Table 3.** Common alkyllysophospholipids used for disease treatment.

### 5.2. Anticancer

The first ALP to be studied in detail, edelfosine was demonstrated to have a cytotoxic effect on a wide range of cell types, both tumour derived and normal [96]. However it was apparent that edelfosine demonstrated a high selectivity towards tumour cells, strongly stimulating apoptosis by an unknown mechanism. Over the next forty years a number of analogues of edelfosine were similarly investigated for their cytotoxic anti-cancer properties. Although the most potent of the ALPs, the clinical use of edelfosine has remained limited to the treatment of acute leukaemia patients in the purging of bone marrow prior to autologous tissue transplantation [102]. Miltefosine, even though it is metabolised in cells unlike the other ALPs, still has potent anti-tumour activity in some animal models [103]. Unfortunately due to its haemolytic properties, its clinical use is restricted as a topical formulation, promising in phase II trials in the treatment of cutaneous metastases of breast cancer [104]. The most recent ALPs, the homologous erucylphosphocholine and erufosine are suitable for intravenous injection having longer 22 carbon chains and a double bond which causes them to associate in aqueous environments as non-haemolytic lamellar rather than micellar structures. They are valued ALPs in the development of cancer treatments as they have the ability to cross the blood-brain barrier, accumulate in the brain and show anti-tumour effects both *in vitro* [105] and *in vivo* [106]. Perhaps the ALP with the most therapeutic potential, perifosine, created by replacing the choline in miltefosine with a heterocyclic piperidine group, demonstrated good pharmacokinetics and strong cytotoxicity against a wide variety of tumours [107]. Its poor performance in single agent phase II trials however, has stimulated its use in successful application in combination with various anti-tumour treatments that affect other pathways in the cell. Perifosine has showed highly promising anticancer therapy in combination with inhibitors of the anti-apoptotic mTOR signalling network. Individually, drugs targeting mTOR are less effective as often the inhibition is overcome through induction of a positive feedback loop by the protein kinase Akt to upregulate mTOR [108]. The additive effect generated with the combinational approach is due to perifosine inhibition of Akt causing suppression of the positive feedback loop.

### 5.3. Antifungal

In the treatment of invasive mycoses, the use of miltefosine has demonstrated some broad spectrum fungicidal activity *in vitro* and in a mouse model of cryptococcosis [109]. In general however the application of ALPs to treat fungal infections in humans has been restricted by the limited therapeutic effect against cryptococcal infections in animals [110]. This may be in part due to their apparent mode of action in inhibiting cytochrome C oxidase in *Saccharomyces cerevisiae* and phospholipase B in *Cryptococcus neoformans*, two non-essential yeast proteins [109,111]. The use of ALPs as potent antifungal agents might be resurrected in part by two recent developments. The synthesis of new analogues based on existing structure–antifungal activity relationship (SAR) information of ALPs has given hope that this class of compounds can have benefit in the treatment of invasive or device-related fungal infections [112]. Furthermore, in a study of combinational therapeutics, some synergy was observed in a number of fungal strains with miltefosine and the broad-spectrum drug voriconazole which may develop with further research into clinical relevance [113].

### 5.4. Antiparasitic

It is in the field of parasitology where the ALPs have shown great promise. Initially, alongside their anti-cancer effects, a range of ALP analogues were found to have strong anti-protozoal activity against the free-living ciliate *Tetrahymena pyriformis* [114] and *Leishmania donovani*, the causative agent of visceral leishmaniasis [115]. Subsequent research demonstrated that different ALPs had varying potency against different protozoan species and lifecycle stage. In general however a range of *Leishmania* species, *Trypanosoma brucei* and *T. cruzi* parasites have showed significant susceptibility to these ALPs with effective dose killing responses in the low micromolar range [reviewed in 116]. The development of ALPs as potential anti-parasitic drugs in a clinical setting came from the discovery that miltefosine completely prevented *L. donovani* infection in mice with very little side effects [117]. Ultimately this research led to the development of a clinically approved formulation of miltefosine, Impavido in 2000, still to date the only approved oral drug for leishmaniasis [118]. Impavido is approved for the treatment of cutaneous and mucosal leishmaniasis but is particularly utilised for the first-line treatment of endemic visceral leishmaniasis in Asia. In addition, the use of miltefosine has been shown to be effective in curing patients infected with *L. donovani* parasites unresponsive or resistant to antimony treatment [119]. Similar to the anti-cancer effects of ALPs, the mode of action of miltefosine against *Leishmania spp.* is not entirely clear. There is a notable structural damage to the plasma membrane of most ALP treated parasites, suggestive of alterations to the lipid content [116]. Recent modern metabolomic approaches have defined cellular changes in miltefosine action against *Leishmania* and indicate disruption of the lipid metabolism of the cells as a primary target [120]. Issues with the development of resistance to miltefosine (partly due to weak therapeutics and rapid metabolism) have led to the development of ALP loaded liposomes. These have proven to be more active than the ALP alone in the treatment of animal models and as in other studies they have shown efficacy against the drug-resistant cell lines [121]. It is clear that the combined use of liposomes and ALPs is a powerful tool, giving a potential dual target approach to combat parasite infection and drug-resistance.

## 6. Lipids and liposomes in health and nutrition

### 6.1. Fatty acids and lipids

It is well documented that omega-3/omega-6 polyunsaturated fatty acids (PUFA) are essential for normal growth and development, especially for visual and neurological development in infants [122, 123]. These fatty acids have also been shown to have numerous beneficial effects on various aspects of human health, and as such the recommended minimal daily intake is set at 250 mg [124]. As humans we are unable to *de novo* synthesise omega-3 PUFA, as we do not have the necessary fatty acid desaturase enzyme(s) and thus rely solely upon dietary intake of these PUFA. Two crucial PUFAs are eicosapentaenoic acid (EPA) and docosahexaenoic acid (DHA), these are primarily accessed via marine sources, i.e. fish or krill oil, while $\alpha$-linolenic acid (ALA), is found in numerous plant sources such as nuts and seeds. The biological activities of omega-3/omega-6 PUFA have been under extensive study for several decades and their beneficial effects on several diseases have been well documented, some of which will be now be discussed.

Dietary changes in fatty acid composition have been show to change the proportion of different types of PUFA in inflammatory and immune cells and thus influencing their function, this is thought to be because they can act as precursors to lipid mediators (eicosanoids/docosanoids) or as ligands for transcription factors [125]. Various omega-3 supplements also seem to boost the effectiveness of anti-inflammatory drugs, several clinical studies have reported that fish oil supplementation has beneficial effects in rheumatoid arthritis, inflammatory bowel disease, and among some asthmatics, supporting the idea that omega-3 PUFA trigger anti-inflammatory and immunomodulatory activities [126]. Along the same lines the PUFA arachidonic acid (AA) is a precursor for prostaglandins, leukotrienes, and related compounds acting as secondary messengers, modulating various roles in inflammation and immunity. Even gamma-linolenic acid a non-essential fatty acid, present in high levels in borage oil has been shown to have several beneficial effects in the treatment of rheumatoid arthritis, atopic eczema and diabetic neuropathy, as well as in the reduction of cholesterol levels [127].

The changing diet of Western societies since industrialisation has been argued to have promoted the pathogenesis of many inflammatory-related diseases, including depressive disorders. Researchers have found a correlation between cultures that eat foods with high levels of omega-3 PUFA also have lower levels of depression [128]. Several epidemiological studies have also shown a significant inverse correlation between intake of oily fish and depression and bipolar disorders [128, 129]. However it has been suggested that the preventive role of omega-3 PUFA may depend on other factors, such as overall diet quality and the social environment. Accordingly, some research suggests that omega-3 PUFAs may be effective in several ways in protecting people against Alzheimer's disease and dementia by reducing the rate of gradual memory loss linked to aging and enhancing the effectiveness of antidepressants [130].

It is common knowledge that fish and fish oil consumption (high in omega-3 PUFA) can significantly reduce the risk of cardiovascular diseases (CVDs) and slow the formation of plaque in the arteries [131]. It is now becoming clear that it is increasingly important to know which fatty acids especially EPA and DHA are attached to which lipid species. This has recently become apparent as no significant statistically correlation is observed between omega-3 PUFAs and the reduced risk of cardiovascular diseases (CVDs) when 20 studies on 68680 patients were re-evaluated. The latest evidence suggests the true biologically active component, or parent lipid species, has a direct influence on its delivery and subsequent usage/*in vivo* activity [132 and references therein]. Despite the various and numerous biological activities of omega-3 PUFA and their corresponding health benefits being extensively studied for several decades. However, the potential different forms in which these could be delivered via dietary intake such as triglycerides (TGs) versus ethyl esters or phospholipids (PLs), has largely been neglected. The fatty acid chain length and unsaturation on the lipids affects their intestinal absorption efficiency, whereas the chemical structure of the lipids (TGs *versus* PLs) determines their digestion products prior to absorption. The enrichment of essential fatty acids in particular phospholipids for increased dietary uptake and nutritional activity in the body is important. Several studies show evidence that dietary PLs have a positive impact in several diseases and potentially reduce side effects of some drugs [133, 134].

Modern diets are often depleted of complex and diverse mixtures of PLs due to increased use of refined oils and purified raw materials, which had led to an overall reduction in the uptake of PLs. Hence, the supplementation of marine PLs may serve three important functions within the functional food segment: (a) emulsifying properties, (b) supplementation of omega-3 PUFAs and (c) beneficial nutritional effects of the PLs themselves [135]. A better understanding of the impact of PL supplementation and its health benefits is required.

The potential anti-obesity effect of conjugated linoleic acid, and its mode of action lowering body fat mass has recently been reviewed by Kennedy *et al* [136]. Conjugated linoleic acid (CLA), a group of conjugated cis and trans isomers of octadecadienoic acid that have been converted from linoleic acid by microbes in the gastrointestinal tract of ruminant animals and often found in beef, dairy foods, and dietary supplements, reduces adiposity in several animal models of obesity and in some humans. CLA was discovered by Pariza and colleagues in 1987, and was first identified as an anti-carcinogen, but subsequently shown to exhibit anti-atherosclerotic and more recently anti-obesity properties [137]. Interest in CLA as an alternative treatment to conventional diabetic and weight loss therapies has increased over the past decade. Supplementation with a mixture of CLA isomers decreased the body fat mass in many animal and some human studies. The major 10,12 isomer of CLA, seems to be responsible for the antiobesity effects. Commercial preparations of CLA are now made from the linoleic acid of safflower or sunflower oils under alkaline conditions. Kennedy *et al* have summarised the recent *in vivo* and *in vitro* findings and propose potential mechanisms by which CLA reduces adiposity including its impact on energy metabolism, adipogenesis, inflammation, lipid metabolism, and apoptosis [136].

### 6.2. Liposomes

Liposomal encapsulation technology used by medical researchers to deliver drugs effectively to specific areas or organs in the body, as discussed earlier, is also being used to target delivery of a number of poorly soluble and high molecular weight bioactive dietary components including natural products such as carotenoids, phytosterol, omega-3 PUFAs, vitamins and other antioxidants to the body. The liposomes provide a number of advantages to other delivery systems and this is why a number of nutritional companies are now utilizing this technique in the oral delivery of dietary supplements and nutrients that are not prematurely decomposed and are pinpointed to specific tissues and organs. This approach has the added bonus that the doses can be reduced by 5 to 15 times less than normal supplement intake, i.e. tablets and capsules. The beneficial action of liposomes in oral delivery of nutrients is due to several modes of their action, including improved nutrient solubilisation and protection against environmental conditions such as moisture, oxygen and degradation by the presence of enzymes in oral and esophageal digestive juices prior to being absorbed into the body [138-140]. The phospholipids of the liposomes are able to repel undesirable activities of the digestive juices of the gastrointestinal tract, until the contents have reached the target tissue and are endocytosed, delivering their cargo into the intra-cellular space. It is important to note that more conventional delivery routes for nutrients, such as tablets, capsules etc., offer different and complementary forms of nutrient bio-availability, however the various food additives used in tablets and capsules, such as binders, fillers, gelatins and sugar affect the absorption process and may cause incomplete disintegration, hence reducing bioavailability of the active components.

More than 50 products and product combinations have been formulated using liposomal delivery systems, some of them are listed in Table 4. A key example of the full potential of using oral liposomal encapsulation is vitamin C, which causes a ~10-fold increase of vitamin C into cellular systems compared to oral tablet/capsule formulations, with no negative effects, such as gastric distress, urinary output or extra load on the liver [141].

| Vitamin/herb/botanical | Active compound(s) | Health benefits |
|---|---|---|
| Vitamin A | Retinol | Retina function, Epithelial tissue growth, Bone growth, Embryonic development |
| Vitamin B2 | Ribofiavin | Essential for metabolizing carbohydrates, fats, and lipids<br>Necessary for the function of vitamins B6, folic acid, and niacin |
| Vitamin B12 | Cyanocobalamine | Deficiency causes pernicious anemia, muscle and nerve paralysis |
| Vitamin C | Ascorbic acid | Antioxidant |

| Vitamin/herb/botanical | Active compound(s) | Health benefits |
|---|---|---|
| Vitamin E | alpha-Tocopherol | Detoxifies free radicals, Prevents damage to cell membranes. Enhances immune response, Antioxidant |
| CoEnzyme Q10 | Ubiquinone-50 | Increased mitochondria function, cofactor in oxidative respiration |
| DHEA | Dihydroepiandrosteindione | Increased libido, Feelings of well being Decreased viral load |
| Echinacea | Echinacosides | Immuno-stimulation |
| Gingko biloba extract | Gingolides | Dementia, Equilibrium disorders,Intermittent claudication |
| Glucosamine sulfate | Glucosamine | Osteoarthritis, Bone, cartilage, and Muscle growth |
| Grape seed extract | Procyanidines | Antioxidant, Inhibits tooth decay, Source of essential oils |
| IGF-1 | Insulin, Growth Factor-1 | Anti-aging |
| Kava kava | Kava lactones | Anxiolytic, insomnia |
| Ma huang | Ephedra | Cough, Bronchitis, Appetite suppression |
| Melatonin | Melatonin | Insomnia, Jet lag |
| Milk thistle | Silymarin | Hepatoprotection, Cirrhosis, Hepatitis, Immunomodulation |
| St. Johns wort | Hypericin, pseudohypercin | Anxiolytic, Depression, Topical inflammation, Wound healing |
| Zinc gluconate, zinc sulfate | Zinc ion | Essential part of more than 200 enzymes involved in digestion, metabolism, reproduction (sperm formation), and wound healing. Involved in sense of taste. Role in function and structure of cell membranes. Major part of the immune system. Component of insulin deficiency |

**Table 4.** Liposomal nutritional products on the market

Dietary polyphenols, including flavonoids, have long been recognized as a source of important molecules involved in the prevention of several diseases, including cancer. However, due to their poor bioavailability, polyphenols remain difficult to be employed clinically. The recent use of liposomes, as a means of improving their pharmacokinetics and pharmacodynamics, hence their bioavailability means there is a renewed interest into the therapeutic benefits of wide range of polyphenols [142, 143].

## 7. Future perspectives

Liposomes are being used in a wide range of applications from drug and gene delivery to diagnostics, cosmetics and food nanotechnology being able to be administrated orally, parenterally or topically. Liposome formation and entrapment of various different types of cargo is now a well established methodology, allowing them to stabilise the encapsulated materials against a range of environmental and chemical changes, including enzymatic and chemical modification, as well as buffering against extreme pH and temperature [144].

There are a rapidly increasing number of new applications for liposomes in the drug and food industry, due to their biocompatibility and biodegradability. The natural composition of the liposomes, which helps in overcoming regulatory hurdles, and if required newly developed formulations can quickly be implemented. However, use of multiple lipid sources (e.g. animal, plant, synthetic sources) often requires additional characterisation and comparability studies. The quality and purity of the lipid starting materials for lipsome formulations are essential to maintain the quality of the later drug or encapsulated product. Therefore the appropriate characterization and specification of the lipid starting material is considered as vital as the product being delivered, as laid out by EU directive 2001/83/EC, along with guidance on process validation CHMP/QWP/848/99 and EMEA/CVMP/598/99 and marketing authorisation of a medicinal product (EMEA/CHMP/QWP/396951/2006).

The remarkable biocompatibility of liposomes probably stems from the fact that they are closely analogous to both naturally occurring endosomes that circulate in the bloodstream before accumulating in specific tissues, and lamellar bodies known to lubricate and protect tissue surfaces and serve in specialist functions, i.e. act a surfactant in the lungs to allow oxygen to pass from the air into the bloodstream. The depletion of lamellar bodies is also implicated in a range of diseases, including serious progressive respiratory conditions, including Cystic Fibrosis and Chronic Obstructive Pulmonary Disease [144]. These are obvious areas of research where liposome technology could be a game changer.

In order to extend and take full advantage of this highly biocompatible and safe biodegradable delivery system, future research should focus on the production of the lipid vesicles through safe, scalable methods, as well as accessing the required high quality/purity of lipids in a cheap and sustainable manner.

## Acknowledgements

TKS research is supported in part by the Wellcome Trust, SUSLA, BBSRC and the European Community's Seventh Framework Programme under grant agreement No.602773 (Project KINDReD). TKS is also an academic consultant for Mylnefield Lipid analysis and Lamellar Biomedical Ltd.

## Author details

Simon A. Young and Terry K. Smith*

*Address all correspondence to: tks1@st-andrews.ac.uk

Biomedical Sciences Research Complex, The North Haugh, The University, St. Andrews, Fife Scotland, U.K

## References

[1] Bangham AD, Horne RW. Negative staining of phospholipids and their structural modification by surface-active agents as observed in the electron microscope. Journal of Molecular Biology 1964;8 660-8.

[2] Bangham AD, Standish MM, Watkins JC. Diffusion of univalent ions across the lamellae of swollen phospholipids. Journal of Molecular Biology 1965;13(1) 238-52.

[3] Bangham AD, Standish MM, Watkins JC, Weissmann G. The diffusion of ions from a phospholipid model membrane system. Protoplasma 1967;63(1) 183-7.

[4] Papahadjopoulos D, Watkins JC. Phospholipid model membranes. II. Permeability properties of hydrated liquid crystals. Biochimica et Biophysica Acta 1967;135(4) 639-52.

[5] Sharma A, Sharma US. Liposomes in drug delivery: progress and limitations. International Journal of Pharmaceutics 1997;154(2) 123–140.

[6] Gregoriadis G, Ryman BE. Liposomes as carriers of enzymes or drugs: a new approach to the treatment of storage diseases. Biochemistry Journal 1971;124(5) 58.

[7] Gregoriadis G, Buckland RA. Enzyme-containing liposomes alleviate a model for storage disease. Nature 1973;244(5412) 170-2.

[8] Nichols JW, Deamer DW. Net proton-hydroxyl permeability of large unilamellar liposomes measured by an acid-base titration technique. Proceedings of the National Academy of Sciences USA 1980;77(4) 2038-42.

[9] Dawson RM, Hemington NL, Miller NG, Bangham AD. On the question of an electrokinetic requirement for phospholipase C action. Journal of Membrane Biology 1976;29(1-2) 179-84.

[10] Guerrieri F, Nelson BD. Studies on the characteristics of a proton pump in phospholipid vesicles inlayed with purified complex III from beef heart mitochondria. FEBS Letters 1975;54(3) 339-42.

[11] Weissmann G, Bloomgarden D, Kaplan R, Cohen C, Hoffstein S, Collins T, Gotlieb A, Nagle D. A general method for the introduction of enzymes, by means of immunoglobulin-coated liposomes, into lysosomes of deficient cells. Proceedings of the National Academy of Sciences USA 1975;72(1) 88-92.

[12] Allison AG, Gregoriadis G. Liposomes as immunological adjuvants. Nature 1974;252(5480) 252.

[13] Straub SX, Garry RF, Magee WE. Interferon induction by poly (I): poly (C) enclosed in phospholipid particles. Infection and Immunity 1974;10(4) 783-92.

[14] Gent MP, Prestegard JH. Interaction of the polyene antibiotics with lipid bilayer vesicles containing cholesterol. Biochimica et Biophysica Acta 1976;426(1) 17-30.

[15] Papahadjopoulos D. Studies on the mechanism of action of local anesthetics with phospholipid model membranes. Biochimica et Biophysica Acta 1972;265(2) 169-86.

[16] Almeida JD, Edwards DC, Brand CM, Heath TD. Formation of virosomes from influenza subunits and liposomes. The Lancet 1975;2(7941) 899-901.

[17] Juliano RL. The role of drug delivery systems in cancer chemotherapy. Progress in clinical and biological research 1976;9 21-32.

[18] Gabizon A, Dagan A, Goren D, Barenholz Y, Fuks Z. Liposomes as in vivo carriers of adriamycin: reduced cardiac uptake and preserved antitumor activity in mice. Cancer Research 1982;42(11) 4734-9.

[19] Gabizon A, Chisin R, Amselem S, Druckmann S, Cohen R, Goren D, Fromer I, Peretz T, Sulkes A, Barenholz Y. Pharmacokinetic and imaging studies in patients receiving a formulation of liposome-associated adriamycin. British Journal of Cancer 1991;64(6) 1125-32.

[20] James JS. DOXIL approved for KS. AIDS Treatment News 1995;(no 236) 6.

[21] Safra T, Muggia F, Jeffers S, Tsao-Wei DD, Groshen S, Lyass O, Henderson R, Berry G, Gabizon A. Pegylated liposomal doxorubicin (doxil): reduced clinical cardiotoxicity in patients reaching or exceeding cumulative doses of 500 $mg/m^2$. Annals of Oncology 2000;11(8) 1029-33.

[22] Lorusso V, Giotta F, Bordonaro R, Maiello E, Del Prete S, Gebbia V, Filippelli G, Pisconti S, Cinieri S, Romito S, Riccardi F, Forcignanò R, Ciccarese M, Petrucelli L, Saracino V, Lupo LI, Gambino A, Leo S. Non-pegylated liposome-encapsulated doxorubicin citrate plus cyclophosphamide or vinorelbine in metastatic breast cancer not previously treated with chemotherapy: A multicenter phase III study. International Journal of Oncology 2014;45(5) 2137-42.

[23] Cabriales S, Bresnahan J, Testa D, Espina BM, Scadden DT, Ross M, Gill PS. Extravasation of liposomal daunorubicin in patients with AIDS-associated Kaposi's sarcoma: a report of four cases. Oncology Nursing Forum 1998;25(1) 67-70.

[24] Glantz MJ, LaFollette S, Jaeckle KA, Shapiro W, Swinnen L, Rozental JR, Phuphanich S, Rogers LR, Gutheil JC, Batchelor T, Lyter D, Chamberlain M, Maria BL, Schiffer C, Bashir R, Thomas D, Cowens W, Howell SB. Randomized trial of a slow-release versus a standard formulation of cytarabine for the intrathecal treatment of lymphomatous meningitis. Journal of Clinical Oncology 1999;17(10) 3110-6.

[25] Harrison TS, Lyseng-Williamson KA. Vincristine sulfate liposome injection: a guide to its use in refractory or relapsed acute lymphoblastic leukemia. BioDrugs 2013;27(1) 69-74.

[26] Kurtz JE, Kaminsky MC, Floquet A, Veillard AS, Kimmig R, Dorum A, Elit L, Buck M, Petru E, Reed N, Scambia G, Varsellona N, Brown C, Pujade-Lauraine E; Gynecologic Cancer Intergroup. Ovarian cancer in elderly patients: carboplatin and pegylated liposomal doxorubicin versus carboplatin and paclitaxel in late relapse: a Gynecologic Cancer Intergroup (GCIG) CALYPSO sub-study. Annals of Oncology 2011;22(11) 2417-23.

[27] Berenson JR, Yellin O, Chen CS, Patel R, Bessudo A, Boccia RV, Yang HH, Vescio R, Yung E, Mapes R, Eades B, Hilger JD, Wirtschafter E, Hilger J, Nassir Y, Swift RA. A modified regimen of pegylated liposomal doxorubicin, bortezomib and dexamethasone (DVD) is effective and well tolerated for previously untreated multiple myeloma patients. British Journal of Haematology 2011;155(5) 580-7.

[28] Pinto AC, Ângelo S, Moreira JN, Simões S. Schedule treatment design and quantitative in vitro evaluation of chemotherapeutic combinations for metastatic prostate cancer therapy. Cancer Chemotherapy and Pharmacology 2011;67(2) 275-84.

[29] Mayer LD, Harasym TO, Tardi PG, Harasym NL, Shew CR, Johnstone SA, Ramsay EC, Bally MB, Janoff AS. Ratiometric dosing of anticancer drug combinations: controlling drug ratios after systemic administration regulates therapeutic activity in tumor-bearing mice. Molecular Cancer Therapeutics 2006;5(7) 1854-63.

[30] Feldman EJ, Lancet JE, Kolitz JE, Ritchie EK, Roboz GJ, List AF, Allen SL, Asatiani E, Mayer LD, Swenson C, Louie AC. First-in-man study of CPX-351: a liposomal carrier containing cytarabine and daunorubicin in a fixed 5:1 molar ratio for the treatment of relapsed and refractory acute myeloid leukemia. Journal of Clinical Oncology 2011;29(8) 979-85.

[31] Tardi P, Johnstone S, Harasym N, Xie S, Harasym T, Zisman N, Harvie P, Bermudes D, Mayer L. In vivo maintenance of synergistic cytarabine:daunorubicin ratios greatly enhances therapeutic efficacy. Leukemia Research 2009;33(1) 129-39.

[32] Caride VJ, Zaret BL. Liposome accumulation in regions of experimental myocardial infarction. Science 1977;198(4318) 735-8.

[33] Freude B, Masters TN, Robicsek F, Fokin A, Kostin S, Zimmermann R, Ullmann C, Lorenz-Meyer S, Schaper J. Apoptosis is initiated by myocardial ischemia and executed during reperfusion. Journal of Molecular and Cellular Cardiology 2000;32(2) 197-208.

[34] Xu GX, Xie XH, Liu FY, Zang DL, Zheng DS, Huang DJ, Huang MX. Adenosine triphosphate liposomes: encapsulation and distribution studies. Pharmaceutical Research 1990;7(5) 553-7.

[35] Verma DD, Levchenko TS, Bernstein EA, Torchilin VP. ATP-loaded liposomes effectively protect mechanical functions of the myocardium from global ischemia in an isolated rat heart model. Journal of Controlled Release 2005;108(2-3) 460–71.

[36] Verma DD, Hartner WC, Levchenko TS, Bernstein EA, Torchilin VP. ATP-loaded liposomes effectively protect the myocardium in rabbits with an acute experimental myocardial infarction. Pharmaceutical Research 2005;22(12) 2115–20.

[37] Sarter B. Coenzyme Q10 and cardiovascular disease: a review. Journal of Cardiovascular Nursing 2002;16(4) 9–20.

[38] Verma DD, Hartner WC, Thakkar V, Levchenko TS, Torchilin VP. Protective effect of coenzyme Q10-loaded liposomes on the myocardium in rabbits with an acute experimental myocardial infarction. Pharmaceutical research 2007;24(11) 2131–7.

[39] Ross AM, Gibbons RJ, Stone GW, Kloner RA, Alexander RW. A randomized double-blinded, placebo-controlled multicenter trial of adenosine as an adjunct to reperfusion in the treatment of acute myocardial infarction (AMISTAD-II). Journal of the American College of Cardiology 2005;45(11) 1775–80.

[40] Takahama H, Minamino T, Asanuma H, Fujita M, Asai T, Wakeno M, et al. Prolonged targeting of ischemic/reperfused myocardium by liposomal adenosine augments cardioprotection in rats. Journal of the American College of Cardiology. 2009;53(8) 709–17.

[41] Kim TD, Kambayashi J, Sakon M, Tsujinaka T, Ohshiro T, Mori T. Metabolism of liposome-encapsulated heparin. Thrombosis Research. 1989;56(3) 369–76.

[42] Bai S, Gupta V, Ahsan F. Cationic liposomes as carriers for aerosolized formulations of an anionic drug: safety and efficacy study. European Journal of Pharmaceutical Sciences 2009;38(2) 165–71.

[43] Meyerhoff A. U S Food and Drug Administration approval of AmBiosome (liposomal amphotericin B) for treatment of visceral leishmaniasis. Clinical Infectious Diseases 1999;28(1) 42-8.

[44] Stauch A, Duerr HP, Dujardin JC, Vanaerschot M, Sundar S, Eichner M. Treatment of visceral leishmaniasis: model-based analyses on the spread of antimony-resistant *L. donovani* in Bihar, India. PLoS Neglected Tropical Diseases 2012;6(12) e1973.

[45] Alving C, Steck E, Chapman Jr W, Waits V, Hendricks L, Swartz Jr G, Hanson W. Therapy of leishmaniasis: superior efficacies of liposome encapsulated drugs. Proceedings of the National Academy of Sciences USA 1978;75(6) 2959–2963.

[46] New RR, Chance ML. Treatment of experimental cutaneous leishmaniasis by liposome-en-trapped Pentostam. Acta Tropica 1980;37(3) 253-6.

[47] Banerjee G, Nandi G, Mahato S, Pakrashi A, Basu M. Drug delivery system: targeting of pentamidines to specific sites using sugar-grafted liposomes. Journal of Antimicrobial Chemotherapy 1996;38(1) 145–150.

[48] Papagiannaros A, Bories C, Demetzos C, Loiseau P. Antileishmanial and trypanocidal activities of new miltefosine liposomal formulations. Biomedicine and Pharmacotherapy 2005;59(10) 545–550.

[49] Yoshihara E, Tachibana H, Nakae T. Trypanocidal activity of the stearylamine-bearing liposome *in vitro*. Life Sciences 1987;40(22) 2153-9.

[50] Tachibana H, Yoshihara E, Kaneda Y, Nakae T. In vitro lysis of the bloodstream forms of *Trypanosoma brucei gambiense* by stearylamine-bearing liposomes. Antimicrobial Agents and Chemotherapy 1988;32(7) 966-70.

[51] Morilla MJ, Montanari JA, Prieto MJ, Lopez MO, Petray PB, Romero EL. Intravenous liposomal benznidazole as trypanocidal agent: increasing drug delivery to liver is not enough. International Journal of Pharmaceutics 2004;278(2) 311-8.

[52] Yardley V, Croft SL. *In vitro* and *in vivo* activity of amphotericin B—lipid formulations against experimental *Trypanosoma cruzi* infections. American Journal of Tropical Medicine and Hygiene 1999;61(2) 193-7.

[53] Gabriëls M, Plaizier-Vercammen J. Physical and chemical evaluation of liposomes, containing Artesunate. Journal of Pharmaceutical and Biomedical Analaysis 2003;31(4) 655-67.

[54] Bayomi MA, Al-Angary AA, Al-Mehsal MA, Al-Dardiri MM. *In vivo* evaluation of arteether liposomes. International Journal of Pharmaceutics 1998;175 1–7.

[55] Owais M, Varshney GC, Choudhury A, Chandra S, Gupta CM. Chloroquine encapsulated in malaria-infected erythrocyte-specific antibody-bearing liposomes effectively controls chloroquine-resistant *Plasmodium berghei* infections in mice. Antimicrobial Agents and Chemotherapy 1995;39(1) 180-4.

[56] Maesaki S. Drug delivery system of anti-fungal and parasitic agents. Current Pharmaceutical Design 2002;8(6) 433-40.

[57] Klemens SP, Cynamon MH, Swenson CE, Ginsberg RS. Liposome-encapsulated-gentamicin therapy of *Mycobacterium avium* complex infection in beige mice. Antimicrobial Agents and Chemotherapy 1990;34(6) 967-70.

[58] Lacerda JF, Oliveira CM. Diagnosis and treatment of invasive fungal infections focus on liposomal amphotericin B. Clinical Drug Investigation 2013;33 Suppl 1 S5-14.

[59] Deol P, Khuller GK. Lung specific liposomes: stability, biodistribution and toxicity of liposomal antitubercular drugs in mice. Biochemica et Biophysica Acta, 1997;1334(2-3) 161-72.

[60] Vyas SP, Kannan ME, Jain S, Mishra V, Singh P. Design of liposomal aerosols for improved delivery of rifampicin to alveolar macrophages International Journal of Pharmaceutics 2004;269(1) 37-49.

[61] Bovier PA. Epaxal: a virosomal vaccine to prevent hepatitis A infection. Expert Review of Vaccines 2008;7(8) 1141-50.

[62] Herzog C, Hartmann K, Künzi V, Kürsteiner O, Mischler R, Lazar H, Glück R. Eleven years of Inflexal V-a virosomal adjuvanted influenza vaccine. Vaccine 2009;27(33) 4381-7.

[63] Kim T, Kim J, Kim S. Extended-release formulation of morphine for subcutaneous administration. Cancer Chemotherapy and Pharmacology 1993;33(3) 187-90.

[64] Cohen SM. Extended pain relief trial utilizing infiltration of Exparel, a long-acting multivesicular liposome formulation of bupivacaine: a Phase IV health economic trial in adult patients undergoing open colectomy. Journal of Pain Research 2012;5 567-72.

[65] Ebrahim S, Peyman GA, Lee PJ. Applications of liposomes in ophthalmology. Survey of Ophthalmology. 2005;50(2) 167-82.

[66] Bourbon JR, Chailley-Heu B, Gautier B. The exogenous surfactant Curosurf enhances phosphatidylcholine content in isolated type II cells. European Respiratory Journal 1997;10(4) 914-9.

[67] Huang Z, Jaafari MR, Szoka FC. Disterolphospholipids: nonexchangeable lipids and their application to liposomal drug delivery. Angewandte Chemie International Edition 2009;48(23) 4146-9.

[68] Lovell JF, Jin CS, Huynh E, Jin H, Kim C, Rubinstein JL, Chan WC, Cao W, Wang LV, Zheng G. Porphysome nanovesicles generated by porphyrin bilayers for use as multimodal biophotonic contrast agents Nature Materials 2011;10(4) 324-32.

[69] Kohli AG, Kierstead PH, Venditto VJ, Walsh CL, Szoka FC. Designer lipids for drug delivery: from heads to tails. Journal of Controlled Release 2014;190C 274-287.

[70] Huang Z, Szoka FC. Sterol-modified phospholipids: cholesterol and phospholipid chimeras with improved biomembrane properties. Journal of the American Chemical Society 2008;130(46) 15702-12.

[71] Khiati S, Luvino D, Oumzil K, Chauffert B, Camplo M, Barthélémy P. Nucleoside-lipid-based nanoparticles for cisplatin delivery. ACS Nano 2011;5(11) 8649-55.

[72] Nobs L, Buchegger F, Gurny R, Allémann E. Current methods for attaching targeting ligands to liposomes and nanoparticles. Journal of Pharmaceutical Sciences 2004;93(8) 1980-92.

[73] Salvati E, Re F, Sesana S, Cambianica I, Sancini G, Masserini M, Gregori M. Liposomes functionalized to overcome the blood-brain barrier and to target amyloid-β peptide: the chemical design affects the permeability across an *in vitro* model. International Journal of Nanomedicine. 2013;8 1749-58.

[74] Kanasty R, Dorkin JR, Vegas A, Anderson D. Delivery materials for siRNA therapeutics. Nature Materials 2013;12(11) 967-77.

[75] Leserman LD, Barbet J, Kourilsky F, Weinstein JN. Targeting to cells of fluorescent liposomes covalently coupled with monoclonal antibody or protein A. Nature 1980;288(5791) 602–604.

[76] Stocker BL, Timmer MS. Chemical tools for studying the biological function of glycolipids. Chembiochem 2013;14(10) 1164-84.

[77] Borborema SE, Schwendener RA, Osso JA Jr, de Andrade HF Jr, do Nascimento N. Uptake and antileishmanial activity of meglumine antimoniate-containing liposomes in *Leishmania* (*Leishmania*) *major*-infected macrophages. International Journal of Antimicrobial Agents 2011;38(4) 341-7.

[78] Lazar AN, Mourtas S, Youssef I, Parizot C, Dauphin A, Delatour B, Antimisiaris SG, Duyckaerts C. Curcumin-conjugated nanoliposomes with high affinity for Aβ deposits: possible applications to Alzheimer disease. Nanomedicine 2013;9(5) 712-21.

[79] Mulder WJ, Strijkers GJ, Habets JW, Bleeker EJ, van der Schaft DW, Storm G, Koning GA, Griffioen AW, Nicolay K. MR molecular imaging and fluorescence microscopy for identification of activated tumor endothelium using a bimodal lipidic nanoparticle. FASEB Journal 2005;19(14) 2008-10.

[80] Strijkers GJ, Kluza E, Van Tilborg GA, van der Schaft DW, Griffioen AW, Mulder WJ, Nicolay K. Paramagnetic and fluorescent liposomes for target-specific imaging and therapy of tumor angiogenesis. Angiogenesis 2010;13(2) 161-73.

[81] Allison AG, Gregoriadis G. Liposomes as immunological adjuvants. Nature 1974;252 252.

[82] Banerji B, Alving CR. Lipid A from endotoxin: antigenic activities of purified fractions in liposomes. Journal of Immunology 1979;123(6) 2558-62.

[83] Alving CR, Rao M, Steers NJ, Matyas GR, Mayorov AV. Liposomes containing lipid A: an effective, safe, generic adjuvant system for synthetic vaccines. Expert Review of Vaccines. 2012;11(6) 733-44.

[84] Liang MT, Davies NM, Blanchfield JT, Toth I. Particulate systems as adjuvants and carriers for peptide and protein antigens. Current Drug Delivery 2006;3(4) 379-88.

[85] Epstein H, Gutman D, Cohen-Sela E, Haber E, Elmalak O, Koroukhov N, Danenberg HD, Golomb G. Preparation of alendronate liposomes for enhanced stability and bioactivity: *in vitro* and *in vivo* characterization. AAPS Journal 2008;10(4) 505-15.

[86] Slegers TP, van Rooijen N, van Rij G, van der Gaag R. Delayed graft rejection in prevascularised corneas after subconjunctival injection of clodronate liposomes. Current Eye Research 2000;20(4) 322-4.

[87] Richards PJ, Williams BD, Williams AS. Suppression of chronic streptococcal cell wall-induced arthritis in Lewis rats by liposomal clodronate. Rheumatology 2001;40(9) 978-87.

[88] Landesman-Milo D, Peer D. Altering the immune response with lipid-based nanoparticles. Journal of Controlled Release 2012;161(2) 600-8.

[89] Felgner PL, Gadek TR, Holm M, Roman R, Chan HW, Wenz M, Northrop JP, Ringold GM, Danielsen M. Lipofection: a highly efficient, lipid-mediated DNA-transfection procedure Proceedings of the National Academy of Sciences USA 1987;84(21) 7413-7.

[90] Lonez C, Vandenbranden M, Ruysschaert JM. Cationic liposomal lipids: from gene carriers to cell signalling. Progress in Lipid Research 2008;47(5) 340-7.

[91] Ozpolat B1, Sood AK2, Lopez-Berestein G3. Liposomal siRNA nanocarriers for cancer therapy. Adv Drug Deliv Rev. 2014 Feb;66:110-6. doi: 10.1016. Epub 2013 Dec 30.

[92] Hendricks GL, Weirich KL, Viswanathan K, Li J, Shriver ZH, Ashour J, Ploegh HL, Kurt-Jones EA, Fygenson DK, Finberg RW, Comolli JC, Wang JP. Sialylneolacto-N-tetraose c (LSTc)-bearing liposomal decoys capture influenza A virus. Journal of Biological Chemistry 2013;288(12) 8061-73.

[93] Burdzy K, Munder PG, Fischer H, Westphal 0. Steigerung der Phagozytose von Peritonealmakrophagen durch Lysolecithin. Zeitung für Naturforschung 1964;19b 111X--1 120.

[94] Munder PG, Modolell M, Bausert W, Oettgen HF, Westphal 0. Alkyl-lysophospholipids in cancer therapy. In: Hersh EM. (ed.) Augmenting Agents in Cancer Therapy. New York; Raven Press; 1981. p441-458.

[95] van Blitterswijk WJ, Verheij M. Anticancer mechanisms and clinical application of alkylphospholipids. Biochimica et Biophysica Acta. 2013;1831(3) 663-74.

[96] Eibl H, Arnold D, Weltzien HU, Westphal O. On the synthesis of alpha and beta lecithins and their ether analogs. Justus Liebigs Annalen der Chemie 1967;709 226-30.

[97] Teshima K, Ikeda K, Hamaguchi K, Hayashi K. Bindings of cobra venom phospholipases A2 to micelles of n-hexadecylphosphorylcholine. Journal of Biochemistry 1983;94(1) 223-32.

[98] Heim ME, Swoboda M, Pahlke W, Edler L, Bicker U. Treatment of autochthonous rat colonic adenocarcinomas with a thioether-lysophospholipid derivative in mono-and combination chemotherapy. Journal of Cancer Research and Clinical Oncology 1984;108(3) 316-20.

[99] Reitz RC, Kötting J, Unger C, Eibl H. Comparison of the tissue distribution of hexadecylphosphocholine and erucylphosphocholine. Progress in Experimental Tumor Research 1992;34 143-52.

[100] Hilgard P, Klenner T, Stekar J, Nössner G, Kutscher B, Engel J. D-21266, a new heterocyclic alkylphospholipid with antitumour activity. European Journal of Cancer 1997;33(3) 442-6.

[101] Konstantinov SM, Georgieva MC, Topashka-Ancheva M, Eibl H, Berger MR. Combination with an antisense oligonucleotide synergistically improves the antileukemic efficacy of erucylphospho-N,N,N-trimethylpropylammonium in chronic myeloid leukemia cell lines. Molecular Cancer Therapeutics 2002;1(10) 877-84.

[102] Vogler WR, Berdel WE, Olson AC, Winton EF, Heffner LT, Gordon DS. Autologous bone marrow transplantation in acute leukemia with marrow purged with alkyl-lysophospholipid. Blood 1992;80(6) 1423-9.

[103] Hilgard P, Stekar J, Voegeli R, Harleman JH. Experimental therapeutic studies with miltefosine in rats and mice. Progress in Experimental Tumor Research 1992;34 116-30.

[104] Leonard R, Hardy J, van Tienhoven G, Houston S, Simmonds P, David M, Mansi J. Randomized, double-blind, placebo-controlled, multicenter trial of 6% miltefosine solution, a topical chemotherapy in cutaneous metastases from breast cancer. Journal of Clinical Oncology 2001;19(21) 4150-9.

[105] Rübel A, Handrick R, Lindner LH, Steiger M, Eibl H, Budach W, Belka C, Jendrossek V. The membrane targeted apoptosis modulators erucylphosphocholine and erucylphosphohomocholine increase the radiation response of human glioblastoma cell lines in vitro. Radiation Oncology 2006;1 6.

[106] Erdlenbruch B, Jendrossek V, Marx M, Hunold A, Eibl H, Lakomek M. Antitumor effects of erucylphosphocholine on brain tumor cells *in vitro* and *in vivo*. Anticancer Research 1998;18(4A) 2551-7.

[107] Vink SR, Schellens JH, van Blitterswijk WJ, Verheij M. Tumor and normal tissue pharmacokinetics of perifosine, an oral anti-cancer alkylphospholipid. Investigational New Drugs 2005;23(4) 279-86.

[108] Cirstea D, Hideshima T, Rodig S, Santo L, Pozzi S, Vallet S, Ikeda H, Perrone G, Gorgun G, Patel K, Desai N, Sportelli P, Kapoor S, Vali S, Mukherjee S, Munshi NC, Anderson KC, Raje N. Dual inhibition of akt/mammalian target of rapamycin pathway by nanoparticle albumin-bound-rapamycin and perifosine induces antitumor activity in multiple myeloma. Molecular Cancer Therapeutics 2010;9(4) 963-75.

[109] Widmer F, Wright LC, Obando D, Handke R, Ganendren R, Ellis DH, Sorrell TC. Hexadecylphosphocholine (miltefosine) has broad-spectrum fungicidal activity and is efficacious in a mouse model of cryptococcosis. Antimicrobial Agents and Chemotherapy. 2006;50(2) 414-21.

[110] Ravu RR, Chen YL, Jacob MR, Pan X, Agarwal AK, Khan SI, Heitman J, Clark AM, Li XC. Synthesis and antifungal activities of miltefosine analogs. Bioorganic and Medicinal Chemistry Letters 2013;23(17) 4828-31.

[111] Wiederhold NP, Najvar LK, Bocanegra R, Kirkpatrick WR, Sorrell TC, Patterson TF. Limited activity of miltefosine in murine models of cryptococcal meningoencephali-

tis and disseminated cryptococcosis. Antimicrobial Agents and Chemotherapy 2013;57(2) 745-50.

[112] Zuo X, Djordjevic JT, Bijosono Oei J, Desmarini D, Schibeci SD, Jolliffe KA, Sorrell TC. Miltefosine induces apoptosis-like cell death in yeast via Cox9p in cytochrome c oxidase. Molecular Pharmacology 2011;80 476.

[113] Imbert S, Palous M, Meyer I, Dannaoui E, Mazier D, Datry A, Fekkar A. *In Vitro* Combination of Voriconazole and Miltefosine Against Clinically Relevant Molds. Antimicrobial Agents and Chemotherapy 2014;pii: AAC.03212-14.

[114] Tsushima S, Yoshioka Y, Tanida S, Nomura H, Nojima S, Hozumi M. Syntheses and antimicrobial activities of alkyl lysophospholipids. Chemical and Pharmaceutical Bulletin 1982;30(9) 3260-70.

[115] Herrmann HO, Gercken G. Metabolism of 1-O-[1′-14C]octadecyl-sn-glycerol in *Leishmania donovani* promastigotes. Ether-lipid synthesis and degradation of the ether bond. Molecular and Biochemical Parasitology 1982;5(2) 65-76.

[116] Croft SL, Seifert K, Duchêne M. Antiprotozoal activities of phospholipid analogues. Molecular and Biochemical Parasitology 2003;126(2) 165-72.

[117] Croft SL, Neal RA, Pendergast W, Chan JH. The activity of alkyl phosphorylcholines and related derivatives against *Leishmania donovani*. Biochemical Pharmacology 1987;36(16) 2633-6.

[118] Sindermann H, Croft SL, Engel KR, Bommer W, Eibl HJ, Unger C, Engel J. Miltefosine (Impavido): the first oral treatment against leishmaniasis. Medical Microbiology and Immunology 2004;193(4) 173-80.

[119] Sundar S, Gupta LB, Makharia MK, Singh MK, Voss A, Rosenkaimer F, Engel J, Murray HW. Oral treatment of visceral leishmaniasis with miltefosine. Annals of Tropical Medicine and Parasitology 1999;93(6) 589-97.

[120] Vincent IM, Weidt S, Rivas L, Burgess K, Smith TK, Ouellette M. Untargeted metabolomic analysis of miltefosine action in *Leishmania infantum* reveals changes to the internal lipid metabolism. International Journal of Parasitology: Drugs and Drug Resistance 2013;4(1) 20-7.

[121] Papagiannaros A, Bories C, Demetzos C, Loiseau PM. Antileishmanial and trypanocidal activities of new miltefosine liposomal formulations. Biomedicine and Pharmacotherapy 2005;59(10) 545-50.

[122] Burri L, Hoem N, Banni S, and Berge K Marine Omega-3 Phospholipids: Metabolism and Biological Activities Int. J. Mol. Sci. 2012, 13, 15401-15419

[123] Kitajka K, Sinclair AJ Weisinger RS, Weisinger HS, Mathai M, Jayasooriya AP, Halver JE and Puskás LG, Effects of dietary omega-3 polyunsaturated fatty acids on

brain gene expression Proceedings of the National Academy of Sciences USA 2014:101 10931-10936

[124] Küllenberg D, Taylor LA, Schneider M and Massing U. Health effects of dietary phospholipids Lipids in Health and Disease, 2012:11:3

[125] Murakami M. Lipid mediators in life science. Exp Anim 2011, 60(1):7-20.

[126] Calder PC Polyunsaturated fatty acids, inflammation, and immunity, Lipids 2001:36:1007-24

[127] Henz BM, Jablonska S, Van De Kerkhof PC, Stingl G, Blaszczyk M, Vandervalk PG, Veenhuizen R, Muggli R and Raederstorff D. Double-blind, multicentre analysis of the efficacy of borage oil in patients with atopic eczema. Br. J. Dermatol. 1999:140, 685-688.

[128] Grosso G, Galvano F, Marventano S, Malaguarnera M, Bucolo C, Drago F, Caraci F. Omega-3 fatty acids and depression: scientific evidence and biological mechanisms. Oxid Med Cell Longev. 2014:313570.

[129] Pepeu G, Pepeu IM, Amaducci L. A review of phosphatidylserine pharmacological and clinical effects. Is phosphatidylserine a drug for the ageing brain? Pharmacol Res 1996, 33(2):73-80.

[130] Kidd PM. Dietary phospholipids as anti-aging nutraceuticals. In Anti-Aging Medical Therapeutics. Volume IV. Edited by: Klatz RAGR. Chicago: American Academy of Anti-Aging Medicine; 2000:282-300.

[131] Wang C, Harris WS, Chung M, Lichtenstein AH, Balk EM, Kupelnick B, Jordan HS, Lau J. n-3 Fatty acids from fish or fish-oil supplements, but not alpha-linolenic acid, benefitcardiovascular disease outcomes in primary- and secondary-prevention studies: A systematic review. Am. J. Clin. Nutr. 2006: 84, 5–17.

[132] Nasopoulou C, Smith TK, Detopoulou M, Tsikrika C, Papaharisis L, Barkas D and Zabetaki I. Structural elucidation of olive pomace fed sea bass *Dicentrarchus labrax* polar lipids with cardioprotective activities Food chemistry 2014:145, 1097-1105

[133] Eros G, Ibrahim S, Siebert N, Boros M, Vollmar B: Oral phosphatidylcholine pretreatment alleviates the signs of experimental rheumatoid arthritis. Arthritis Res Ther 2009, 11(2):R43.

[134] Cohn JS, Wat E, Kamili A, Tandy S.Dietary phospholipids, hepatic lipid metabolism and cardiovascular disease. Curr Opin Lipidol 2008, 19(3):257-262.

[135] Cohn J, Kamili A, Wat E, Chung RW, Tandy S. Dietary Phospholipids and Intestinal Cholesterol Absorption. Nutrients 2010, 2(2):116-127.

[136] Kennedy A, Martinez K, Schmidt S, Mandrup S, LaPoint K and McIntosh M. Antiobesity Mechanisms of Action of Conjugated Linoleic Acid J Nutr Biochem. 2010: 21(3): 171–179.

[137] Ha YL, Grimm NK, Pariza MW. Anticarcinogens from fried ground beef: heat-altered derivatives of linoleic acid. Carcinogenesis 1987;8:1881–1887.

[138] Keller BC. Liposomes in nutrition Trends in Food Science & Technology. 2001:12 25–31.

[139] Gibbs BF, Kermasha S, Alii I, Mulligan CN.Encapsulation in the food industry: a review. Int J Food Sci Nut1999: 50:213–224.

[140] Kirby CJ, Whittle CJ, Rigby N, Coxon DT, Law BA. Stabilization of ascorbic acid by microencapsulation in liposomes. Int J Food Sci Technol 1991: 26:437–449.

[141] Tan C, Xue J, Lou X, Abbas S, Guan Y, Feng B, Zhanga X and Xia S. Liposomes as delivery systems for carotenoids: comparative studies of loading ability, storage stability and in vitro release. Food Funct. 2014:5, 1232

[142] Mignet N, Seguin J and Chabot GC Bioavailability of Polyphenol Liposomes: A Challenge Ahead Pharmaceutics 2013, 5, 457-471

[143] Lasic DD Novel applications of liposomes. TIBTECH 1998:16: 307-321

[144] Marcil PV, Drouin E and Levy E. Mechanisms of lipid malabsorption in Cystic Fibrosis: the impact of essential fatty acids deficiency Nutrition & Metabolism, 2005:2:11

# 6

# Clinical Trials in Paediatrics — Regulatory and Methodological Aspects

Adriana Ceci, Viviana Giannuzzi, Donato Bonifazi, Mariagrazia Felisi, Fedele Bonifazi and Lucia Ruggieri

## 1. Introduction

Until very recently, decisions about the medical treatment of children with acute or chronic health conditions were based on the results of research conducted almost exclusively in adults. Although differences in treatment effects between young and adult patients are well known (e.g. regarding mechanism of action and metabolism), there were less clinical trials (CTs) than needed to adequately evaluate the effects of new medicines in children. This was mainly due to:

- the lack of appropriate rules for the conduct of paediatric CTs, especially with regard to ethical considerations;
- the lack of an adequate methodology enabling to provide powered evidences while taking into account the paediatric specificities [1];
- the lack of economic interest of the industrial developers due to the limited market offered by children.

Starting from 1994, Food and Drug Administration (FDA) adopts different measures to promote, incentive or oblige to conduct paediatric trials. More recently, for effect of the Paediatric Regulation (EC) No 1901/2006 [2] requiring a sound scientific evidence for treatment benefits in children and adolescents, the conduct of CTs testing medications for their use in children and adolescents becomes mandatory in the European Union (EU).

Despite the high number,,(more than 1000) of Paediatric Investigation Plans (PIPs) applied to receive an opinion by the Paediatric Committee (PDCO) at the European Medicines Agency

(EMA) since the Regulation entry into force very few advancements have been done in terms of new studies, new trials and new paediatric approved medicines on the market. [3]. At the same time, looking at the American side, we can observe that the implementation of the existing rules has been and are still strongly problematic and under debate, allowing to recent modifications of rules and guidelines.

The aim of this chapter is to describe the requisites for implementing paediatric CTs in compliance with the principles of good clinical practice (Good Clinical Practice, GCP), and with the regulatory standards in order to be part of an agreed PIP in EU or of a Pediatric Study Plan (PSP) in the United States (U.S.).

It will include the following topics:

**1.** Paediatric trial regulatory aspects

*Currently covered by the CTs Directive 2001/20/EC* [4], *rules on paediatric trials are changing for effect of the recently approved CT Regulation that will enter into force by 2016* [5]. *The transition phase and the new context deriving by this transition will be considered in this chapter mainly in terms of a) trial authorisation, b) rules and competencies of Ethics Committees, c) consent and assent from parents and children, d) children privacy and confidentiality.*

**2.** Paediatric Plans and paediatric trials methodology

*The traditional drug development approaches do not satisfy the requirements of research in the paediatric population. In particular, in paediatrics the following issues are challenging: large population needed for Randomised Controlled Trials (RCTs), randomisation procedure, placebo use, validate paediatric endpoint, appropriate outcomes, long-term effects evaluations, etc.*

*In the last years, the main activities performed at scientific and regulatory levels to cover these gaps have been aimed to identify innovative methods of research to overcome the existing paediatric limitations.*

**3.** Paediatric trial incentives and main results of the existing legislation

*By many years the U.S. legislation provides financial incentives to study medicines in children. This has produced a significant increase in the number of paediatric trials conducted since 1997. The EU paediatric medicines Regulation, which was adopted in 2007* [2] *is also based on a series of incentives and requirements and will lead to a further stimulation of paediatric drug development. This chapter explores the distribution and other characteristics of recently conducted paediatric trials in EU and US also providing a comparison between the two areas.*

## 2. Paediatric trial regulatory aspects

### 2.1. The legislative framework to promote paediatric medicines and research

To overcome the lack of paediatric trials, many initiatives have been promoted both in U.S. and in Europe.

The first rule came from FDA in 1994 [1]. It was an attempt to use existing data (may be extrapolated from adults) and additional pharmacokinetic (PK), pharmacodynamic (PD), and safety studies, if the course of the disease and the response to the drug are similar in children and adults. The 1994 law did not impose a general requirement to the manufacturers to carry out studies when existing information was not sufficient and was not successful to obtain its aim.

In 1997, for the first time, the FDA Modernisation Act [6] introduced incentives for conducting paediatric studies on drugs for which exclusivity or patent protection exists, while off-patent drugs were excluded. At that time it was not accepted that FDA would mandate timing and other paediatric studies provisions to the manufacturers.

Today, the current U.S. regulatory framework includes:

- The Best Pharmaceuticals for Children Act **(BPCA)** [7], that provides incentives for drug companies to conduct (after FDA Written Request) paediatric studies by granting additional six months of marketing exclusivity.
- The Paediatric Research Equity Act (**PREA**) [8] that requires drug companies to study their products in children under certain circumstances. When paediatric studies are required, they must be conducted with the same drug and for the same use for which they were approved in adults.[1]

Noticeably, BPCA provided mechanisms for studying on- and off-patent drugs and to test off-patent drugs by:

- Identifying and prioritising drugs which need to be studied;
- Developing study requests in collaboration with experts at National Institutes of Health (NIH), FDA and other organisations;
- Conducting studies on priority drugs after manufacturers decline to do so.

On the other hand, under the **PREA** as originally enacted, a proposed timeline and plan for the submission of paediatric studies were not required to be submitted during the New Drug Application (NDA).By July 9th 2012, for the first time PREA includes a provision that requires manufacturers to submit a Pediatric Study Plan **(PSP)** early in the drug development process. Pediatric Review Committee (PeRC) is a consultative body which reviews all activities under PREA (the same committee is in charge for the activities foreseen under BPCA).

A similar intervention in the EU arrived almost 10 years later. In fact, the EU Paediatric Regulation [2] entered into force in January 2007. After the Paediatric Regulation approval, relevant changes have been implemented not only in Europe but also in the U.S.

The main pillars of the EU Paediatric Regulation are:

- to set up a new Committee at EMA named the Paediatric Committee (PDCO);

1 More details at: Drugs/DevelopmentApprovalProcess/DevelopmentResources/ucm049867.htm

- to rule a new type of Marketing Authorisation, the Paediatric Use Marketing Authorisation (PUMA) only accessible to off-patent drugs;
- to introduce the obligation for the manufacturers to apply for a PIP early in the drug developmental process;
- the obligation to conduct the paediatric studies in compliance with an approved PIP that can also include waiver (exemption to conduct any paediatric studies) or deferral (the right for the manufacturer to delay the paediatric study respect to the adults MA);
- to state that dedicated incentives should be provided under the European Research Framework to develop off-patent drugs if included in a 'Priority List' published by the PDCO-EMA

### 2.2. The current regulatory framework for approving clinical trials

The introduction of specific rules devoted to implement the paediatric research in the paediatric population allowed an increased attention to the CT approval and conduct.

For many years, the traditional approach to diagnosis and treatment has been based on symptoms and signs, which reflect, in the majority of the cases, the patient phenotype. Accordingly, trials have been conducted by grouping patients into broad groups with similar symptoms. Pharmaceutical and biotechnology companies have developed medicines for these broad populations, and the regulatory assessment of risk and benefit has been based on the average clinical response across these groups. This model has been strongly regulated with the aim of performing ethically and methodologically well-conducted CTs.

In Europe several guidelines, directives and regulations have been released, including Directives 2005/28/EC [9] and 2001/20/EC [4], GCP Guidelines (CPMP/ICH/135/95) [10], Reg. (EC) No 726/2004 [11]. In particular, Directive 2001/20/EC has established specific provisions regarding the conduct of CTs on human subjects involving medicinal products and recognises GCP principles. As internationally agreed and in accordance with GCP [10], a CT may not commence in EU if an Ethics Committee has not approved the study. The Directive 2001/20/EC also introduced the concept of "Competent Authority", adding the legal obligation to obtain an "authorisation" in addition to the positive opinion of the Ethic Committee.

However, the above mentioned provisions in Europe have never considered the paediatric specificity until the approval of the CT Directive. In fact, the main novelty of the Directive has been represented by the introduction of a dedicated article (art. 4) that refers to differences in the ethical and methodological approaches between paediatric and adult trials and provides the basis for including paediatric trials in the developmental process of adult drugs. Moreover, following the approval of the Paediatric Regulation, destined to increase the number of paediatric trials, the art. 4 of Directive 2001/20/EC was considered insufficient to protect children involved in a trial [12]. The '*Ethical Recommendations on paediatric trials*' issued in 2008 by the EU Commission [13], represent the more advanced regulatory framework for paediatric research in Europe.

In U.S. the ethics framework for approval of CTs is quite similar. Every CT must be approved and monitored by an **Institutional Review Board** (IRB) to make sure the risks are as low as possible and potential benefits are valuable. An IRB is an independent committee of physicians, statisticians, community advocates, and others people ensuring that a clinical trial is ethical and the rights of study participants are protected. All institutions that conduct or support biomedical research involving people must, have an IRB that initially approves and periodically reviews the research.

In the U.S. legislation, details on how to conduct trials in the paediatric population are included into Subpart D (401-409) of the *'Code of Federal Regulations TITLE 45 PUBLIC WELFARE, PART 46 PROTECTION OF HUMAN SUBJECTS'*: Additional Protections for Children Involved as Subjects in Research [14]. In the code different provisions are identified on the basis of the risk level of the trial such as: 1- Research not involving greater than minimal risk; 2- Research involving greater than minimal risk but presenting the prospect of direct benefit to the individual subjects; 3- Research involving greater than minimal risk and no prospect of direct benefit to individual subjects, but likely to yield general knowledge about the subject's disorder or condition.

In addition, research that presents a reasonable opportunity to advance the understanding, prevention, or alleviation of a serious problem affecting the health or welfare of children can be also approved under special conditions.

A great relevance is given to the procedures to obtain the children assent. The permission to include a child in the trial is given by both parents in case of researches involving greater than minimal risk, and by only one parent if only a minimal risk is concerned.

### *2.2.1. What is changing in the regulatory framework*

After its entry into force, the EU Directive 2001/20/EC has been the object of many concerns and debates leading to a new legislative process aimed to change and consolidate a EU framework by the means of a *Regulation*[2] instead of a *Directive*. In line with different reports and publications [15] the main problems dealing with the Directive were:

**1.** *The need for harmonisation of aspects and procedures aimed at providing ethical protection*

In contrast with the U.S. where only one Federal rule applies, in Europe Directive 2001/20/EC, given its 'non-binding' nature, needed to be implemented by all the different Member States (MSs). Therefore, the harmonisation of ethical issues and the authorisation procedures in different countries were faced but not solved in the context of Directive 2001/20/EC, and this holds true in the case of paediatric trials [16]. In addition, Directive 2001/20/EC does not provide information on how competent authorities and Ethics Committees of each MS should act in case of multi-centre and multi-national studies, while these studies prevail among the trials aimed to a MA approval.

**2.** *The increased burden of administrative and authoritative procedures causing delay in conducting clinical trials in Europe*

---

2*Regulation, unlike Directive, supersedes national laws and it is directly implemented throughout Europe without the need for transposition into national laws.*

The main cause for the decreasing number of trials conducted in Europe and for the increasing of costs is due to the double obligation to obtain an "authorisation" from the Ethic Committees and the Concerned Authorities to be repeated in all the concerned member states. As reported in the EC Explanatory Memorandum preparing a new Regulation [15]: *'The number of applications for clinical trials fell by 25% from 2007 to 2011. For non-commercial sponsors, the increase in administrative requirements due to the Directive 2001/20/EC has led to a 98% increase in administrative costs; the insurance fees have increased by 800% for industry sponsors; the average delay for launching a clinical trial has increased by 90%, to 152 days'.*

From 2016, with the application of the new EU Regulation on CTs (Regulation 536/2014) [5], a unique central procedure will be applied to be carried out through a single EU CT portal, where an homogeneous submission package (valid for all MSs) will be submitted in order to obtain the CT authorisation. The centralised submission will include also the ethical assessment, both for adults and paediatric trials.

Noticeable, the principal duty of the centralised assessment will consist in confirming or not the nature of trial that could be 'interventional' 'low-risk interventional' or 'non-interventional'.

The category of 'non-interventional trial is a novelty in the EU context and is based on a recognised 'minimal risk' of the trial (e.g. only limited procedures added to the current therapy) to which a lower level of requirements (including insurance coverage) is needed.

A "Reporting Member State", in charge to draw up an "assessment report" and the release of the authorisation, will be proposed by the sponsor corresponding to the country where it intends to carry out the Clinical Trial Application (CTA) at first. In case of multi-national trials, the other involved MSs follow a simplified procedure of assessment focused on national and ethical aspects (e.g. informed consent, recruitment of subjects, data protection, suitability of investigators and trial sites, mechanisms of insurance compensation collection of biological samples, submission fees, arrangements for rewarding/compensating investigators and subjects) for their own territory compliance.

In case of paediatric trials, for effect of a large consultation process and after relevant amendments provided by different stakeholders, in particular by the Paediatric Research Networks (such as EnPREMA[3], TEDDY[4] and GRiP[5]), the new Regulation represents a potential positive step in the process to increase the number and the quality of paediatric trials.

In more details, the Regulation states that:

- The application should refer to the PDCO opinions and related approved PIPs: The Reporting MS shall assess the application with regard to the relevance of the CT, including PDCO' opinions on PIPs.

---

3 EnPREMA is the Network of the existing Paediatric Network, stated in the Paediatric Regulation and set up at EMA

4 TEDDY is a European Network of Excellence for Paediatric Clinical Research. For more information, http://www.teddyoung.net/

5 GRiP amendments are available here http://www.grip-network.org/index.php/sfPropelFileStorage/download/name/GRiP+on+CT+regulation.pdf

- As stated in the Paediatric Regulation [2], all paediatric studies should be registered in the EU register of CTs, including studies that are part of an agreed PIP and carried out in third countries.

With regards to the preparation of submission documents, besides the rules applying for every type of trials, issues specifically dealing with paediatrics have been established as follow:

- the cover letter shall indicate the reference to trial population (minors), and a statement that the trial is part of an agreed PIP.
- the link to the Decision of the Agency on its website must be indicated in order to demonstrate that at the time of the Ethic Committee application, the Agency will have already issued the Decision about the PIP;
- the protocol shall include a justification for including minors and detail the procedures for inclusion of single subjects;
- the summary of the results of the CT shall include paediatric regulatory details (information whether the CT is a part of a PIP).

Finally, some important requirements, already stated in previous non-mandatory documents, such as the need for paediatric expertise or advice in Ethics Committees, become mandatory, such as the involvement of minors in the informed consent procedure according to their age and mental maturity. The table below shows the comparison between EU and U.S. rules on specific key topics of paediatric trials.

| **TOPICS** | **Europe (Regulation 536/2014)** | **U.S. (Subpart D (401-409) - Code of Federal Regulations title 45-46)** |
|---|---|---|
| **Trial authorisation/ approval** | The Reporting Member State and other MSs involved authorise the trial.<br>The assessment includes the Ethics Committees review.<br>The reporting Member State shall assess the application with regard to the relevance of the clinical trial, including PDCO' opinions on PIPs. | An Institutional Review Board (IRB) approves and monitors the trial. |
| **Ethics Committee rules and competencies** | Experts in paediatric research are members of Ethics Committees reviewing the protocol. Alternatively the Ethics Committees take advice from external experts on clinical, ethical and psychosocial issues in the field of paediatrics. | IRBs are also allowed to invite individuals with special expertise or knowledge to provide consultation and information on individual protocols, where needed. |

| TOPICS | Europe<br>(Regulation 536/2014) | U.S.<br>(Subpart D (401-409) - Code of Federal Regulations title 45-46) |
|---|---|---|
| **Research involving neonates** | No specific rules. All rules intended to paediatric research apply. Research on non viable or of uncertain viability neonates are not cited. | Specific rules apply to neonates: a) non viable, b) of uncertain viability, c) viable (general rules apply). |
| **Risk/Benefit** | No specific rules for paediatric population. | Each IRB shall approve only Paediatric Research not involving greater than minimal risk or involving greater than minimal risk if:<br>- presenting the prospect of direct benefit to the individual subjects<br>- likely to yield general knowledge about the subject's disorder or condition (if minimal risk increase)<br>- research not otherwise approvable which presents an opportunity to understand, prevent, or alleviate a serious problem affecting the health or welfare of children (under special conditions). |
| **Minimal Risk definition** | Minimal risk could be defined as the probability of harm or discomfort not greater than that ordinarily encountered in daily life or during the performance of routine physical or psychological examinations or tests. | Minimal risk means that the probability and magnitude of harm or discomfort anticipated in the research are not greater than those ordinarily encountered in daily life or during the performance of routine physical or psychological examinations or tests (this rule is not a specific paediatric rule). |
| **Consent and assent from parents and children** | Informed consent of the parents or legal representative. Assent of the children, that are entitled to receive information according their age and maturity.<br>No minimum age is defined for providing assent.<br>Need to obtain the consent if the subject reaches the age of legal competence during the trial | Parents (both or only one, according the level of risk) or guardians provide permission before children can be enrolled in research. Researchers must seek a child's assent unless the IRB determines that the children to be involved are not capable of providing assent, given their age, maturity, and psychological state.<br>The regulations do not describe the information that must be provided to children but rely on IRBs to use their discretion in judging assent provisions. |
| **Children privacy and confidentiality** | No specific rules for children issued in Reg. 536/2014 (as well as in the Privacy Directive 95/46/EC) | Children confidentiality and privacy is not mentioned in FDA code. |

| TOPICS | Europe (Regulation 536/2014) | U.S. (Subpart D (401-409) - Code of Federal Regulations title 45-46) |
|---|---|---|
| | The only reference is present in the EC Ethical Recommendation,2008 | FDA regulation (50.25(a)(5)) states that in seeking parents' informed consent, (5) a statement describing the extent, if any, to which confidentiality of records identifying the subject will be maintained (including the possibility of FDA inspection) must be provided. However, this point is not cited with reference to children's assent. |

**Table 1.** EU and U.S. regulations on paediatric research

## 3. Paediatric plans and paediatric trials methodology

### 3.1. Paediatric plans

As detailed before, both EU and U.S. legislation currently require that a developmental plan (i.e. the PIP in EU and the PSP in U.S.) is approved by the responsible Official Bodies before the paediatric studies will start.

PSP is required for each drug or biological product that includes a new active ingredient, new indication, new dosage form, new dosing regimen, or new route of administration (including a biosimilar product that has not been determined to be interchangeable with the reference product).

FDA strongly regulates the timing to which the **PSP** should be presented (not later than 60 calendar days after the date of the end-of-phase 2 meeting or equivalent timing if the meeting would not have place. A PSP should include;"(i) an outline of the paediatric study or studies that the sponsor plans to conduct (including, to the extent practicable study objectives and design, age groups, relevant endpoints, and statistical approach); (ii) any request for a deferral, partial waiver, or waiver if applicable, along with any supporting information; and (iii) other information specified in the regulations"

In EU the Paediatric Regulation [2] requires **PIPs** to be submitted to the Agency early, wherever possible and the PIPs should:

- include a description of the studies and of the measures to adapt the medicineformulation to make its use more acceptable in children, such as use of a liquid formulation rather than large tablets;
- cover the needs of all age groups of children, from birth to adolescence;
- define the timing of studies in children compared to adults[6].

The table below describes the main measures included in the EMA-PDCO and FDA guidance.

| TOPICS | EMA provisions (PIP)[17] | FDA provisions (PSP) [18] |
|---|---|---|
| **WHO** | The sponsor of a 'product not yet authorised' (that NOT includes variations) (art.7).<br>The sponsor of a marketed patented drug willing to introduce variations (art. 8).<br>The sponsor (even different from the MAH) willing to develop a paediatric study on an old off-patent drug (art. 30. This is voluntary and lead to a PUMA). | The sponsor of a 'new active ingredient' (that includes variations) (this is an obligation under PREA). |
| **WHEN** | Early, wherever possible (in time for studies to be conducted in the paediatric population, where appropriate, before MAAs are submitted).<br>PDCO requires: "not later than upon completion of the human PK studies and initial tolerability studies, or the initiation of the adult phase-II studies (proof-of-concept studies), but before pivotal trials or confirmatory (phase-III) trials are initiated.<br>Applications during confirmatory or phase-III trials in adults, or after starting CTs in children, are likely to be considered unjustified. | Not later than 60 calendar days after the date of the end-of-phase 2 meeting (special rules apply according with the FDA meetings timing).<br>For products for life-threatening diseases, at the end-of-phase 1 meetings. |
| **which AGE TO COVER** | All the paediatric population's groups (birth to 18 years). | All relevant paediatric populations (birth to 16 years). |
| **CONTENTS** | **Administrative and product information** also including:<br>- A.5: Regulatory information on CTs related to the<br>condition (EAA).<br>A.6: Marketing authorisation status of the medicinal product.<br>A.7: Advice from any regulatory authorities.<br>A.8: Orphan drug status in the EEA. | n.a. |
| | Overview of the **Disease Condition** in the Paediatric Population:<br>- pathophysiology of the disease, | Overview of the **Disease Condition** in the Pediatric Population:<br>- pathophysiology of the disease, |

6 EMA website: http://www.ema.europa.eu/ema/index.jsp?curl=pages/regulation/document_listing/document_listing_000293.jsp&mid=WC0b01ac0580025b91

| TOPICS | EMA provisions (PIP)[17] | FDA provisions (PSP) [18] |
|---|---|---|
| | - diagnosis,<br>- currently available treatments and/or prevention<br>- incidence and prevalence of the disease. | - diagnosis,<br>-currently available treatments and/or prevention<br>- incidence and prevalence of the disease. |
| | Overview of the **Drug or Biological Product:**<br>- mechanism of action<br>- potential therapeutic benefits<br>- Other possible therapeutic uses of the drug | Overview of the **Drug or Biological Product:**<br>- mechanism of action<br>- potential therapeutic benefits<br>- Other possible therapeutic uses of the drug |
| | **Extrapolation** could include:<br>- efficacy from adults to children or from older to younger children,<br>- safety information from adults to children can also be included,<br>- modelling of PK and/or PD if used for decision-making. | Overview of Planned **extrapolation** to Specific Paediatric Populations:<br>- any plans to extrapolate efficacy from adult or from one paediatric age group to another including neonates,<br>- extrapolation for other drugs in the same class, can be considered as supportive information, |
| | **Request for Drug-specific waivers (global or partial):**<br>The requirement to submit a PIP shall be waived for specific medicinal products or classes of medicinal products that:<br>are likely to be ineffective or unsafe in part or all of the paediatric population;<br>are intended for conditions that occur only in adult populations;<br>do not represent a significant therapeutic benefit over existing treatments for paediatric patients. | **Request for Drug-Specific Waiver(s):**<br>(a) Necessary studies are impossible or highly impracticable (because, for example, the number of patients is so small or the patients are geographically dispersed).<br>(b) There is evidence strongly suggesting that the drug or biological product would be ineffective or unsafe in all paediatric age groups.<br>(c) The drug or biological product (1) does not represent a meaningful therapeutic benefit and (2) is not likely to be used in a substantial number of paediatric patients<br>Partial waiver provision also apply:<br>-if attempts to produce a paediatric formulation failed<br>- for a specific age group. |
| | Planned **Nonclinical and Clinical Studies and timeline** | **Planned Nonclinical and Clinical Studies and timeline** |
| | **Paediatric Formulation Development** | **Pediatric Formulation Development** |

**Table 2.** Main provision to apply for PIP and PSP

Considering the two described systems, we noted some interesting differences. In particular, while the EU Paediatric Regulation covers all the paediatric medicines (in-patent, off-patent, under development) and deserves incentives only to the off-patent drugs, in U.S. two different regimens apply for: a) medicines to be granted a paediatric exclusivity after a solicited request (Written Request) as stated in BPCA, and b) medicines for which a PSP is mandatory under PREA. Noticeably, the medicines that are under PREA can also be granted a Written Request, allowing to receive a paediatric exclusivity (see also Fig.1).

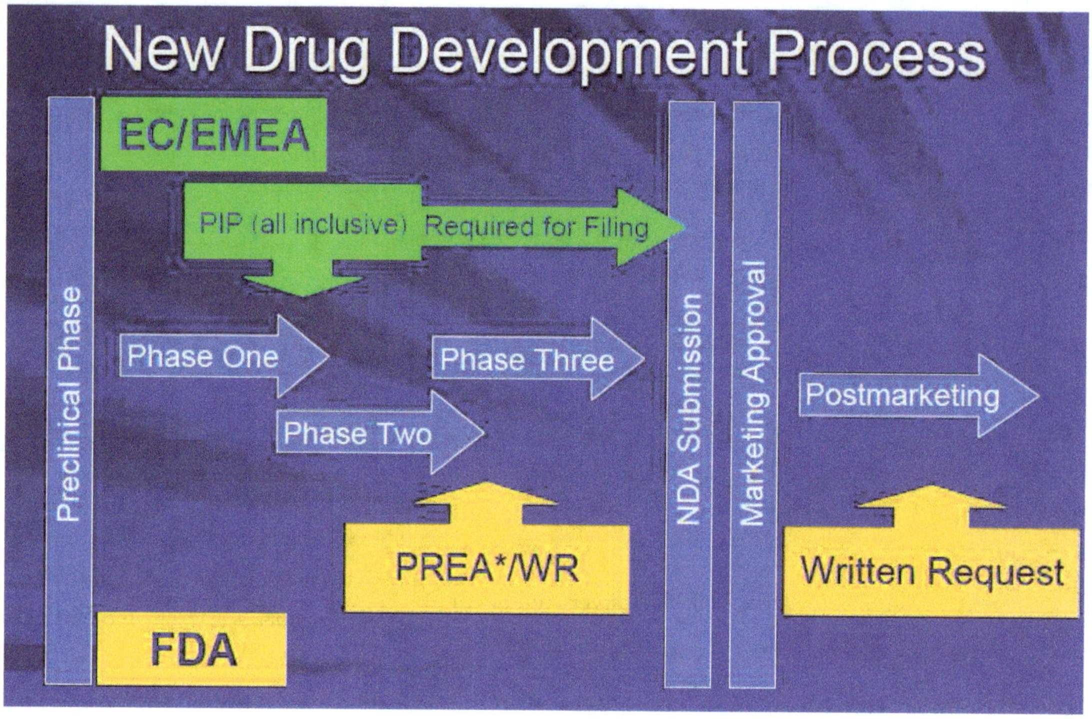


**Figure 1.** Paediatric drug regulatory process in EU and U.S. (source: FDA and EMA Paediatric Regulatory Process: J Temek, MD, FDA website)

Moreover, the paediatric developmental plan procedures of the two Agencies are not completely aligned mainly due to the different regulatory status provided by the different regulations and the different approaches of the two Committees. In particular:

- In EU, unlike in the U.S., a MAA (Marketing Authorisation Application) (equivalent to NDA in U.S.) must contain the results of the paediatric studies conducted in compliance with the agreed PIP (or waiver or deferral). In lack of this, the MA cannot be granted.
- In EU, the paediatric product development is requested earlier in the regulatory process than in U.S.
- In EU, the PDCO, the counter part to the PeRC in the U.S, unlike the PeRC, makes binding decisions.
- FDA "feasibility " criteria for waivers do not exist in the EU legislation. Thus, a study may be required in EU but waived in the U.S. under PREA.
- FDA may request or grant paediatric studies under BPCA, using the voluntary financial incentive, even during the PSP process, while in Europe patented drugs do not have access to financial incentives.

- Finally, unlike the U.S., the EU does not have a public process whereby paediatric focused post-marketing safety reviews are presented to an Advisory Committee.

These differences still represent an obstacle to a prompt development of paediatric drugs in a global context. An intensive work aimed at merging the paediatric efforts at the two levels is highly required and desirable. To this aim, currently a process of 'Information Exchange' is in place to discuss product-specific paediatric development issues and general scientific/ regulatory/safety issues. The Japan Pharmaceuticals and Medical Devices Act (PMDA) has recently joined this initiative as observer.

## 3.2. Paediatric trials methodology

### *3.2.1. The ICH-E11 guideline*

Before specific paediatric legislations were in place, regulators, companies and clinicians were well aware that the current methodological approach, based on well-designed RCTs, could result difficult to apply in selected cases such as the paediatric population.

In particular, in paediatrics the following issues are challenging large population available for RCTs, randomisation procedure, placebo use, availability of validate paediatric endpoints, appropriate outcomes, long-term effects evaluations, etc.

The ICH-E11 Guideline, issued in 2000 at international level [19], has represented the main international reference for paediatric CTs and the methodological standard to perform paediatric CTs scientifically correct, and ethical in the same time. It still represents the only standard acceptable by the Regulatory Authorities.

The guideline milestones are:

- Paediatric patients should be given medicines that are properly evaluated for their use in the intended population.
- Product development programs should include paediatric studies when paediatric use is anticipated.
- Development of appropriated products in paediatric patients should be timely and, often requires the development of paediatric formulations.
- The rights of paediatric participants should be protected and they should be shielded from undue risks.
- Responsibility should be shared among companies, regulatory authorities, health professionals and society as a whole.
- Marketing Authorisation Holders (MAHs), and competent authorities/medicine regulatory agencies are the two major stakeholders responsible for medicine safety at the time of authorisation.

The approach to the clinical programme needs to be clearly addressed with the regulatory authorities at an early stage and then periodically during the development process. To this aim, the guideline has provided specific indications on trial characteristics, including:

- when initiating a paediatric program for a medicinal product (need of a medicinal products, therapeutic benefits, lack of alternatives);
- timing of initiation of paediatric studies during medicinal product development (need that preliminary safety/tolerability data are known in adults);
- types of studies (PK, PK/PD, efficacy, safety); according to the principle to avoid unnecessary studies in all paediatric age groups, large efficacy studies should be considered only when extrapolation of results from adults (or from older children to younger) is not feasible; on the contrary, PK studies and short and long term safety evaluations are always required.
- age categories: five paediatric ages have been identified from neonates to adolescents and each paediatric group should be given medicines that have been appropriately evaluated for their use;
- special rules for ethic approval of paediatric clinical investigation (including children right to be informed and privacy).

#### *3.2.2. The ICH-E11 modification process*

Currently, a revision of the ICH-E11 guideline is ongoing. It derives by the relevant changes occurred in the last years, both at scientific and regulatory levels. **Innovative methods of research are in progress** to overcome the existing paediatric studies limitations and are having a profound impact on the assessment procedures at the regulatory agencies level. The main novelties in the field are:

- use of innovative PK/PD methodologies for dosing and efficacy extrapolation exercises [20];
- use of population PK PD (pop PKPD) models to assess different clinical scenarios without exposing children to any risk to explore new drug [21];
- use of alternative statistical approaches to reduce the size of the experimental population and the number of the trials needed in the clinical phase [22].

The updated E11 Guideline as proposed in August 2014, aims to include the new scientific and technical knowledge advances in paediatric drug development in a new regulatory guidance. To this aim, an addendum to the ICH Topic E11 guideline will be finalised by November 2015 with the following revised topics:

- Timing of paediatric development: need for more harmonisation and clarity to guide the developers of paediatric medicines; it is proposed to focus on the multi-national/multi-regional status of many paediatric trials for which the requirements of multiple regulatory authorities should be satisfied.
- Age classification and paediatric subsets including neonates: there is the need for better understanding the developmental process in paediatric subsets, especially neonates and infants.
- Ethical considerations in paediatric studies: there is the need for enhance the ethical considerations in paediatric studies.

- Types of studies and methodology of CTs: the advances in paediatric CTs design and conduct should be incorporated in the ICH-E11 guidance including: innovative study designs, development of clinical outcome assessments, development of validated age-appropriate clinical endpoints and surrogate markers (biomarkers), specific scales for measuring outcomes particularly in case of younger age groups,
- Common rules to apply appropriate principles for extrapolation of data (from adult to paediatric populations or older children or different indication). This last point could possibly lead both the Agencies to agree a Paediatric Algorithm firstly proposed at FDA level and still now not regularly adopted at EMA level.
- Formulation challenges in paediatric drug development: need for developing specific comprehensive guidance on formulation development for children.

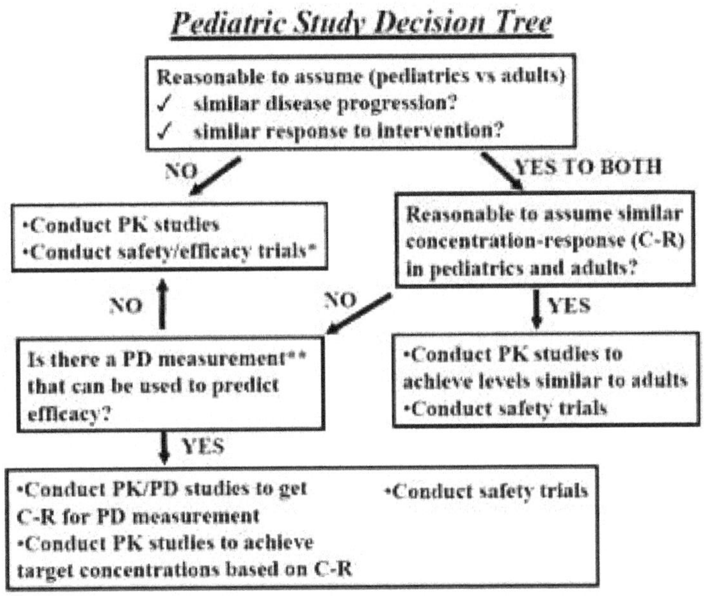


**Figure 2.** Paediatric Study decision tree for bridging efficacy data in an adult population to a paediatric population (source: FDA)

## 4. Paediatric trial incentives and main results of the existing legislation

As stated before, important changes both in U.S. and EU legislations both imposed the pharmaceutical industry to study medicines in children, with the aim to increase the number of paediatric trials to be conducted, to reduce the existing gap. A comparison between the two regulations in terms of impact on paediatric trials is difficult, because of the existing differences on requirements and incentives provided in the two contexts, as well as the very limited amount of published data on the regulations results. As a general finding, it seems that public funding provisions and active strategies both in Europe and US have a strong relevance in improving the current situation through the conduction of studies in children and adolescent in the world.

### 4.1. Impact of paediatric regulation on paediatric trials

In Europe, the most recent available document summarising the main results of the Paediatric Regulation has been released by the EC covering the period 2007-2012. It provides relevant information on PIPs and paediatric trials approved in Europe. It states that:

By the end of 2012, the Agency had agreed 600 PIPs (more than 1.000 presented). Of these, 453 were for medicines that were not yet authorised in the EU (Article 7), while the remaining ones are related to new indications for patent-protected products (Article 8) or PUMA (Article 30).These plans cover a broad range of therapeutic areas, as shown in the figure below and all the paediatric ages including neonates.

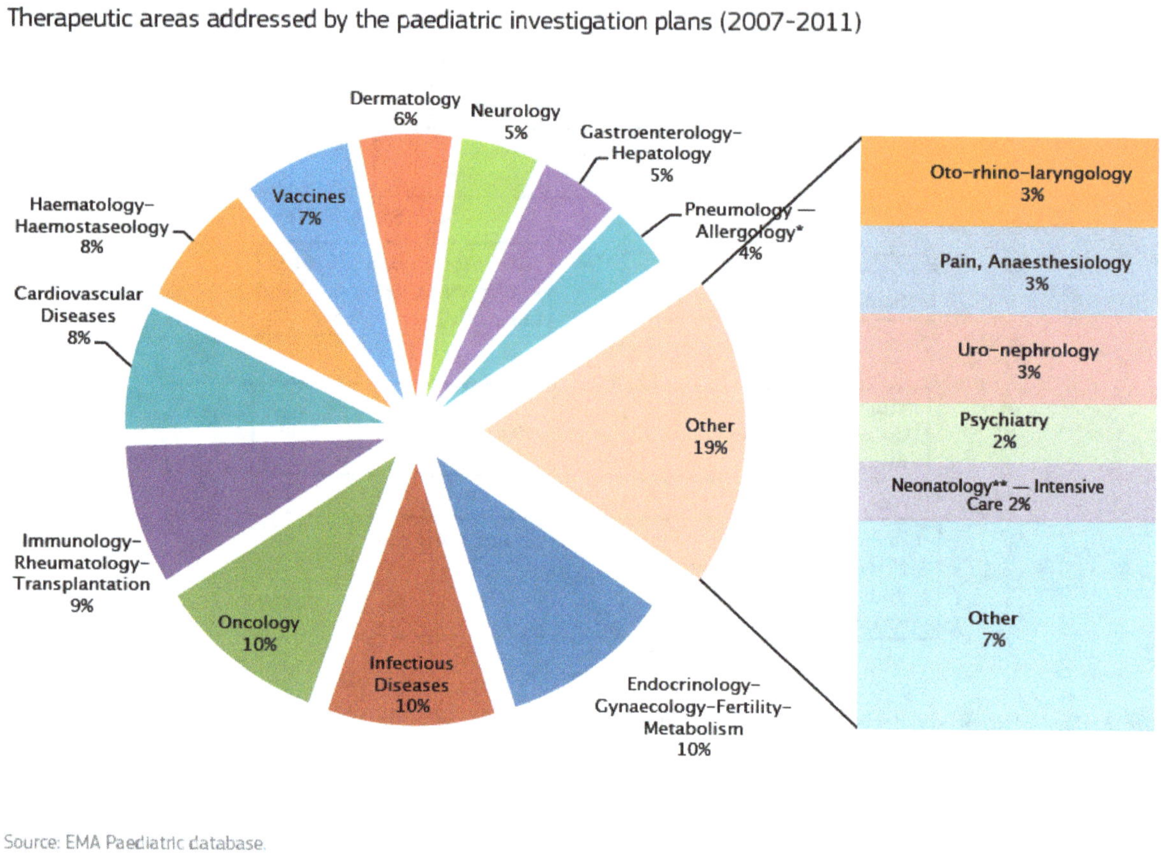


**Figure 3.** Therapeutic areas addressed by the PIPs (2007-2011).[7]

Regarding the number of paediatric trials, the reference derived by the official source EudraCT[8] demonstrates that the number of trials in children did not increase after the approval of the Regulation but remained stable between 2006 and 2012, corresponding to an average of 350 trials per year. However, until recently EudraCT was limited to paediatric trials com-

7 Progress Report on the Paediatric Regulation COM (2013) 443 Final

8 EUDRACT is the EU register of all (ongoing, completed, prematurely terminated) trials with medicinal products taking place in the European Union and those studying medicines for paediatric use contained in an agreed PIP carried out in third countries.

mencing in the EU, while data on paediatric trials that are part of a PIP and conducted outside the EU have only become available since spring 2011.

| | 2005 | 2006 | 2007 | 2008 | 2009 | 2010 | 2011 | 2012 |
|---|---|---|---|---|---|---|---|---|
| Paediatric trials (number) | 254 | 316 | 355 | 342 | 404 | 379 | 334 | 332 |
| Paediatric trials that are part of an agreed PIP* | 2 | 1 | 2 | 6 | 16 | 30 | 76 | 76 |
| Proportion of paediatric trials that are part of an agreed PIP among paediatric trials* | 1 % | 0 % | 1 % | 2 % | 4 % | 8 % | 23 % | 23 % |
| Total number of trials (adults and/or children) | 3 350 | 3 979 | 4 749 | 4 512 | 4 445 | 4 026 | 3 809 | 3 698 |
| Proportion of paediatric trials of all trials | 8 % | 8 % | 7 % | 8 % | 9 % | 10 % | 9 % | 9 % |

Source: EudraCT Data Warehouse using a predefined query on 6 March 2013 and counting the first authorised trial only, in the case of more than one Member State

**Table 3.** Paediatric Clinical Trials by year of authorisation.

Of the total number of trials conducted in the last years after the approval of the Paediatric Regulation, only a few have been included in the Marketing Authorisation documentation, in order to obtain a paediatric indication.

In particular, data from TEDDY-EPMD[9], a database including information on the paediatric medicines approved by EMA, demonstrate that, after the implementation of the Paediatric Regulation, on a total of almost 70 new active substances approved for children by EMA, 33 applications include a paediatric plan (all available in 'COM (2013) 443 Final' at www.ema.europa.eu). Additional 12 medicines received a paediatric indication using results of the existing studies after reviewing all the studies at central level (art.45-46 of the Paediatric Regulation) (26).

### 4.2. Impact of FDA rules on paediatric trials

Between the 1998 and 2011the FDA issued ~340 Written Requests for new paediatric studies, today 533 labelling changes associated with BPCA and PREA acts have been approved (BPCA only = 161; BPCA + PREA = 73; PREA only = 249; Rule = 49; None = 1), which is significantly higher if compared to the number of labelling changes approved in Europe.

On the basis of these data, according to Lynn Yao it is possible to affirm that: 'Before BPCA and PREA became law, more than 80% of the drugs approved for adult use were being used

9 www.teddyoung.net

in children, even though their safety and effectiveness had not been established in children. Today that number has been reduced to about 50%. (http://blogs.fda.gov/fdavoice/index).

| **With New Pediatric Studies** | **N°484** |
|---|---|
| PK | 122 |
| Efficacy | 133 |
| Safety | 281 |
| With no New Pediatric Studies | N°49 |
| TOTAL | N°533 |

**Table 4.** FDA- New Pediatric Labelling Information Database (1998-2014)

An analysis performed on 174 CTs completed for Pediatric Exclusivity published in May 2010 [23], demonstrated that the U.S. is the most frequent site for conducting CTs, followed by Europe. However, 65% of paediatric trials were conducted in at least 1 country outside the U.S. and 11% did not include any sites in the U.S. Fifty-four countries were represented, and 38% of trials enrolled patients in more than 1 site located in a developing/transition country.

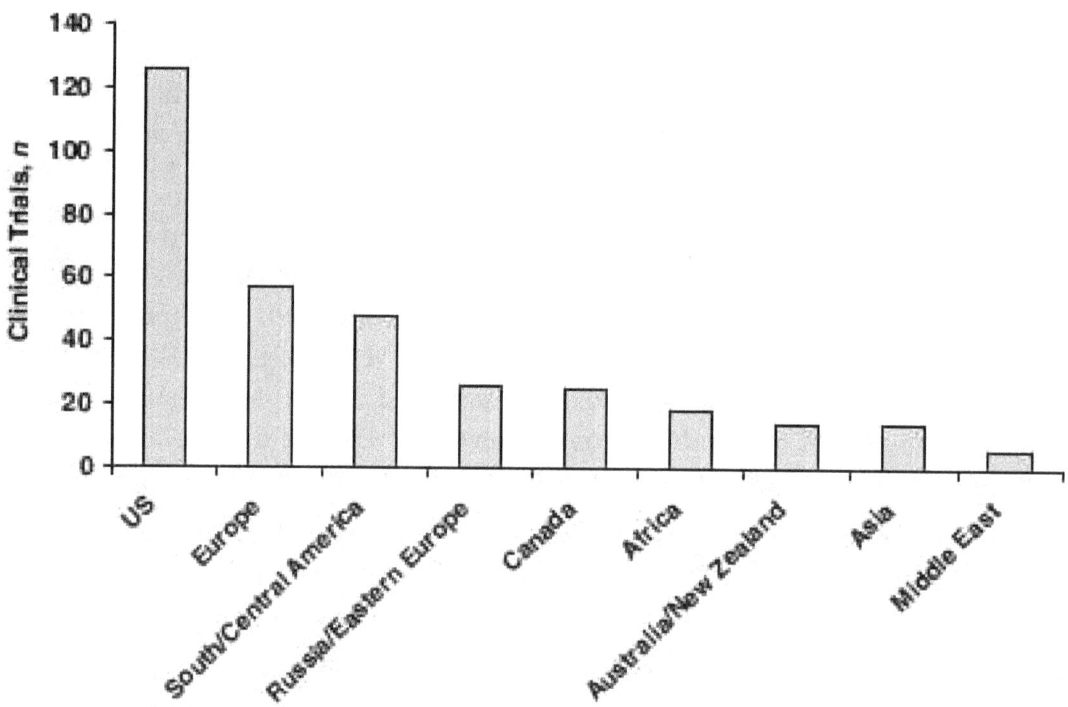


**Figure 4.** Location of 174 trials included in BPCA act.

Under these programs, ~436 separate studies that enrolled ~56,000 children were performed over a 5-years period. An example of results achieved by public incentives to paediatric research is provided by an extensive study evaluating outcomes of BPCA procedures granted from 2002 to 2007 [24]. This study, analysing 99 Written Request[10] applications submitted to FDA, reports that:

- 257 paediatric CTs (average 2.6 trials per application) have been conducted, covering approximately 60 indications. The most commonly studied indications were bacterial infections;
- the paediatric trials enrolled at least 46,000 subjects in 5,850 clinical centres;
- all paediatric ages have been addressed, but most of patients were aged 12-17 years old;
- in contrast with the sponsors' trend to shift the location of adult trials away from the country, the U.S. remains the dominant location for paediatric trials (54%), although most paediatric drug programmes are global;
- The trials were distributed across more than 60 countries and the EU contributed 11% of the centres and 7% of patients

### 4.3. Funded studies for paediatric medicines in EU and US

Both in EU and in U.S., funding is devoted to better support paediatric drugs development. Initiatives in this direction are justified under many points of view such as:

Relatively few trials specifically studying the younger age groups, (neonates, infants and toddlers) were approved. In fact it has been demonstrated [23] that from 1998 through 2010, only 23 (6 percent) of the 365 labelling changes, after the submission of new paediatric studies, included the addition of information from studies with neonates.

The most commonly studied indications do not necessarily reflect greatest paediatric therapeutic needs but closely matched the distribution of these drugs over the adult market, and not the drug utilization by children [23].

Off-label drugs are poorly studied. Neither the financial benefit for the pharmaceutical companies in USA, neither the new MA, the PUMA, ad hoc created in EU, demonstrated to be attractive for the commercial sponsors.

Strategies have put in place to overcome this limitation mainly based on funding ad hoc studies and promoting non-commercial, research-driven paediatric trial. Positive examples of these strategies in EU and in US are described below.

1. *FP7 Research Framework provisions to develop off-patent drugs currently used off-label in children*

The EU supports research into paediatric medicinal products through its multi-annual Framework Programme for Research and Technological Development.

According to article 40 of the Regulation, the European Research Framework Programs should reserve funds to support PUMAs in case of off-patent drugs recognised as of high therapeutic interest for children and included in a 'Priority List' (PL) adopted, on annual basis, by the EMA (European Medicines Agency) through its Paediatric Committee.

10 A Written Request may be initiated by FDA or in response to a Proposed Pediatric Study Request (PPSR).

In the last 6 years such EC funds have been delivered through the Seventh Framework Programme for Research (FP7-FRP). In particular, with reference to HEALTH-(2007-2013) Programme area, five calls for proposal have been released with reference to the topic 4.2-1 'to develop off-patent medicinal products for the paediatric population'.

From 2007 to 2013, 20 projects were granted with funds. The total amount awarded to these projects is 98.6 million Euros.

The twenty approved projects are investigating a total of 24 active substances, in 10 therapeutic areas (see tab. 5). In particular a total of 71 studies have been funded, involving almost 400 investigational sites in EU and non-EU countries, 246 partners of whom 51 are private companies and around 7000 children (representing 23% of all the paediatric patients included in clinical trials in Europe from 2007 to 2011) were recruited. Eighty percent of the projects include studies to develop new age-appropriate formulations or dosage form and all paediatric subgroups are represented in the clinical trials with particular reference to preterm and/or term newborns.

| Project | Active Substance(S) | Addressed paediatric indication(s) | Therapeutic area |
|---|---|---|---|
| TINN | Ciprofloxacin* | treatment of infections in preterm and term newborns | Infections |
| | Fluconazole | | |
| TINN2 | Azithromycin | treatment of infections in preterm and term newborns | |
| NeoMero | Meropenem | treatment of late-onset sepsis in neonates and infants aged <3 months<br>treatment of bacterial meningitis in neonates and infants aged <3 months | |
| NeoVanc | Vancomycin | treatment of late onset bacterial sepsis caused by vancomycin susceptible bacteria in neonates and infants aged under three months | |
| NeoOpioid | Morphine | treatment of acute pain | Pain |
| | Fentanyl | | |
| GAPP | Gabapentin | treatment of chronic pain | |
| Loulla & Philla | Methotrexate* | treatment of Acute Lymphoblastic Leukemia | Malignant neoplasms |
| | 6-Mercaptopurine* | | |
| 03K | Cyclophosphamide | treatment of paediatric malignancies | |
| | Temozolomide | | |
| EPOC | Doxorubicin* | treatment of childhood cancer | |
| HIP trial | Dopamine | management of hypotension in preterm newborns | Cardiology |
| NeoCirc | Dobutamine | treatment of systemic hypotension in infants | |
| LENA | Enalapril | cardiac failure in children | |

| Project | Active Substance(S) | Addressed paediatric indication(s) | Therapeutic area |
|---|---|---|---|
| NEMO | Bumetanide | treatment of neonatal seizures in babies with hypoxic ischemic encephalopathy | Neurology |
| KIEKIDS | Ethosuximide | treatment of absence and myoclonic epilepsy | |
| TAIN | Hydrocortisone* | treatment of adrenal insufficiency in neonates and infants | Endocrinology |
| METFIZZ | Metformin | treatment of polycystic ovary syndrome | |
| CloSed | Clonidine* | Sedation in intensive care | Intensive care/ anaesthesiology |
| DEEP | Deferiprone* | treatment of chronic iron overload | Haematology |
| PERS | Risperidone | treatment of conduct disorder<br>treatment of schizophrenia | Child & adolescent psychiatry |
| NEuroSIS | Budesonide* | prevention of bronchopulmonary dysplasia | Respiratory and cardiovascular disorders |

* received an Orphan Drug designation (four in the same indication addressed by the project)

**Table 5.** FP7 approved projects in Europe ([25]

These data demonstrated that paediatric studies receiving support from the EU institutions are attractive even outside Europe and also for the private companies engaged in view of the final PUMA approval.

Furthermore, to date, 22% of the planned enrolment for these trials is completed, that is in contrast with the reported low recruitment capacity and difficulties with the conduct of paediatric trials in Europe.

**2.** *The Pediatric Trials Network (PTN)*

Sponsored by the Eunice Kennedy Shriver National Institute of Child Health and by the Human Development (NICHD), the Pediatric Trials Network (PTN) is an alliance of clinical research sites located around the United States that are cooperating in the design and conduct of paediatric CTs. PTN relates to BPCA since funds are devoted to develop research driven studies in the area where the investments of private companies are very limited and the FDA incentives resulted insufficient.

As European Consortia, the PTN is studying the formulation, dosing, efficacy, and safety of drugs used in paediatric patients. In keeping with the goals of the Best Pharmaceuticals for Children Act, data collected from PTN trials will help regulators to revise drug labels for safer and more effective use in infants and children.

Currently 20 PTN trials are in progress, the results of 4 of them have been published. Noticeably, 3 active substances funded within PTN are also funded under EU FP7 projects. The list of the projects is available on the FDA website and results are continuously updated.

| Trial | Status |
|---|---|
| Metronidazole | Enrolment and analysis completed, clinical study report submitted to FDA, results published |
| TAPE | Enrolment completed in less than 2 months, results published |
| Acyclovir | Enrolment complete, analysis in progress, results published |
| Hydroxyurea | Enrolment completed |
| POPS | Enrolment ongoing |
| Lisinopril PK | Database locked; analyses in progress |
| Midazolam | Data analysis in progress |
| Ampicillin | Results published |
| Obesity informatics | Analysis in progress |
| Anti-staph trio | Enrolment ongoing |
| Sildenafil | Enrolment ongoing, interim PK analysis |
| Clindamycin obesity | Enrolment ongoing |
| Fluconazole safety | Meta-analysis ongoing |
| Midazolam obesity | Protocol in development |
| Acyclovir phase II | Protocol complete, opening sites |
| Pantoprazole | Enrolment ongoing |
| Pediatrix meta-analysis | Protocol complete, analysis ongoing |
| Antibiotic safety (SCAMP) | Protocol complete, selecting sites |
| Diuretic safety | Protocol complete, opening sites |
| Methadone pharmacokinetics | Enrolment ongoing |

**Table 6.** PTN trials

Taking into account these results, we consider that the problems issued by paediatric drug development are only partially solved. Regulations are now quite similar both with reference to the requirements and the incentives provided but profound differences still exist in the practical application.

The U.S. remains the dominant location for paediatric trials but the balance may change in the future. EU results in increasing the numbers of paediatric approved drugs are still disappointing but in EU the number of studies in specific categories (neonates) and of projects responding to real therapeutic need (off-label) is higher than in US. However the approved drugs in this category still remain very few (on a total of 533 labelling changes in U.S. only 19 off-patent drugs have been the object of a FDA Written Request while in EU only 2 PUMA have been granted till now).

## 5. Conclusive remarks

Despite many regulatory provisions have globally focused, in EU and in US, the attention on the paediatric themes, some significant issues have to be further improved in order to fill in the existing gaps. Some of the most relevant criticisms are summarised below.

1. Especially in EU, it has been recognised that paediatric development strategy is still often perceived as a regulatory obligation, more than an integral part of the whole medicinal development process [26].

2. Paediatric provisions demonstrated not to be able to specifically address the paediatric needs. For example, in Europe most of the therapeutic needs periodically identified by expert groups at EMA/PDCO are still uncovered by PIPs and/or PUMAs. In the U.S. there is a discrepancy between the drug prescription pattern in children and the drugs granted paediatric exclusivity. Actually, the majority of drugs granted paediatric exclusivity is rarely used by children and drugs frequently used by children are underrepresented in the paediatric studies aimed to obtain exclusivity [27].

3. The field of neonatology is quite critical. In Europe, the number of neonates included in clinical trials substantially increasedafter the Paed. Reg. entered into force [3]. However many neonatal therapeutic needs recognised by EMA/PDCO are still unmet [28]. Similarly, in the U.S. only a small percentage (6%) of the labelling changes involving the submission of new paediatric studies included the addition of information from studies with neonates [29].

4. With reference to the availability of drug formulations suitable for children, a lack of age-appropriate formulations, in terms of safety of excipients, palatability, acceptability, dosing flexibility, accuracy and practical handling still exists [3]. In U.S., a public-funded Pediatric Formulations Platform[11] is trying to fill this gap but no similar initiatives have been identified in Europe.

5. Deferral measures have been introduced in both regions to avoid delays, provoked by paediatric development, to the availability of drugs for adults. As a negative counterpart, deferrals are deeply impairing paediatric drug development: 63% of new medicines intended for both adults and children have a deferral in the agreed PIP [3]. In the U.S, despite nearly all (98%) of the rationales for deferrals were consistent with the law, the amount of deferred studies delayed and/or pending is relevant (78%). It has been estimated that the number of pending studies grew by 50%, while the number of delayed studied increased by more than 80% [30].

6. Another example of criticism in paediatric drugs availability deals with rare diseases: both in EU and in the U.S, very few medicinal products for rare diseases affecting children have a paediatric indication[12]. As a consequence, in the U.S. (but not in EU), specific orphan

11 http://bpca.nichd.nih.gov/collaborativeefforts/initiatives/pages/index.aspx

12 data deriving from EuOrphan, a database of EU and U.S. orphan drugs hosted by Gianni Benzi Foundation

programs for paediatrics have been recently proposed (Rare Pediatric Disease Priority Review Voucher Program). The first voucher was awarded under this program in February 2014, but it is still too early to measure the impact.

7. Finally, a lack of appropriate measures to incentive paediatric research has been observed especially in EU. As already mentioned, the PUMA has been unsuccessful until now and, despite the positive results achieved by the projects for the development of off-patent drugs, the specific funding programme setup from 2007 to 2013 under the EU Seventh Framework Programme has not been renewed in Horizon 2020.

On the basis of these few considerations, EU and U.S. regulators should continue to discuss coordinated approaches and to share results.

In particular, these efforts should be concentrate to minimize unnecessary paediatric trials and to optimize trial design, so that the limited paediatric populations available are enrolled only in ethically implemented, scientifically important trials.

## Acknowledgements

This project has received funding from the European Union's Seventh Framework Programme for research, technological development and demonstration under grant agreement n° 261060 - GRiP (Global Research in Paediatrics).

## Author details

Adriana Ceci[1*], Viviana Giannuzzi[1], Donato Bonifazi[2], Mariagrazia Felisi[2], Fedele Bonifazi[2] and Lucia Ruggieri[3]

*Address all correspondence to: adriceci.uni@gmail.com

1 Fondazione per la Ricerca Farmacologica Gianni Benzi onlus, Valenzano, Italy

2 Consorzio per Valutazioni Biologiche e Farmacologiche, Pavia, Italy

3 Gruppo Italiano per gli Studi di Farmacoeconomia, Pavia, Italy

## References

[1] U.S. Code 21 CFR Part 201, Specific Requirements on Content and Format of Labeling for Human Prescription Drugs; Revision of "Pediatric Use" Subsection in the Labeling; Final Rule, December 13, 1994 (FR 59 64240).

[2] European Parliament and Council of the European Union. Regulation (EC) No 1901/2006 of 12 December 2006 on medicinal products for paediatric use and amending Regulation (EEC) No 1768/92, Directive 2001/20/EC, Directive 2001/83/EC and Regulation (EC) No 726/2004. Official Journal of the European Union, 2006,L 378/1.

[3] EMA/PDCO 5-year Report to the European Commission General report on the experience acquired as a result of the application of the Paediatric Regulation (2012) EMA/428172/2012.

[4] European Parliament and the Council of the European Union. Directive 2001/20/EC of 4 April 2001 on the approximation of the laws, regulations and administrative provisions of the Member States relating to the implementation of good clinical practice in the conduct of clinical trials on medicinal products for human use. Official Journal L121, 01/05/2001.

[5] European Parliament and Council of the European Union. Regulation (Eu) No 536/2014 Of The European Parliament And Of The Council of 16 April 2014 on clinical trials on medicinal products for human use, and repealing Directive 2001/20/EC. Official Journal of the European Union, 2014, L158.

[6] Food and Drugs Administration, Food Safety Modernization Act (FSMA) of 1997 P.L. 105-115 111 Stat. 2296

[7] Food and Drugs Administration, Best Pharmaceuticals for Children Act (BPCA) of 2002 P. L. 107-109. Stat. 1789

[8] Food and Drugs Administration, Paediatric Research Equity Act (PREA) of 2003 P. L. 108-155. Stat. S 650

[9] European Parliament and Council of the European Union. Directive 2005/28/EC of 8 April 2005 laying down principles and detailed guidelines for good clinical practice as regards investigational medicinal products for human use, as well as the requirements for authorisation of the manufacturing or importation of such products. Official Journal of the European Union, 2005, L91.

[10] European Medicines Agency. ICH Topic E 6 (R1): Guideline for Good Clinical Practice. CPMP/ICH/135/95. July 2002.

[11] European Parliament and Council of the European Union. Regulation (EC) No 726/2004 of 31 March 2004 laying down Community procedures for the authorisation and supervision of medicinal products for human and veterinary use and establishing a European Medicines Agency. Official Journal of the European Union, 2006,L 136/1.

[12] Altavilla A, Giaquinto C, Giocanti D, Manfredi C, Aboulker JP, Bartoloni F, et al. Activity of ethics committees in Europe on issues related to clinical trials in paediatrics: Results of a survey. Pharmaceuticals Policy and Law. 2009; 11(1.2):79-87.

[13] European Commission. Ethical Considerations for Clinical Trials on medicinal products conducted with the paediatric population - Recommendations of the Ad Hoc

Group for the development of implementing guidelines for Directive 2001/20/EC relating to good clinical practice in the conduct of clinical trials on medicinal products for human use, 2008.

[14] Code of Federal Regulations, Title 45 Public Welfare Department of Health and Human Services Part 46 Protection of Human Subjects, 2009.

[15] European Commission, Proposal for a Regulation of the European Parliament and of the Council on clinical trials on medicinal products for human use, and repealing Directive 2001/20/EC (COM(2012) 369 final), 17.7.2012

[16] Altavilla A, Giaquinto C, Ceci A. European survey on ethical and legal framework of clinical trials in paediatrics: results and perspectives. J Int Bioethique. 2008; 19(3): p. 17-48.

[17] European Commission. Communication from the Commission — Guideline on the format and content of applications for agreement or modification of a paediatric investigation plan and requests for waivers or deferrals and concerning the operation of the compliance check and on criteria for assessing significant studies (2014/C 338/01).

[18] Food and Drugs Administration, Guidance for Industry Pediatric Study Plans: FDA, July 2013.

[19] European Medicines Agency. ICH Topic E 11. Clinical Investigation of Medicinal Products in the Paediatric Population Note for guidance on clinical investigation of medicinal products in the paediatric population (CPMP/ICH/2711/99).

[20] De Cock RF, Piana C, Krekels EH, Danhof M, Allegaert K, Knibbe CA. The role of population PK-PD modelling in paediatric clinical research. Eur J Clin Pharmacol. 2011 May;67 Suppl 1:5-16.

[21] Knibbe C, Della Pasqua O, Danhof M. Personal communication: Introduction to population PKPD modelling in paediatric paediatric clinical pharmacology. Available at: http://www.ema.europa.eu/docs/en_GB/document_library/Presentation/2009/11/WC500009645.pdf

[22] Ceci A, Catapano M, Manfredi C, Wong I et al. Drug Development – A Case Study Based Insight into Modern Strategies, edited by Chris Rundfeldt, p.cm. ISBN 978-953-307-257-9.

[23] Dunne J. et al. Globalization Facilitates Pediatric Drug Development in the 21st Century, Drug Information Journal, Vol. 44, pp. 757–765, 2010.

[24] Pasquali S. et al. Globalization of Paediatric Research, Paediatrics Vol 126: September 2010.

[25] Ruggieri L, Giannuzzi V, Baiardi P, Bonifazi F, Davies EH, Giaquinto C, Bonifazi D, Felisi M, Chiron C, Pressler R, Rabe H, Whitaker MJ, Neubert A, Jacqz-Aigrain E, Eichler I, Turner MA, Ceci A; on behalf of the GRiP Consortium. Successful private-

public funding of paediatric medicines research: lessons from the EU programme to fund research into off-patent medicines. Eur J Pediatr. 2014 Sep 23.

[26] General report on experience acquired as a result of the application of the Paediatric Regulation, summary of the replies to the public consultation, Brussels, SANCO/D5/FS/ci D(2013) 27105

[27] Boots I, Sukhai RN, Klein RH, Holl RA, Wit JM, Cohen AF, Burggraaf J.Stimulation programs for pediatric drug research – do children really benefit? Eur J Pediatr. 2007 Aug;166(8):849-55. Epub 2007 Jan 17.

[28] European Medicines Agency/Paediatric Committee (2007-2013) priority list for studies on off-patent paediatric medicinal products

[29] Institute of Medicine. Safe and Effective Medicines for Children: Studies Conducted Under the Best Pharmaceuticals for Children Act and the Pediatric Research Equity Act. Washington, DC: National Academies Press; 2012.

[30] Outcomes of Written Requests, Requirements, Studies, and Labeling Changes Cover of Safe and Effective Medicines for Children in "Safe and Effective Medicines for Children: Pediatric Studies Conducted Under the Best Pharmaceuticals for Children Act and the Pediatric Research Equity Act." Committee on Pediatric Studies Conducted Under the Best Pharmaceuticals for Children Act (BPCA) and the Pediatric Research Equity Act (PREA); Board on Health Sciences Policy; Institute of Medicine; Field MJ, Boat TF, editors. Washington (DC): National Academies Press (US); 2012 Feb 29

7

# Targeting Bacterial Persistence to Develop Therapeutics Against Infectious Disease

Elizabeth Hong-Geller and Sofiya N. Micheva-Viteva

## 1. Introduction

The application of the prototype antibiotics penicillin and streptomycin to bacterial infection in the 1940's marked a historic milestone in medicine and heralded a new era of antimicrobial therapy as the modern standard for infectious disease management. Yet, even in those early days of discovery, scientist Joseph Bigger noted an unexplained phenomenon. Although penicillin treatment of *Staphylococcus aureus* infection killed the great majority of the bacterial population, a small subset of cells (~1 in $10^5$) continued to persist and remained recalcitrant to antibiotic-mediated killing.[1] When re-grown in the absence of antibiotic, the bacterial community once again became sensitive to antibiotic-mediated killing and resembled the original culture (~1 in $10^5$ persisters), providing conclusive proof that these organisms were not drug-resistant strains that had evolved via genetic mutations (in which case all bacteria in the final population would be drug-resistant). (Fig. 1) Instead, persister cells are phenotypic variants that are genetically identical to the susceptible bacterial population, but have modified their physiology to survive environmental stress. These bacteria exhibit antibiotic tolerance that is non-heritable and reversible upon removal of the antibiotic, a completely different phenomenon than the more well-studied antibiotic resistance mechanisms mediated by genetic mutation. Persistence is akin to a community "insurance policy" in which surviving persister cells hedge against unlikely but catastrophic events, while still maintaining near optimal growth at the population level.[2, 3]

In this review, we will discuss the known molecular mechanisms that underlie bacterial persistence, the impact of persistence on infectious disease, and the different strategies that are being developed to target persisters in disease. The human toll of pathogen infection has been compounded by the rampant use of antibiotics in the last half-century, leading to the rapid evolution of drug-resistant strains to practically every approved antibiotic. There is a

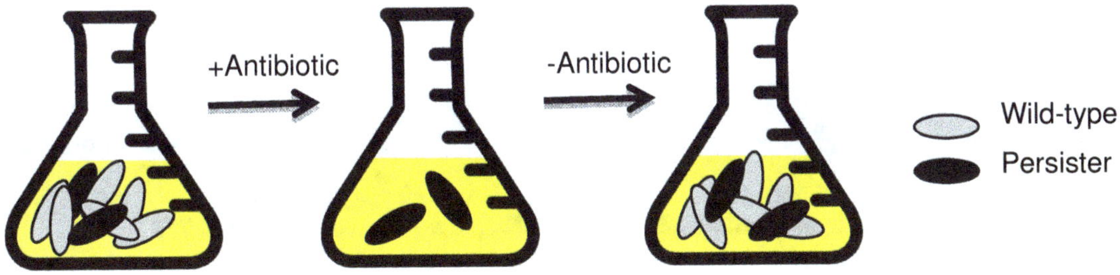


**Figure 1.** Bacterial persisters are recalcitrant to antiiotic killing. After removal of antibiotic, bacterial community expands to contain both wild-type and persister sub-groups, indicating that the persisters are phenotypic variants instead of containing genetic mutations.

great public health need to identify novel strategies for development of therapeutics to treat pathogen infection. Development of novel therapies that either kill persisters directly or stimulate their reversion to logarithmic growth may effectively reduce disease relapse and shorten the treatment period.[4] It may be the case that a combination therapy comprised of conventional antibiotics that kill replicating pathogens and new drugs that target the metabolically-inactive persisters can also reduce the rate of emergence of antibiotic resistance.

## 2. Impact of bacterial persistence on infectious disease

Without question, bacterial persistence greatly contributes to the burden of infectious disease, where persisters survive antibiotic treatment to re-infect patients in a frustrating cycle of chronic infection. Many antibiotics have been shown to be only active against dividing bacteria.[5] Persisters are thought to be dormant cells that greatly slow down essential cellular functions that antibiotics generally target, including trancription, translation, cell wall synthesis, and DNA replication. Persisters are found at relatively higher levels in stationary phase compared to logarithmic cultures, consistent with a dormant state. The persistence state has been found in many different bacterial species, including *E. coli*, *Mycobacterium tuberculosis*, and *Pseudomonas aeruginosa*, underscoring the evolution of persistence as a survival strategy in different stressful environments.[6]

There is also increasing evidence that persisters mediate drug tolerance in biofilm formation associated with chronic diseases, including endocarditis, gingivitis, and osteomyelitis.[7] Biofilms form a protective environment for persisters, shielding them from the host immune system.[8] (Fig. 2) Biofilms can form readily on in-dwelling devices, such as catheters and prostheses, or on physiological surfaces, such as *P. aeruginosa* infection of the lung in cystic fibrosis patients. The dormancy of persisters and the different pathways that lead to their formation contribute to the unique challenge in treatment of chronic infections, especially in immunocompromised patients where biofilms can form deep in the soft tissues. In addition, the presence of different subpopulations of persistent pathogens with varying antiobiotic susceptibilities further complicates treatment with optimizing drug efficiencies.

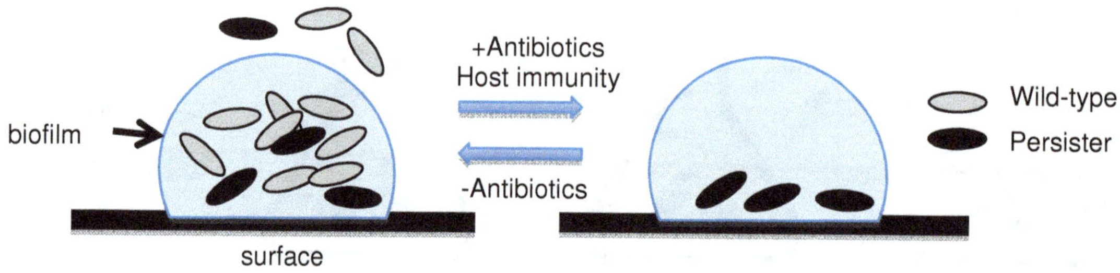


**Figure 2.** Biofilm formation with persisters. Biofilms can contain both wild-type replicating and persister cells. Addition of antibiotics and host immunity can kill both wild-type and persister cells in the biofilm and extracellular milieu. The biofilm matrix can protect persisters from killing and can lead to re-population of pathogen in the biofilm after antibiotics are removed.

## 3. Molecular mechanisms of bacterial persistence

Despite observance of the persister phenotype since the 1940's, the genetic regulatory pathways that switch bacteria into the persister phenotype remain poorly understood. Further research on bacterial persistence rapidly declined with the availability of potent antibiotics. Furthermore, there were technical difficulties in obtaining sufficient numbers of persister cells for analysis and a lack of sophisticated and sensitive methods to study rare biological events at single cell resolution. With the recent emergence of antibiotic-resistant bacterial strains, interest in the mechanisms of bacterial persistence has slowly resurged, amid rapid advances in microfluidics and advanced imaging that can be applied to single cell analysis. [9, 10] A list of genes and pathways linked to persistence is listed in Table 1.

In the 1980's, a genetic screen was performed to select for *E. coli* mutants that exhibited increased persistence in response to ampicillin exposure.[11] *hipA* (high persistence) was the first gene identified that modulated the frequency of persister formation, with the gain-of-function allele *hipA7* inducing ~1% persisters in culture, an ~1000 fold increase in persisters compared to a wild-type strain. HipA is a component of a toxin-antitoxin (TA) module that plays a role in inhibition of protein and nucleic acid synthesis in response to stress. HipA functions as a kinase that phosphorylates the essential translation factor Elongation Factor Tu (EF-Tu) to inhibit translation.[12]

The increased level of persister cells has led to the use of *hipA* mutants in multiple studies on bacterial persistence, including integration of microfluidics and single cell microscopy[13] and microarray analysis.[14] These types of studies can enable quantitative analysis of single cell behavior and gene expression dynamics to measure cell-to-cell heterogeneity in a clonal cell population. For example, growth patterns of fluorescently-labeled *E. coli hipA* mutants in the channels of a microfluidic device suggested that slow-growing persister cells were already present in the bacterial culture prior to antibiotic exposure, suggesting that the persistent state may partially stem from stochastic mechanisms.[13] This study led to the identification of two different persister types. Type I persisters are non-growing cells that enter at stationary phase, a dormant state that protects them from the lethal action of several antibiotics known to affect mainly actively growing cells. Type II persisters do not require a starvation signal to enter the persister state and are continuously generated during exponential growth in a fashion that seems to depend on the population size. Although Type I and II persisters exist in wild-type populations of *E. coli*, their differentiation has only been achieved using time lapse single cell microscopy. Bacterial cells were also shown to still express proteins for a short period of time prior to entering into full dormancy, indicating a gradual downregulation of essential cellular processes during switching to the persistence state.[15]

While HipA contributes to persistence in *E. coli*, the absence or poor conservation of *hipA* in other bacteria that have exhibited persistence suggested the existence of other persistence mechanisms. Several other genetic screens have led to identification of additional metabolic genes that function in cell dormancy, including GlpD[16], an enzyme that functions in glycerol-3-phosphate metabolism, PhoU[17], a negative regulator that inhibits energy metabolism and nutrient transport, the global regulators DksA and DnaKJ[18], and the HipA-like toxin proteins RelE and MazF.[19 - 21] Transient ectopic overexpression of chaperone DnaJ and PmrC were also shown to increase the number of persisters by up to 1000-fold.[19]

There is also increasing evidence that bacterial communication via chemical signaling may play a role in establishing persistence. Recently, indole signaling has been implicated in triggering persistence, leading to enhancement of persister formation in *E. coli* by ~10-fold in response to multiple antibiotics.[22] This indole signaling is dependent on activation of the OxyR and phage-shock pathways and enables the bacterial community to alter its frequency of persistence as a survival mechanism. Another mediator of bacterial cell-cell communications, the quorum-sensing peptide CSP pheromone was also implicated in the formation of stress-induced multidrug-tolerant persisters in the oral pathogen *Streptococcus mutans*, the leading etiological agent of dental biofilm.[23] In addition, gaseous ammonia released by stationary phase bacterial cultures was found to modify the antibiotic resistance spectrum of bacterial neighbors.[24] Ammonia release increases the level of intracellular polyamines, which modulates membrane permeability to different antibiotics.

These results suggest that persisters may form through independent parallel mechanisms and do not follow a single linear regulatory pathway. The underlying commonality is that each of these mechanisms leads to a small subset of quiescent or slowly-dividing cells within an otherwise rapidly dividing population. The fact that the great majority of candidate persister genes have been identified in *E. coli* leaves open the question of whether persistence mechanisms are universal or species-specific. For example, *P. aeruginosa* infection in cystic fibrosis patients is thought to be exacerbated by persister cells in biofilm formation and subsequent recalcitrance to antibiotic treatment.[25] However, the majority the *E. coli* persister gene candidates do not have confirmed homologs in *P. aeruginosa*. An independent screen of a transposon insertion library from *P. aeruginosa* identified a separate list of genes, including a putative DNA helicase and type IV pilus response regulator, as putative persister genes.[26] Another study developed computational algorithms based on systems biology data such as transcriptomics profiles and functional interactions networks to predict novel *M. tuberculosis* genes required for long-term persistence in mouse lungs.[27] In this study, 18 novel genes were experimentally validated to play a role in persistence. To date, clear understanding of the molecular mechanisms that regulate persister formation has yet to emerge.

| Key gene/pathway | Mechanism | Ref |
|---|---|---|
| Toxin/antitoxin | | |
| HipA/B | Kinase that phosphorylates EF-Tu | [11-12] |
| RelE | Ribosome-dependent endonuclease | [20] |
| RelA | (p)ppGpp synthetase | [35-36] |
| TisB | Antimicrobial peptide that opens membrane channel | [38-40] |
| MazF | Endonuclease | [21] |
| Other genes | | |
| GlpD | Glycerol-3-phosphate metabolism | [16] |
| PhoU | Negative regulator of energy metabolism | [17] |
| DksA | Transcriptional regulator of rRNA | [18] |
| DnaKJ | Chaperone | [18] |
| PmrC | Transfer of phosphoethanolamine to lipidA | [19] |
| DinG | DNA helicase in *P. aeruginosa* | [26] |
| PilH | Type IV pilus response regulator in *P. aeruginosa* | [26] |
| Other molecules | | |
| Indole | Activation of OxyR and phage-shock pathways | [22] |
| CSP | Quorom-sensing peptide | [23] |
| Ammonia gas | Increase in intracellular polyamines | [24] |

**Table 1.** Selected molecular pathways that lead to bacterial persistence

## 4. Toxin/Anti-toxin (TA) modules

One common gene family that has been linked to bacterial persistence is the TA loci, which function in adaptation to rapidly changing environmental conditions in many bacteria and Archaea.[28] TA modules are present in the genome of diverse bacteria, with more than 50 modules in *Mycobacterium tuberculosis*, a pathogen that enters dormancy as part of its disease lifecycle. Type II TA modules typically encode for a pair of co-transcribed stress-inducible proteins, a stable toxin that inhibits cell growth, and a more labile anti-toxin that regulates the activity of its cognate toxin. (Fig. 3) The toxin and anti-toxin form a tight complex and repress their own expression. Depletion of the anti-toxin leads to release of its cognate toxin, which interferes with an essential cellular target, such as mRNA, DNA gyrase, or DNA helicase, to induce cell cycle arrest or inhibit metabolic functions. There are three types of antitoxins: type I TA antitoxins encode small antisense RNAs that repress toxin gene translation, type II loci encode protein antitoxins, and type III loci express small RNA antitoxins.[29 - 31] It should be noted that the term 'toxin' can be considered a misnomer, since the toxin genes do not kill the bacteria, but rather repress cell growth.

Since the initial mapping of the *hipA* toxin to a TA locus, several other studies have linked TA function to bacterial persistence. *E. coli* becomes dormant if toxin levels exceed a specific threshold, with the amount determining the length of time bacteria remains in dormancy.[32] Persister cells increased their TA expression levels, and deletion of ten TA loci that encoded for mRNA endonucleases in *E. coli* led to a marked reduction in frequency of persister formation.[33] Furthermore, overexpression of the toxin can induce a persistence state from which cells can be resuscitated by expression of anti-toxin gene transcription.[34] This evidence supports a model in which TA loci play a key role in switching on the persistence state in response to environmental stressors.

Other TA loci, in addition to *hipA/B*, have been implicated in mediating persistence. For example, the toxin RelA has been shown to be required for the long-term survival and persistence of *M. tuberculosis* in mice.[35] Interestingly, RelA encodes for (p)ppGpp synthetase, which functions in the synthesis of (p)ppGpp, or guanosine tetra-and pentaphosphate, a signaling molecule that has been shown to be indicative of the persistent state.[36] (p)ppGpp is a central mediator of the stringent response, which modulates cell expression to survive stress and nutrient limitations.[37] Persisters exhibit relatively higher levels of (p)ppGpp, which is consistent with the slowed growth rate and metabolically inactive state in persisters. Damage of DNA induces the SOS response and expression of the TisB toxin, an endogenous antimicrobial peptide that causes persister formation by opening an ion channel.[38 - 40] This decreases the proton motive force and ATP levels, leading to target shutdown and a dormant, drug-tolerant state.

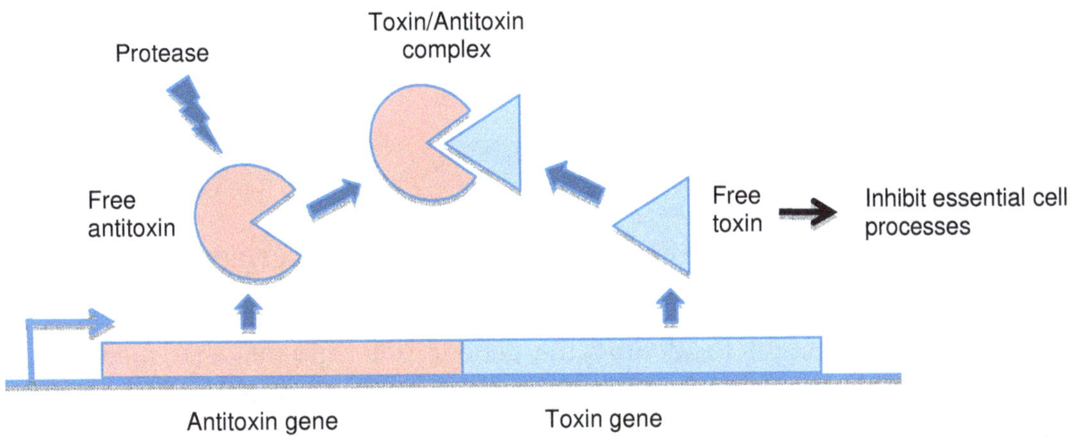


**Figure 3.** Co-expression and regulation of the TA loci. The anti-toxin regulates toxin activity by forming a tight complex with the toxin. The antitoxin is generally produced at a higher rate than the toxin and is degraded by cellular proteases.

Since both toxin and anti-toxin transcripts are co-expressed from a single promoter, the imbalance between the two transcripts is primarily caused by accumulation of specific proteases, such as the Lon protease in *E. coli*, that target the anti-toxin for degradation. Deletion of *lon*, but not other protease-encoding genes, led to a decrease in persistence, indicating that Lon plays in specific role in induction of persistence.[33] Lon was also identified in a screen of a *P. aeruginosa* PAO1 luciferase fusion library as a differentially-regulated gene upon exposure to a sub-inhibitory concentration of gentamicin and was shown to be essential for biofilm formation.[41]

## 5. Isolation of bulk and single cell persisters

Persisters are a difficult cell population to manipulate, due to their transient nature, low frequency, and mechanistic heterogeneity. A variety of methods have been utilized for persister enrichment and have leveraged *hipA* mutant *E. coli* strains as the starting material to maximize persister numbers. Persister cells have been isolated based on sedimentation of surviving cells following antibiotic treatment.[3, 14] Transcriptomics profiling from the persister population indicated that genes involved in energy production were downregulated, consistent with a dormant phenotype. However, since each antibiotic and microbe exhibits unique killing and survival kinetics, respectively, treatment to isolate persisters is highly dependent on the individual system. Prolonged exposure to antibiotic agents may also activate stress response mechansims, which have been recently linked to induction of persistence. Another isolation method utilized an *E. coli* strain expressing a green fluorescent protein (GFP) reporter fused to a ribosomal RNA promoter *rrnBP1*.[42] Since persisters display low metabolic activty, sorting of dimly green cells by FACS will concentrate persisters that exhibit little of no transcription from the *rrnBP1* promoter. Finally, persisters have also been isolated by using a combination of alkaline and enzymatic lysis that targets the cell membrane and kills normally growing cells.[43] This strategy took 25 min compared to >3 hrs for previous methods and hence is less likely to induce a stable stress response. Furthermore, persisters isolated with this protocol did not exhibit activation of the SOS response, indicating that stress response was not activated.

## 6. Therapeutic strategies that target bacterial persistence

Initially, investigators sought to identify the genetic determinants that mediate persister formation as potential targets to prevent or reverse persistence. Given the number of disparate genes that appear to be involved in persistence, such an approach may prove to be difficult. Nevertheless, identification of bacterial proteins that are essential even in persisters can provide novel targets for drug development. Since persisters exist in a slowed metabolic state, it is likely that changes in environmental parameters can shift pathogen metabolism from persistence to a replicating state. In the last several years, compounds have been identified that have exhibited promise in the switching of persisters into growing cells susceptible to antibiotic killing or in the direct killing of persisters. (Table 2) These strategies can be integrated with current antibiotics regimens to develop novel viable therapies for treatment of infectious disease.

### 6.1. Metabolite stimulation of aminoglycoside-mediated bacterial killing

A promising strategy for the eradication of persistent bacteria is the combination of an antibiotic that kills actively replicating bacteria with a metabolite that may enhance the susceptibility of the persistent bacteria to antibiotics. An elegant example of this strategy was the addition of metabolites to stimulate cellular metabolism and switch *E. coli* and *S. aureus* persisters back to the wild-type state to be susceptible to aminoglycosides.[44] Multiple carbon sources that maximize coverage of glycolysis, the pentose-phosphate pathway and the Entner-Doudoroff pathway were tested for their ability to potentiate aminoglycosides against *E. coli* persisters. Metabolites that enter upper glycolysis, including glucose, mannitol, and fructose, and one that enters lower glycolysis, pyruvate, led to a reduction in persister viability in response to the aminoglycoside gentamicin, by three orders of magnitude. Other metabolites that enter the latter two pathways (e.g. arabinose and ribose) did not have a significant effect on persister death. This potentiation was found to be specific to aminoglycosides, and did not occur in persisters exposed to quinolone or β-lactam antibiotics, which target DNA and the cell wall, respectively. The metabolic stimuli were found to generate a proton-motive force (PMF), which facilitates aminoglycoside uptake and subsequent bacterial killing. Treatment of persisters with an inhibitor of PMF, the ionophore CCCP, abolished aminoglycoside potentiation by the metabolite/gentamicin treatment. These results indicate that persisters, although dormant, are nevertheless primed for metabolic uptake and energy metabolism.

In both an *E. coli* biofilm model and a chronic biofilm-associated infection in mice, a combination of mannitol and gentamicin reduced biofilm viability by several orders of magnitude compared to antibiotic alone. In the infected mice, the dual treatment inhibited bacterial spread to the kidneys, compared to no treatment or antibiotic alone, demonstrating the feasibility for potential clinical use. Metabolite-enabled killing of persisters was also shown to be effective in the Gram-positive pathogen *Staphylococcus aureus*, although with fructose as the most effective metabolite, due to the differential expression of metabolite transporters in *S. aureus*. Thus, delivery of PMF-stimulating metabolites may be a novel strategy to complement current aminoglycoside treatments to generate more effective antibacterial therapies.

### 6.2. Hyperactivation of ClpP protease kills persisters

Modulation of target protein function that is lethal for microbes is a novel approach for persister cell elimination. In a recent paper, activation of the ClpP protease by the antibiotic acyldepsipeptide 4 (ADEP4) was shown to kill persister cells by degrading over 400 cellular proteins.[45] ADEP exhibits anti-bacterial activity against Gram-positive bacteria *in vitro* and in several rodent models of bacterial infection.[46] ClpP is a proteolytic subunit that normally pairs with different ATPase regulatory subunits to degrade misfolded proteins in the bacterial cytoplasm. Binding of ADEP to ClpP maintains the catalytic chamber of ClpP in an open configuration to enable promiscuous cleavage of proteins and decouple protein degradation from dependence on ATP hydrolysis. Null mutants of *clpP* were resistant to ADEP4, but were found to be highly resistant to killing by multiple antibiotics. This uncontrolled proteolysis ultimately resulted in bacterial autolysis and cell death. Treatment with ADEP4 exhibited a decrease in cell count of *S. aureus* stationary cells by 4 $\log_{10}$ in two days. Conventional antibiotics, including rifampicin, linezolid, and ciprofloxacin, were inactive against stationary phase *S. aureus*. However, treatment with a combination of ADEP4 and a conventional antibiotic led to eradication of *S. aureus* persisters in growing and stationary cultures. Furthermore, this combination treatment cleared a chronic biofilm infection in a mouse model that was previously untreatable with just conventional antibiotics.[45] These studies demonstrate that persisters are not invulnerable to killing and that ADEP4 is an effective antibiotic against persisters in a deep-seated biofilm infection. Conventional antibiotics were likely not effective against persisters due to pathogen tolerance rather than the inability to diffuse within the biofilm.

| Compound | Mechanism | Ref |
|---|---|---|
| Metabolites (e.g. mannitol, fructose) | Metabolite stimulation to generate a proton-motive force for aminoglycoside-mediated killing | [44] |
| ADEP4 | Activation of the Clp protease to promiscuously cleave target proteins in persisters | [45] |
| HT61 | Drug compound depolarizes and breaks down bacterial cell wall | [47] |
| C10 | Drug compound killed persisters in combination with antibiotics | [48] |
| Pyrazinamide | Byproduct pyrazinoic acid activates multiple essential cellular processes | [53] |
| Diarlyquinolines (TMC207) | Inhibitor of ATP synthase to block energy metabolism in TB | [55] |
| Imidazopyridines<br>Benzimidazoles<br>Thiopenes | Drug compounds that reduced ATP content in both replicating and persistent Mycobacteria | [58] |
| Muropeptides | Activation of PrkC to stimulate translation | [60] |
| Rpf (Resuscitation promotion factor) | Degradation of peptidoglycan as mediators to induce cell growth | [61] |

**Table 2.** Strategies to defeat bacterial persistence

### 6.3. Drug screening against metabolically-inactive bacteria

Small molecule library screens have been performed to identify compounds that specifically target persisters. A quinolone-derived library was screened against non-multiplying *S. aureus* using a long-term stationary phase culture.[47] One compound in particular, termed HT61, exhibited 6 logs killing compared to 1 log for commercially-available antibiotics, such as amoxicillin and linezolid, in *S. aureus* persisters and clinical methillicin-resistant *S. aureus* strains. HT61 acts via depolarization of the bacterial cell membrane and subsequent breakdown of the cell wall. HT61 also displayed significant bactericidal effects against other Gram positive pathogens, including *Streptococcus pyogenes* and *Streptococcus agalactiae*, but was less potent for actively-replicating *S. aureus* and not effective against Gram negative bacteria such as *E. coli* and *Klebsiella aerogenes*. In a mouse skin bacterial colonization model, HT61 effectively killed surface *S. aureus* and did not induce adverse effects in a minipig skin model. Importantly, HT61-resistant *S. aureus* were not detected even after 50 passages of exposure, suggesting that compounds that target persisters may bypass development of antibiotic resistance in normally replicating bacteria.

Another screen was performed to identify compounds from a library composed of 6800 chemicals, based on scaffolds and physicochemical properties, that can effectively kill persisters.[48] Compounds were downselected based on enhanced killing of *E. coli* K-12 in combination with both ampicillin and norfloxacin, two antibiotics with different mechanisms of action. In particular, one compound denoted C10, 3-[4-(4-methoxyphenyl)piperazin-1-yl]piperidin-4-yl biphenyl-4-carboxylate, exhibited a marked decrease in *E. coli* and *Pseudomonas aeroginosa* persistence frequency in combination with fluoroquinolone antibiotics, but did not affect normal antibiotic-sensitive cells. While persisters were killed when treated with a combination of C10 and norfloxacin, they also exhibited fast re-growth in the presence of C10 alone, suggesting that C10 may induce reversion of dormant persisters into replicating antibiotic-sensitive cells. It will be necessary to identify the binding target of C10 to more fully understand the mechanism of action on bacterial persistence.

### 6.4. Combination therapy to treat tuberculosis

Combination treatments that target both replicating and persistent bacteria will likely prove to be an effective strategy to combat chronic infections. A good example of this approach is the multiple drug treatment of tuberculosis (TB), a global disease mediated by *Mycobacterium tuberculosis,* that causes ~2 million deaths per year. Dormant TB can survive within a host for decades, thus requiring long-term treatment. Treatment of active *M. tuberculosis* by a front-line cocktail of four drugs, isozianid, rifampicin, pyrazinamide, and ethambutol, can be effective in controlling the disease in the first several months. Isoniazid is effective against rapidly growing bacilli in lesions, whereas rifampicin and pyrazinamide are thought to be more effective in killing persistent bacilli.[49] These persistent bacilli localize in macrophages within tissue cavities. Upon exposure in a low $O_2$ (hypoxic) and nutrient environment, they enter a low-metabolic, dormant state by downregulation of protein and nucleic acid synthesis and formation of a thick cell wall. TB persister cells escape both host immune detection and killing by isoniazid, which can lead to disease relapse upon exit out of the dormant state in the host.

Interestingly, the mechanism of action of the front-line drug pyrazinamide, known for >50 yrs, has only recently been deciphered. Pyrazinamide is activated by a mycobacterial amidase to yield the bioactive compound pyrazinoic acid, which has been linked to multiple essential cellular processes, including ribosome function[50], fatty acid synthase II[51], and respiratory activity.[52] Trapping of pyrazinoic acid in the cell leads to a rise in acidity, which kills the pathogen.[53] Other existing antibiotics, such as moxifloxacin and gatifloxacin, have also been shown to enhance rates of *M. tuberculosis* persister death when combined with conventional drug treatments.[54]

Although in a latent state, *M. tuberculosis* still performs respiratory energy conversion to maintain requisite metabolic functions, providing a potential target for novel drug development. Dormant mycobacteria were found to express a functional ATP synthase to generate energy that drives basal cellular reactions. A newly-discovered inhibitor of ATP synthase, diarylquinoline TMC207, was recently identified as a potent anti-mycobacterial compound against replicating *M. tuberculosis*.[55] Significantly, nanomolar concentrations of TMC207 were able to kill dormant pathogen by blocking ATP synthase activity at a higher efficacy than observed for replicating mycobacteria, despite ATP synthase being transcriptionally downregulated in latent *M. tuberculosis*.[56] TMC207 also exhibited potent sterilization in an infected lung mouse model, comparable to the triple drug combination of rifampicin, isozianid, and pyrazinamide. The high efficacy of TMC207 may stem from killing of both actively-growing and dormant pathogen. These results suggest that basal ATP synthase activity is essential for the survival of dormant *M. tuberculosis,* and ATP homeostasis may represent a viable target for development of persister-directed drugs. TMC207 is presently in Phase II clinical trials for TB treatment. Furthermore, medicinal chemistry optimization efforts led to generation of novel diarylquinoline chemotypes that targeted Gram-positive pathogens, including *S. aureus* in replicating planktonic and metabolically resting biofilm states, potentially broadening the antibacterial spectrum of diarylquinoline-based antibiotics.[57]

To further identify novel inhibitors against dormant mycobacteria, a hypoxic model system was established to screen >600,000 compounds for those that lowered ATP content in a non-replicating *M. bovis* BCG recombinant strain.[58] The screen yielded 140 non-cytotoxic compounds, including imidazopyridines, benzimidazoles, and thiopenes, which modulated respiratory function against both replicating and non-replicating mycobacteria. Reduction of cellular ATP levels was shown to correlate with cell death in bacteria treated with the three compound clusters. Thus, these clusters may form the basis of antibiotic compound development against mycobacteria.

### 6.5. Bacterial factors that trigger exit from dormancy

Sporulation is another form of persistence in which both pathogen and environmental microbes enter a metabolically-inactive state and become resistant spores under unfavorable conditions. For example, in nutrient-poor environments, *Bacillus* and *Clostridium* species undergo tightly regulated transcriptional and morphological changes to form a dormant but robust spore that is resistant to extreme stress conditions, such as high temperatures, desiccation, and toxicity. In the laboratory, *Bacillus subtilis* spores have been shown to germinate and exit the spore state in response to treatment with various nutrients, such as amino acids.[59] Binding of these nutrients to receptors on the inner membrane of the spore leads to rehydration of the cell interior and breakdown of the peptidoglycan spore layer. *B. subtilis* has also been shown to exit dormancy in response to peptidoglycan-derived muropeptides, consisting of a disaccharide-tripeptide with a meso-diaminopimelic acid (m-DAP) residue in the third position.[60] Peptidoglycan from growing cells, but not stationary cells, have been shown to more effectively induce germination, suggesting that these muropeptides may function as signaling molecules that can stimulate dormant cells. In response to muropeptide binding to its extracellular domain, the serine/threonine kinase PrkC has been shown to phosphorylate elongation factor G (EF-G), which modulates ribosomal activity and initiation of translation to induce microbial exit from dormancy.[60]

Other protein factors expressed by microbes have been reported to stimulate growth of dormant cells. The environmental microbe, *Micrococcus luteus*, secretes a resuscitation-promoting factor (Rpf), which can stimulate exit from dormancy when added to *M. luteus* cultures.[61] *M. luteus* Rpf has been shown to hydrolyze peptidoglycan at picomolar concentrations and stimulate aged cultures of *M. tuberculosis*, thus exhibiting cross-species activity.[62, 63] *M. tuberculosis* expresses five endogenous Rpfs that function in reactivation of chronic tuberculosis in animal models.[64] Although the exact function of Rpfs remains unclear, it has been suggested that Rpf-mediated proteolysis of peptidoglycan can generate muropeptides for PrkC-like kinases to activate protein translation.[65]

## 7. Conclusion

The rise in antimicrobial drug resistance, alongside the failure of conventional research efforts to discover new antibiotics, will eventually lead to a public health crisis that can drastically curtail our ability to combat infectious disease. Bacterial persistence is an underexplored mechanism by which to develop novel treatments to complement or extend the current repertoire of antibiotics.[66 - 68] Although persisters do not cause overt disease, they act as a pool from which bacteria can emerge from dormancy to cause recurrent infection. Mechanisms of persister formation appear to be highly redundant across different bacterial species, which contributes to the difficulty in identification of universal mechanisms to target and eradicate persistence. To date, the more successful strategies in the lab have been to target cell functions, such as basal energy metabolism and cell wall integrity, that are also essential for persister cell maintenance.[69] Of particular note, addition of metabolites such as mannitol or fructose was shown to potentiate aminoglycoside-mediated killing by generating a proton motive force to stimulate aminoglycoside uptake.[44] Several medicinal chemistry strategies to screen for small molecules effective against persisters have also identified lead targets for potential optimization and rational drug design.

By developing treatments against both persisters and replicating pathogens, it may be possible to shorten antibiotic regimens, especially for deep-seated diseases such as tuberculosis, and reduce relapse rates in patients. Another advantage to combination therapies is potential extension of the useful life of current antibiotics to kill pathogen at a faster rate, and thus slow down the further emergence of antibiotic resistance. Additional strategies to optimize pulse-dosing regimens using multiple antibiotics that include anti-persister drugs may be able to sterilize particularly recalcitrant chronic infections. These types of therapies may be designed for the individual patient as part of an increasingly personalized approach to medicine. Aside from the clinical relevance of bacterial persisters, non-genetic heterogeneity has been found to play important roles in other systems, including susceptibility of cancer cells to treatment[70], host response to viral infection[71], and bacterial responses to other stresses.[72] Thus, understanding the mechanisms of cell-to-cell variability will provide insights into the general adaptation of life to variable environments.

## Acknowledgements

The writing of this review was supported by a Defense Threat Reduction Agency (DTRA) grant to EH-G to study molecular mechanisms of bacterial persistence and develop therapeutics stratagies to defeat persistence.

## Author details

Elizabeth Hong-Geller* and Sofiya N. Micheva-Viteva

*Address all correspondence to: ehong@lanl.gov

Los Alamos National Laboratory, Bioscience Division, Los Alamos, NM, USA

## References

[1] Bigger J. Treatment of staphylococcal infections with penicillin by intermittent sterilisation. Lancet 1944;244 497-500.

[2] Levin B, Rozen D. Non-inherited antibiotic resistance. Nat Rev Microbiol 2006;4 556-62.

[3] Lewis K. Persister cells. Annual review of microbiology 2010;64 357-72.

[4] Coates A, Hu Y. Targeting non-multiplying organisms as a way to develop novel antimicrobials. Trends Pharmacol Sci 2008;29 143-50.

[5] Gilbert P, Collier P, Brown M. Influence of growth rate on susceptibility to antimicrobial agents: biofilm, cell cycle, dormancy, and stringent response. Antimicrob Agents Chemo 1990;34 1865-8.

[6] Dhar N, McKinney J. Microbial phenotypic heterogeneity and antibiotic tolerance. Cur Opin Microbiol 2007;10 30-8.

[7] Hall-Stoodley I, Costerton J, Stoodley P. Bacterial biofilms: from the natural environment to infectious disease. Nature Rev Microbiol 2004;2 95-108.

[8] Mah T. Biofilm-specific antibiotic resistance. Future Microbiol 2012;7 1061-72.

[9] Bennett M, Hasty J. Microfluidic devices for measuring gene network dynamics in single cells. Nat Rev Genet 2009;10 628-38.

[10] Young J, Locke J, Altinok A, Rosenfeild N, Bacarian T, Swain P, Mjolsness E, Elowitz M. Measuring single-cell gene expression dynamics in bacteria using fluorescence time-lapse microscopy. Nat Protoc 2012;7 80-8.

[11] Moyed HS, Bertrand KP. hipA, a newly recognized gene of *Escherichia coli* K-12 that affects frequency of persistence after inhibition of murein synthesis. J Bacteriol 1983;155 768-75.

[12] Schumacher M, Piro R, Xu W, Hansen S, Lewis K, Brennan R. Molecular mechanisms of HipA-mediated multidrug tolerance and its neutralization by HipB. Science 2009;323 396-401.

[13] Balaban N, Merrin J, Chait R, Kowalik L, Leibler S. Bacterial persistence as a phenotypic switch. Science 2004;305 1622-162.

[14] Keren I, Shah D, Spoering A, Kaldalu N, Lewis K. Specialized persister cells and the mechanism of multidrug tolerance in *E. coli*. J Bacteriol 2004;186 8172-80.

[15] Gefen O, Gabay C, Mumcuoglu M, Engel G, Balaban N. Single-cell protein induction dynamics reveals a period of vulnerability to antibiotics in persister bacteria. Proc Natl Acad Sci 2008;105 6145-9.

[16] Spoering A, Vulic M, Lewis K. GlpD and PlsB participate in persister cell formation in *E. coli*. J Bacteriol 2006;188 5136-44.

[17] Li Y, Zhang Y. PhoU is a persistence switch involved in persister formation and tolerance to multiple antibiotics and stresses in *E. coli*. Antimicrob Agents Chemother 2007;51 2092-9.

[18] Hansen S, Lewis K, Vulic M. Role of global regulators and nucleotide metabolism in antibiotic tolerance in *E. coli*. Antimicrob Agents Chemo 2008;52 2718-26.

[19] Vasquez-Laslop N, Lee H, Neyfakh A. Increased persistence in *E. coli* caused by controlled expression of toxins or other unrelated proteins. J Bacteriol 2006;188 3494-7.

[20] Griffin M, Davis J, Strobel S. Bacterial toxin RelE: a highly efficient ribonuclease with exquisite specificity using atypical catalytic residues. Biochem 2013;52 8633-42.

[21] Aizenman E, Engelberg-Kulka H, Glaser G. An *E. coli* chromosomal "addiction module" regulated by guanosine 3',5'-bispyrophosphate: a model for programmed bacterial cell death. Proc Natl Acad Sci 1996;93 6059-63.

[22] Vega N, Allison K, Khalil A, Collins J. Signaling-mediated bacterial persister formation. Nat Chem Biol 2012;8 431-3.

[23] Leung V, Levesque C. A stress-inducible quorum-sensing peptide mediates the formation of persister cells with noninherited multidrug tolerance. J Bacteriol 2012;194 2265-74.

[24] Bernier S, Letoffe S, Delepierre M, Ghigo J. Biogenic ammonia modifies antibiotic resistance at a distance in physically separated bacteria. Mol Microbiol 2011;81 705-16.

[25] Spoering A, Lewis K. Biofilms and planktonic cells of *Pseudomonas aeruginosa* have similar resistance to killing by antimicrobials. J Bacteriol 2001;183 6746-51.

[26] De Groote V, Verstraeten N, Fauvart M, Kint C, Verbeeck A, Beullens S, Cornelis P, Michiels J. Novel persistence genes in *Pseudomonas aeruginosa* identified by high-throughput screening. FEMS Microbiol Lett 2009;297 73-9.

[27] Dutta N, Bandyopadhyay N, Veeramani B, Lamichhane G, Karakousis P, Bader J. Systems-biology-based identification of *Mycobacterium tuberculosis* persistence genes in mouse lungs. mBio 2014;5 e01066-13.

[28] Gerdes K, Maisonneuve E. Bacterial persistence and toxin-antitoxin loci. Annu Rev Microbiol 2012;66 103-23.

[29] Fozo E, Hemm M, Storz G. Small toxic proteins and the antisense RNAs that repress them. Microbiol Mol Biol Rev 2008;72 579-89.

[30] Gerdes K, Christensen S, Lebner-Olesen A. Prokaryotic toxin-antitoxin stress response loci. Nat Rev Microbiol 2005;3 371-82.

[31] Fineran P, Blower T, Folds I, Humphreys D, Lilley K, Salmond G. The phage abortive infection system, ToxIN, functions as a protein-RNA toxin-antitoxin pair. Proc Natl Acad Sci 2009;106 894-9.

[32] Rotem E, Loinger A, Ronin I, Levin-Reisman I, Gabay C, Shoresh N, Biham O, Balaban N. Regulation of phenotypic variability by a threshold-based mechanism underlies bacterial persistence. Proc Natl Acad Sci 2010;107 12541-6.

[33] Maisonneuve E, Shakespeare L, Jorgensen M, Gerdes K. Bacterial persistence by RNA endonucleases. Proc Natl Acad Sci 2011;108 13206-11.

[34] Pedersen K, Christensen SK, Gerdes K. Rapid induction and reversal of a bacteriostatic condition by controlled expression of toxins and antitoxins. Mol Microbiol 2002;45 501-10.

[35] Dahl J, Kraus C, Boshoff H, Doan B, Foley K, Avarbock D, Kaplan G, Mizrahi V, Rubin H, Barry C. The role of RelMtb-mediated adaptation to stationary phase in long-

term persistence of *Mycobacterium tuberculosis* in mice. Proc Natl Acad Sci 2003;100 10026-31.

[36] Korch S, Henderson T, Hill T. Characterization of the hipA7 allele of *E. coli* and evidence that high persistence is governed by (p)ppGpp synthesis. Mol Microbiol 2003;50 1199-213.

[37] Baracchini F, Bremer H. Stringent and growth control of rRNA synthesis in *E. coli* are both mediated by ppGpp. J Biol Chem 1988;263 2597-602.

[38] Dorr T, Vulic M, Lewis K. Ciprofloxacin causes persister formation by inducing the TisB toxin in *Escherichia coli*. PLoS Biol 2010;8 e1000317.

[39] Unoson C, Wager E. A small SOS-induced toxin is targeted against the inner membrane in *Escherichia coli*. Mol Microbiol 2008;70 258-70.

[40] Gurnev P, Ortenberg R, Dorr T, Lewis K, Bezrukov S. Persister-promoting bacterial toxin TisB produces anion-selective pores in planar lipid bilayers. FEBS Lett 2012;586 2529-34.

[41] Marr A, Overhage H, Bains M, Hancock R. The Lon protease of *Pseudomonas aeruginosa* is induced by aminoglycosides and is involved in biofilm formation and motility. Microbiol 2007;153 474-82.

[42] Shah D, Zhang Z, Khodursky A, Kaldalu N, Kurg K, Lewis K. Persisters: a distinct physiological state of *E. coli*. BMC Microbiol 2006;6 53.

[43] Canas-Duarte S, Restrepo S, Pedraza J. Novel protocol for persister cells isolation. PLoS One 2014;9 e88660.

[44] Allison KR, Brynildsen MP, Collins JJ. Metabolite-enabled eradication of bacterial persisters by aminoglycosides. Nature 2011;473 216-20.

[45] Conlon B, Nakayasu E, Fleck L, LaFleur M, Isabella V, Coleman K, Leonard S, Smith R, Adkins J, Lewis K. Activated ClpP kills persisters and eradicates a chronic biofilm infection. Nature 2013;503 365-70.

[46] Brotz-Oesterhelt H, Beyer D, Kroll H, Endermann R, Ladel C, Schroeder W, Hinzen B, Raddatz S, Paulsen H, Henninger K, Bandow J, Sahl H, Labischinski H. Dysregulation of bacterial proteolytic machinery by a new class of antibiotics. Nat Med 2005;11 1082-7.

[47] Hu Y, Shamaei-Tousi A, Liu Y, Coates A. A new approach for the discovery of antibiotics by targeting non-multiplying bacteria: a novel topical antibiotic for staphylococcal infections. PLos One 2010;5 e11818.

[48] Kim J, Heo P, Yang T, Lee K, Cho D, Kim B, Suh J, Lim H, Shin D, Kim S, Kweon D. Selective killing of bacterial persisters by a single chemical compound without affecting normal antibiotic-sensitive cells. Antimicrob Agents Chemo 2011;55 5380-3.

[49] Mitchison D. Pyrazinamide-on the antituberculosis drug frontline. Nat Med 1996;6 635-6.

[50] Shi W, Zhang X, Jiang X, Yuan H, Lee J, Barry C, Wang H, Zhang W, Zhang Y. Pyrazinamide inhibits trans-translation in *Mycobacterium tuberculosis*. Science 2011;333 1630-2.

[51] Sayahi H, Zimhony O, Jacobs W, Shekhtman A, Welch J. Pyrazinamide, but not pyrazinoic acid, is a competitive inhibitor of NADPH binding to *Mycobacterium tuberculosis* fatty acid synthase I. Bioorg Med Chem Lett 2011;21 4804-7.

[52] Lu P, Haagsma A, Pham H, Maaskant J, Mol S, Lili H, Bald D. Pyrazinoic acid decreases the proton motive force, respiratory ATP synthesis activity, and cellular ATP levels. Antimicrob Agents Chemo 2011;55 5354-7.

[53] Zhang Y, Mitchison D. The curious characteristics of pyrazinamide: a review. Int J Tuber Lung Dis 2003;7 6-21.

[54] Hu Y, Coates A, Mitchison D. Sterilizing activities of fluoroquinolones against rifampicin-tolerant populations of *Mycobacterium tuberculosis*. Antimicrob Agents Chemo 2003;47 653-7.

[55] Andries K, Verhasselt P, Guillemont J, Gohlmann H, Neefs J, Winkler H, Van Gestel J, Timmerman P, Zhu M, Lee E, Williams P, de Chaffoy D, Huitric E, Hoffner S, Cambau E, Truffot-Pernot C, Lounis N, Jarlier V. A diarylquinoline drug active on the ATP synthase of *Mycobacterium tuberculosis*. Science 2005;307 223-7.

[56] Koul A, Vranckx L, Dendouga N, Balemans W, Van den Wyngaert I, Vergauwen K, Gohlmann H, Willebrords R, Poncelet A, Guillemont J, Bald D, Andries K. Diarylquinolines are bactericidal for dormant mycobacteria as a result of disturbed ATP homeostasis. J Biol Chem 2008;283 25273-80.

[57] Balemans W, Vranckx L, Lounis N, Pop A, Guillemont J, Vergauwen K, Mol S, Gilissen R, Motte M, Lancois D, De Bolle M, Bonroy K, H L, Andries K, Bald D, Koul A. Novel antibiotics targeting respiratory ATP synthesis in Gram-positive pathogenic bacteria. Antimicrob Agents Chemo 2012;56 4131-9.

[58] Mak P, Rao S, Tan M, Lin X, Chyba J, Tay J, Ng S, Tan B, Cherian J, Duraiswamy J, Bifani P, Lim V, Lee B, Ma N, Beer D, Thayalan P, Kuhen K, Chatterjee A, Supek F, Glynne R, Zheng J, Boshoff H, Barry C, Dick T, Pethe K, Camacho L. A high-throughput screen to identify inhibitors of ATP homeostasis in non-replicating *Mycobacterium tuberculosis*. ACS Chem Biol 2012;7 1190-7.

[59] Setlow P. Spore germination. Curr Opin Microbiol 2003;6 550-6.

[60] Shah I, Laaberki M, Popham D, Dworkin J. A eukaryotic-like Ser/Thr kinase signals bacteria to exit dormancy in response to peptidoglycan fragments. Cell 2008;135 486-96.

[61] Mukamolova G, Kaprelyants A, Young D, Young M, Kell D. A bacterial cytokine. Proc Natl Acad Sci 1998;95 8916-21.

[62] Mukamolova G, Murzin A, Salina E, Demina G, Kell D, Kaprelyants A, Young M. Muralytic activity of *Micrococcus luteus* Rpf and its relationship to physiological activity in promoting bacterial growth and resuscitation. Mol Microbiol 2006;59 84-98.

[63] Shieeva M, Bagramyan K, Telkov M, Mukamolova G, Young M, Kell D, Kaprelyants A. Formation and resuscitation of "non-culturable" cells of *Rhodococcus rhodochrous* and *Mycobacterium tuberculosis* in prolonged stationary phase. Microbiol 2002;148 1581-91.

[64] Russell-Goldman E, Xu J, Wang X, Chan J, Tufariello J. *Mycobacterium tuberculosis* Rpf double-knockout strain exhibits profound defects in reactivation from chronic tuberculosis and innate immunity phenotypes. Microbiol 2008;148 1581-91.

[65] Kana B, Mizrahi V. Resuscitation-promoting factors as lytic enzymes for bacterial growth and signaling. FEMS Immunol Med Microbiol 2010;58 39-50.

[66] Bald D, Koul A. Advances and strategies in discovery of new antibacterials for combating metabolically resting bacteria. Drug Disc Today 2013;18 250-5.

[67] Smith P, Romesberg F. Combating bacteria and drug resistance by inhibiting mechanisms of persistence and adaptation. Nat Chem Biol 2007;3 549-56.

[68] Allison K, Brynildsen M, Collins J. Heterologous bacterial persisters and engineering approaches to eliminate them. Cur Opin Microbiol 2011;14 593-8.

[69] Hurdle J, O'Neill A, Chopra I, Lee R. Targeting bacterial membrane function: an underexploited mechanism for treating persistence infections. Nat Rev Microbiol 2011;9 62-75.

[70] Kessler D, Austin R, Levine H. Resistance to chemotherapy: patient variability and cellular heterogeneity. Cancer Res 2014;74 4663-70.

[71] Snidjer B, Sacher R, Ramo P, Damm E, Liberali P, Pelkmans L. Population context determines cell-to-cell variability in endocytosis and virus infection. Nature 2009;461 520-3.

[72] Booth I. Stress and the single cell: intrapopulation diverisity is a mechanism to ensure survivial upon exposure to stress. Int J Food Microbiol 2002;78 19-30.

# 8

# Advanced Human *In vitro* Models for the Discovery and Development of Lung Cancer Therapies

Samuel Constant, Song Huang,
Ludovic Wisniewski and Christophe Mas

## 1. Introduction

Lung cancer is the leading cause of cancer deaths in both men and women, with more than 1 million deaths worldwide each year [1]. Unfortunately, this difficult therapeutic area has shown the highest failure rate in clinical trials over the last 30 years [2] and hitherto, there is no effective treatment for patients with lung cancer. The reasons for this drug attrition are multiple, but one major explanation is considered to be the lack of relevant preclinical models to appropriately validate potential drug targets and rank novel therapeutic agents before engaging in clinical trials [3].

Genetically engineered mice, ectopic and orthotopic xenotransplantation of tumors into immunodeficient mice are common models used as surrogate of patients to evaluate drug candidates before clinical testing. Although animal models can recapitulate important facets of human responses, their limitations as preclinical cancer models have now been widely documented [4-7]. Fundamental differences in transcriptional regulation [8], telomerase activity [9], neoplastic transformation mechanisms [10], cytokines production [11] as well as matrix metalloproteinases biology [12] are but a few features which compromise the design of efficient cancer therapies. Even the patient derived xenograft model (PDX), which better recapitulate the phenotypic features of the human tumor, displays a number of inherent limitations [13]. In this system, the tumorgraft established from primary tumor fragments has to be maintained through serial transplantations into mice, which will lead to the loss of the human stroma environment after 2-3 passages [14]. Clearly, such a replacement of the original tumor microenvironment by murine host components has significant consequences on growth features as well as response to therapies. Indeed, a number of oncogenic mouse ligands fail to cross-activate their related human receptors [15, 16] while stromal mediators have been identified as a critical source triggering tumour cells resistance to treatment [17, 18]. These observations highlight the importance of considering tumor-extracellular matrix interactions in the design of *in vitro* cancer models. Modern tumor biology has moved away from the traditionalist view conveyed for years by 2D cultures saturated with growth factors by revealing that the many varieties of cells that compose a tumor don't just grow on their own but constantly integrate and react to signals coming from the extracellular matrix components. Solid tumors are now regarded as complex organs able to instruct the surrounding tissue to promote their own growth and progression, but also dependent on both molecular and mechanical signals coming from the adjacent healthy environment [19, 20]. Therefore, experimental models recapitulating true human cancer biology are mandatory for the validation of therapeutic agents in order to keep away from the risk of studying no more than adaptive cancer biology in a wrong environment that will eventually result in translation failure.

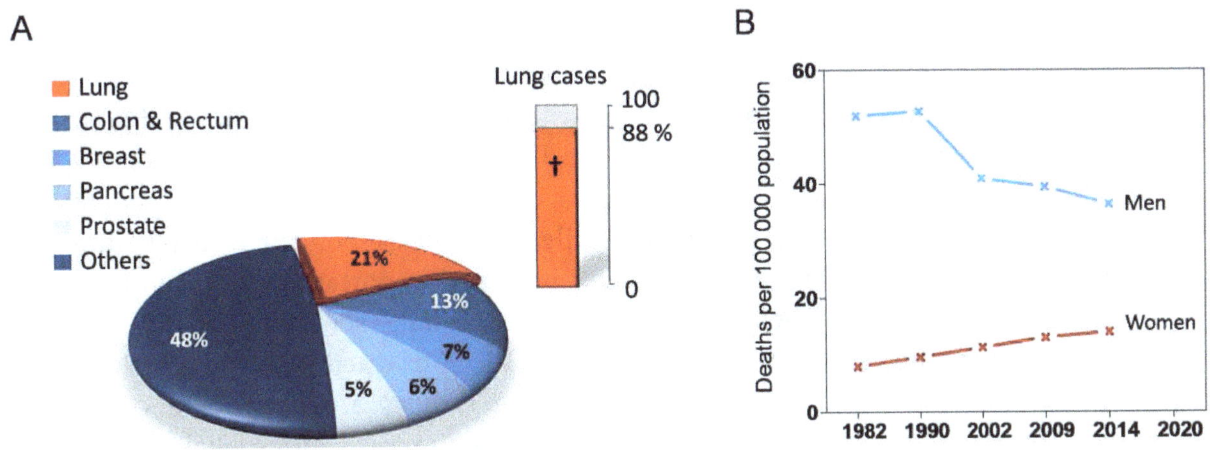


**Figure 1.** (A) Cancer deaths anticipated in 2014. Estimated leading cancer sites mortality in European Union for the year 2014 expressed as percent of total cancer deaths. Column diagram highlights the mortality rate within the population specifically affected by lung cancer. (B) Age-standardized (world population) EU male (blue) and female (red) lung cancer death rates per 100,000 from 1982 to 2014. The graph shows the unfavourable trend for female lung cancer with a regular increase in case numbers over the last 30 years. Source: Malvezzi et al, Annals of oncology, 2014; 25(8): 1650-6. and Bosetti et al, Annals of oncology, 19: 631–640, 2008.

In this article we report the significant efforts ongoing within academia and industry to developing *in vitro* novel complex human tumor models that should improve the identification and selection of efficient lung cancer therapies. We first focus on the human lung cancer cell lines currently available, their contribution to lung cancer biology and their use in research. Then, we will move from cell monolayers to three-dimensional (3D) cultures, exploring at first the function of natural and synthetic extracellular matrix before to document some recent advances in the field, including spheroids, bioscaffolds, decellularized lung matrix models and precision-cut lung tumor slices. Finally, we will present the bioengineering of a new generation of lung cancer models: OncoCilAir™. These 100% human models, which combine *in vitro* both tumor nodules surrounded by a functional airway epithelium and stroma, open new ways to test simultaneously drug efficacy, side toxicity and tumor recurrence in a single, integrated and accessible 3D model.

## 2. Lung cancer, current treatments and perspectives

Lung cancer (LC) is one of the major health concerns in the western world. LC is the most frequently diagnosed cancer in men and women and represents the most common cause of cancer-related deaths, both in the United States and in Europe, with a significant rate of 27% and 21% of total cancer deaths, respectively [21] (Fig.1A). The LC epidemic has been clearly linked to tobacco smoking [22], and while mortality rate in men has regularly fallen over the last decades (53 lung cancer deaths for every 100,000 European males in the late 1980s to 41.1/100,000 in 2009) thanks to strong measures for smoking control and prevention in middle-aged men, female LC rates are predicted to rise 8% in 2015 [1] (Fig.1B). There are two main types of lung cancer: non-small lung cancer (NSCLC) which account for about 85% of all lung cancers and small cell lung cancer (SCLC, 15%). SCLC is the most aggressive form of LC, with fast growing cells leading to large tumors. Histologically, NSCLC includes 3 subgroups: adenocarcinoma, squamous cell and large cell carcinoma [23]. As in many other forms of cancer, LC does not display too many symptoms, develops slowly over a period of several years, and only manifests itself in advanced stages (III or IV), where five-year survival rates are less than 10% because of high degree of metastasis. The overall median survival in stage IV is only about 8-10 months [24]. Platinum and taxane based chemotherapies (cisplatin, paclitaxel) has remained for years the treatments of choice, but more recently LC patients have been selected based on their tumor mutation profile. In most cases, oncogene driver mutations are exclusives (EGFR, ALK/EML4, KRAS, PTEN, etc...) and importantly, they divided patient populations into molecular subsets that do not show the same sensitivity to different treatments [25]. This patient stratification has enabled the introduction of targeted therapies directed against specific signaling pathways whose tumors are dependent on. Indeed, humanized recombinant antibodies directed against the vascular endothelial growth factor (VEGF) (bevacizumab) or small molecule inhibitors of EGFR-TK (erlotinib, gefitinib and afatinib), ALK and MET (crizotinib, ceritinib) have recently been used as a promising new line of therapies to treat lung cancer. Unfortunately, this drug portfolio extends survival only by a few months (Table 1) since most of the patients develop resistance to treatments, leading invariably to the recurrence of the disease [26-32]. Huge efforts are now undertaken to understand and circumvent drug resistance mechanisms. First observations have pointed out two main mechanisms for drug resistance acquisition: the selection of another pre-existing oncogene mutation or the activation of a bypass track, i.e. the deregulation of an alternative growth signaling pathway to maintain cell proliferation and tumor progression [33]. In *EGFR*-mutant lung cancer treated with the EGFR-TK inhibitors erlotinib and gefitinib, resistance is generally mediated by the T790M EGFR second-site mutation (~50% of the cases) [34] or phosphatidylinositol 3-kinase PI3K–AKT pathway activation via focal amplification of MET as second signaling pathway (~5%) [35]. For *ALK*-mutant lung cancer treated with crizotinib, mechanisms of resistance include the gatekeeper mutation L1196M (~30% of the cases) and KIT and EGFR signaling pathways activation as bypass track (~45%) [36]. Overall, these findings argue for the use of combined therapies in a manageable way. But recent data based on the analysis of tumor specimens at the time of acquired resistance suggest a much more complex landscape. In fact, multiple mechanisms, as diverse as epigenetic changes [37], epithelial to mesenchyme transition (EMT) or conversion from a LC histological type to another (EGFR-dependent NSCLC to SCLC), are induced under the selective pressure of targeted therapies [38, 39]. These observations imply the arrival of a personalized medicine, where a careful profiling of patient tumor's mutation status (germline and somatic) and epigenetic signature will be mandatory all along the therapy to identify and adapt the correct treatment strategy. However, such scheduled combinatorial regimen would require the development of multiple-generation inhibitors to overcome specific subsets of resistance mutations and induce durable remissions. But the ability to escape multiple types of treatment could well be a hallmark of cancer cells. With this in mind, alternative strategies are worth considering. Instead of constraining tumor cells signalling through exogenous therapies making them overreact, a different approach might be to restrict tumor progression through its own microenvironment. The original 1975's experiment of teratocarcinoma injection into blastocysts from Mintz and Illmensee was the first example of tumor repression by the microenvironment [40]. Today, tumor reprogramming through stroma instruction is emerging as a new treatment paradigm [41-43]. From this perspective, advanced human three-dimensional (3D) cell culture approaches modelling tumor-stroma communication could be key to accelerate the development of new lung cancer therapeutics.

| Generic | Trade Name | Indication | Type | Class | Target | PFS | Ref |
|---|---|---|---|---|---|---|---|
| ▶ Afatinib | Gilotrif | NSCLC | small molecule | antineoplastic antiangiogenesis | EGFR HER2-4 | 3.3-13.6 | [32] |
| ▶ Crizotinib | Xalkori | NSCLC | small molecule | antineoplastic | ALK MET, ROS1 | 9.7 | [29] |
| ▶ Ceritinib | Zykadia | NSCLC | small molecule | antineoplastic | ALK IGF1R | 7 | [31] |
| ▶ Erlotinib | Tarceva | NSCLC | small molecule | antineoplastic antiangiogenesis | EGFR | 12-14 | [26;27] |
| ▶ Gefitinib | Iressa | NSCLC | small molecule | antineoplastic antiangiogenesis | EGFR | 7.7-12.9 | [26] |
| ▶ Bevacizumab | Avastin | NSCLC | rHMAb | antiangiogenesis | VEGF | 6.2 | [28] |

**Table 1.** Targeted therapies approved by the Food and Drug Administration in the treatment of lung cancer. The median time to progression on targeted therapy (Progression Free Survival - PFS) is given in months. rHMAb: recombinant human monoclonal antibody. Source: National Cancer Institute database, 2014.

## 3. Lung cancer cell lines

Cell lines derived from human tumors provide an unlimited, self-replicating source of malignant cells that can be studied by investigators throughout the world. Therefore, even if cell lines represent only a highly selected fraction of the original tumor, their ease of access has resulted in the production of a very large body of literature. Indeed, it is acknowledged that most of our understanding of the molecular mechanisms involved in LC comes from studies done on mouse or human cell lines [44].

### 3.1. Lung cancer cell lines collection

To date, more than 250 LC cell lines have been established, mainly from Western population. Currently, the American Type Culture Collection (ATCC, Manassas, VA) catalog lists 121 human lung tumor cell lines. Among this panel, SCLC is less represented, first due to the lower frequency of the disease, and second because SCLC tumors are rarely surgically resected. Indeed, only small tissue samples from biopsy examinations, malignant aspirates, and rare malignant effusions are available for research use. Moreover, the fact that SCLC tumor cells lack the ability to adhere to culture dishes and required to be grown *in vitro* as floating cell aggregates or spheroids has precluded for a long time their expansion as cell lines. SCLC was first successfully cultured in Japan in 1971 [45].

Regarding NSCLC, primary and metastatic tumor materials are more easily accessible, even through routine bronchoscopy [38, 39]. However, although cells from metastatic tumors, especially from malignant effusions, are relatively easy to culture, cell cultures from primary solid tumor are not obvious to establish, with success rates ranging from 2.6 to 5% [46, 47]. Various protocols are in use, but on the whole, tumor tissues minced in small pieces are either directly cultured as fragments in a matrix (e.g. Matrigel®) or subjected to enzymatic dissociation (collagenase/hyaluronidase) and then suspended in culture medium. Clearly, positive results are higher when starting from material corresponding to advanced stages as MHC III and IV [46]. The culture medium composition is also critical and the development of serum-free chemically defined media (e.g. ACL4) has significantly improved success rates [48].

The resulting current LC cell lines depository represent therefore a unique resource that can be extremely valuable in term of genetic manipulation, high-throughput screening and development of more complex co-culture models.

### 3.2. Lung cancer cell lines as *in vitro* model

LC cell lines have been used for decades in functional studies with the aim to identify new oncogene drivers or tumor suppressors. Thus, LC cell lines compared to normal human bronchial epithelial cells were instrumental to generate list of differentially expressed genes that could account for tumorigenicity and represent therefore new therapeutic targets. As an example, this strategy lead to the detection of *ERBB3*, a gene associated with the EGF signaling pathway, among the genes over-expressed in LC cell lines [49]. Interestingly, this result was validated later on by another study that identified the activation of ERBB3 signaling as a mechanism of resistance to gefitinib [35]. Since these initial findings, ERBB3 has been recognized as a key node of LC progression and several humanized anti-ErbB3 antibodies are currently in pre-clinical development [50].

However, cell lines limitations have emerged as our knowledge about the disease increased. As an example, several studies have shown that differences in genetic background are important in defining cancer biology as well as in drug sensitivity [51]. Thus, a potential shortcoming of the current LC collection may reside in its under-representation of some populations, like the East Asian population, possibly introducing bias in research and drug discovery. Indeed, epidemiologic surveys have revealed that in the US, 10% of patients with NSCLC have tumour associated with EGFR mutations, while this number increases to 35% in

East Asia, suggesting different selection mechanisms or sensitivity for lung cancer subtypes among different ethnic groups.

Accordingly, the recent classification of lung cancers into genetic subsets based on mutations in driver oncogenes (*see previous section*) prompted the community to accurately characterize the LC cell lines collection at the genomic and genetic levels. In this perspective, the Sanger Cancer Institute has initiated the genetic characterization of a panel of cancer cell lines (The Cancer Genome Project, http://cancer.sanger.ac.uk/cancergenome/projects/cell_lines/). Using current high throughput techniques this program provides information on mutations, copy number variations, single nucleotide polymorphisms (SNPs) and microsatellite instability of 136 cell lines representative of the different type of lung cancers (adenocarcinoma, small cell carcinoma, etc...) with the aim to define a genetic profile predictive of drug sensitivity. Such a signature should contribute to stratify patient population and to identify efficient targeted therapies.

Another emerging use of LC cell line is related to the identification of resistance mechanisms. As documented in section 2, so far all the approaches used in the treatment of lung cancer have resulted in the acquisition of resistance by the patients. One successful approach to discovering resistance mechanisms has been to culture sensitive cell lines with increasing concentrations of the drug until resistance emerges. The resistant cell line can subsequently be analysed to identify the resistance mechanisms, leading to the identification of resistance biomarkers and new strategies to overcome resistance [36].

Undoubtedly, cell lines have proven to be useful in elucidating important aspect of lung cancer biology. However, thanks to modern deep-sequencing technologies, we now know that lung tumors are composed of population of cells with distinct molecular and phenotypic properties [52] and consequently, that cell lines do not fully recapitulate human tumor biology. Clearly, the scientific community has taken into account these limitations, as shown by the growing interest for the establishment of complex *in vitro* cell models intended to bridge the gap between animal models and human studies.

## 4. Biocompatible matrices for 3D cell culture

In this section, we will try to briefly resume different ways and techniques used to culture the cells in 3D. Maintaining a 3D structure is critical to reproduce the tumour-stroma environment, communication between tumour cells, and the interaction with other surrounding cell types such as epithelial cells or fibroblasts [19]. Advances in materials chemistry and processing technologies, as well as developmental biology have led to the design of 3D cell culture matrices and bioscaffolds that better represent the geometry, chemistry, and signaling environment of natural extracellular matrix.

To obtain 3D cell cultures, cells are generally seeded onto/into biocompatible scaffolds or matrices. The 3D differentiation of cells depends on various parameters but it is generally accepted that best results are obtained when the natural environment is closely imitated [53]. Natural extracellular matrices are mainly composed of fibrous network made of collagen, elastic fibers, water and other materials like glycosaminoglycans, proteoglycans and glycoproteins [54]. To mimic the natural extracellular environment of the cells important parameters have to be taken into account [55]:

1. The matrix composition (collagen, fibrin, alginate, etc.)
2. The structure (pore size, pore distribution, pore geometry, etc.)
3. The manufacturing method (electrospinning, 3D printing, inverted colloidal crystal, spontaneous polymerization, etc.)
4. The biocompatibility

As the fate of a cell is largely determined by its environment, the elaboration of the right extracellular context is critical to promote the correct differentiation of a cell population.

For example, it is well known that epithelial cells have to be cultured at the air-liquid interface to differentiate. This could be easily obtained by seeding cells onto micro porous supports or scaffolds allowing nutrients to come from the back. The apical side of the cells remains generally exposed to the air [56]. This basic principle of air-liquid interface cultivation can be transposed to most of epithelial cells such as airway, vaginal, buccal, intestinal, etc. However, this approach is no more suitable when the cells are not from epithelial origin [57, 58].

It is typically the case for fibroblasts that are not able to survive when directly exposed to the air. To culture fibroblasts in 3D, a different type of environment is required. Cells can be embedded into a biocompatible matrix based on various components [53]. Among the most used we find collagen and fibrin. Collagen is the major component of connective tissues, it is naturally produced by fibroblasts and can be easily isolated from many type of tissues such as dermis, bone, tendon, etc...

Whereas collagen is easily obtained, applications for human therapies and 3D cell culture remain limited because of contamination risks between animals and humans (e.g. Creutzfeldt-Jakob). Moreover, the gel polymerization can be difficult to control thus reducing the field of applicability. Another drawback is the variation between batches to batches. These weaknesses have led to the development of new generations of synthetic matrices and scaffolds where polymerization as well as intrinsic properties of materials (elasticity, porosity, permeability, hydration, etc.) can be more easily controlled. The matrices used today for 3D cell culture can be divided into 3 groups:

a. Natural compounds: collagen, gelatin, hyaluronate, glycosaminoglycan, chitosan, alginate, silk, fibrin, dextran, matrigel®, etc...
b. Synthetic compounds: polyglycolic acid (PGA), polylactic acid (PLA), polylactic-co-glycolic acid (PLGA), polycarpolactone (PCL), polyethylene glycol (PEG), polyvinyl alcohol (PVA), polypropylene fumarate (PPF), polyacrylic acid (PAA), etc...
c. Mixed compounds, made of natural compounds synthetically modified. These included peptide-coupled alginates, chitosan, hyluranan, tyrosine-derived polymers, etc...

Each material has its own strengths and weaknesses and therefore it is fundamental to select matrix components in function of the needs. In the context of lung tumor cell model, it is pertinent to determine the final end-point studied. For example, if cells invasion has to be studied, it is necessary to use matrix components where cells are able to adhere, migrate and proliferate [59]. Moreover, some cells have the ability to digest and transform the scaffold and elaborate a new environment adapted to their needs. In that case it will be valuable to select a natural matrix component like collagen or fibrin. If the goal of the experiment is to obtain a 3D scaffold for human therapy, the best choice will be the use of synthetic matrices where all components can be defined and controlled [60]. If the sensitivity of a cancer cell to a drug has to be studied, a relevant choice could be the use of cell spheroids embedded into a non degradable matrix component, like alginate [61]. In that case, cells are immobilized and their drug susceptibility can be determined using a simple viability test. Alginate scaffold has been optimized for 3D tumor modeling using H460, A549 and H1650 NSCLC cell lines [62]. In this study the anticancer effects of various chemotherapeutic agents were studied and compared with conventional 2D cell culture models. Results have shown that cells grown in 3D demonstrated a more realistic drug response with higher resistance to chemotherapy [62].

Clearly, there is a tremendous flexibility to reconstitute a scaffold and the choice of synthesis should be guided by the type of cells, the application and the desired physical properties [53]. In addition, new perspectives are offered by bioprinting technologies. The possibility to organize extracellular matrix into precise geometries should help engineering 3D complex tumor tissues for *in vitro* assays [63].

## 5. Tumor spheroid models for lung cancer research

Numerous anchorage-independent assays have been developed for drug discovery. The most popular is the spheroid model because it allows both 3D self-organization of tumor cells and drug screening in high-throughput format. Many normal and malignant cell types can be grown as sphere-shaped cell colonies, so called spheroids. Cells that don't form spheroids spontaneously can be induced to do so by co-culturing with spheroid-forming non-clonogenic feeder cells [64]. As spheroid environment can be controlled, effects on tumor cell viability can be carefully examined. This model is particularly adapted to high throughput screening in 96-well plate assays, and numerous solutions are commercially available.

Phenotypic and functional differences between lung tumor cells grown as 2D monolayer cultures, versus cells grown as 3D spheroids have been observed. Indeed, the 3D spheroid culture changed the cellular response to drugs and growth factors suggesting to be more accurately mimicking the natural tumor microenvironment than classical culture of lung cell line [65]. Multi-cell type tumor spheroids are a valuable model to reproduce cellular heterogeneity and provide more comprehensive assessment of tumor response to therapeutic strategies. 3D co-culture model using NSCLC cell lines in combination with lung fibroblasts can be prepared [66]. To date, co-cultures involving up to three different cell types in a single spheroid (tumor cells, fibroblasts and endothelial cells) have been established, but without any proof of micro-capillary functionality [67]. Recent studies report that NSCLC can acquire epithelial-mesenchymal transition and cancer stem-like phenotypes within chitosan-hyaluronan membrane-derived 3D tumor spheroids [68].

## 6. Microfluidic chip-based 3D co-cultures

In the continuity of the pioneering work of Donald Ingber (organ on chip), a series of 3D lung-on-a-chip microfluidic devices have been developed. Briefly, lung-on-a-chip is a biomimetic microsystem that reconstitutes the critical functional alveolar-capillary interface of the human lung, with periodic mechanical stretching and flow of the medium carrying immune cells. Using this micro-fluidic device, the authors were able to replicating the immune responses against bacterial infections *in vitro* [69]. Afterwards, devices were optimized as a drug screening platform to select individualized treatment for lung cancer. In these systems, lung cancer and stromal cell lines were co-cultured as 3D spheroids under continuous media supplementation, mimicking the circulation of nutrients and metabolic waste out of the cultures [70]. Another similar model has been developed for chemoresistive testing of pleural mesothelioma cancer spheroids. Interestingly, growth inhibitory concentration of cisplatin showed higher concentration in perfused tumor spheroids compared with spheroids cultured under static conditions [71]. These systems represent therefore valuable tools to get information about the efficacy of chemotherapeutic drugs in a dynamic microenvironment which recapitulate the actual *in vivo* situation, but they do not address side-toxicity on normal lung physiology. The challenge will be to improve the model so that it incorporates normal and functional tissues. That could be achieved by connecting such devices with other microphysiological organotypic chips, representative of healthy lung tissues.

## 7. *Ex vivo* 3D lung cancer model based on decellularized matrix

As it is not obvious to identify the ideal matrix components and conditions suitable for the development of various lung tumor types, an alternative strategy is to take advantage of existing natural matrices. This methodology relies on the initial work of Ott and colleagues that first succeed in regenerating a bioartificial organ from a rat cadaveric lung [72]. Briefly, in this model the organ of interest is perfused with a detergent in order to remove donor cells and leave the components of the extracellular matrix. The resulting decellularized matrix is then reloaded with human lung adenocarcinoma tumor cells. In addition to their well-adapted composition, decellularized matrices also display specific elasticity which has been pointed out as critical for tumor cell growth. To date, rat decellularized lung matrix [73] and porcine decellularized intestinal submucosa [17] have been used as scaffold. Interestingly, tumor cell lines (A549, H460 and H1299) engrafted in this microenvironment formed 3D lung tumor nodules and displayed histological features reminiscent of the original primary tumor [74]. They also recovered functionalities (e.g. MMP-9 production) that were lost in 2D culture [73]. These ex vivo 3D models can be kept in culture for up to 28 days and exhibit sensitivity to treatment comparable to what is observed in clinic [17]. Although relevant for fundamental research, current *ex vivo* 3D lung models clearly show limitations. First, they are difficult to produce, the cultivation of the cells must take place in a special incubator, and consequently they cannot be used for high-throughput screening. Second, they do not recapitulate the human – human interactions between tumor and stroma. Indeed, epithelial and mesenchymal cells have been removed from epithelial space by the decellularization process. Third, they necessitate large amount of tumor cells (~25 millions) in order to colonize the matrix, precluding personalized medicine. And finally, they required the sacrifice of animals for matrix supply. However, *ex vivo* 3D lung models must be seen as the gold standard to be reached by 3D bioprinting technologies combined to synthetic matrices.

## 8. Precision-cut lung tumor slices

As previously mentioned, the tumor microenvironment provides essential signaling necessary for establishing and maintaining tumor specific morphogenic programs. Precision-cut lung slices (PCLS) obtained from freshly isolated human lung cancer tissues maintain both the original cancer microenvironment and preserve the complexity of the tumor-stroma interaction [75, 76]. Usually thin tissue slices (~200 μM) are prepared with a vibratome and cultured submerged into medium for several days. PCLS constitute a valid tool for the *in vitro* evaluation of tumor morphology, proliferation, viability and resistance to therapy [75]. Moreover, a major advantage of this model is the preparation of multiple experimental replicates from a single tumor, allowing performing drug efficacy studies. Indeed, dose-response experiments with the PIK3 inhibitor LY294002 have shown that PCLS cultures from lung cancer may be used to predict tumor sensitivity to drugs in a patient-specific manner [75]. In a different study, tumor PCLS were used to investigate nanoparticles delivery of antisense as lung cancer treatment. The model was instrumental to demonstrate that nanoparticles could penetrate into tumor tissue and target telomerase activity, without disturbing adjacent tissue architecture or inducing significant side-toxicity [76]. PCLS established from human lung tumor tissue represent therefore a useful *in vitro* tumor model that has the potential to enhance preclinical drug evaluation studies. However, an obvious limitation of PCLS is their short lifespan, ~5 days, which prevents long-term exposure, and therefore chronic treatment evaluation.

## 9. Engineered 3D lung tumor tissues: The OncoCilAir™ model

Tissue engineering is an innovative technology designed at first to produce artificial functional tissues to repair or replace portion of injured tissues. While initially seen as unrealistic, this field has made tremendous progress over the past decade, and regenerative medicine will soon become a routine technique [77]. Today, it is possible by combining human cells with suitable bioscaffolds to produce *in vitro* tissue equivalents from many sources (e.g. corneal, cartilage, intestinal, muscle, respiratory, skin, etc...). More recently, this promising technology has been applied to the field of oncology with some attempts to develop engineered tumor tissues for pre-clinical research (e.g. human melanoma model) [78]. Here we took advantage of our tissue engineering know-how in the respiratory field [79] to develop a complex, but accessible, 3D lung cancer model: OncoCilAir™ [80, 81]. To this purpose, human primary bronchial cells, lung fibroblasts and lung adenocarcinoma cell lines were co-cultured at the air-liquid interface in a transwell insert (Fig.2). After appropriate differentiation, the system closely reproduces malignant pulmonary nodules invading a human functional airway epithelium (Fig.3).

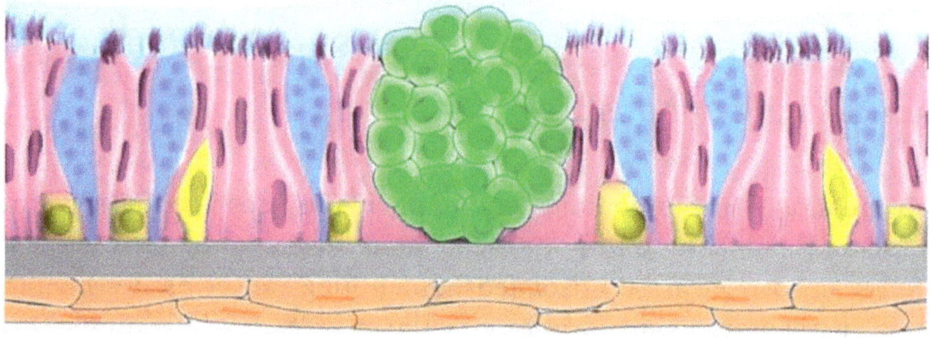

**Figure 2. Schematic representation of the OncoCilAir™ lung cancer model.** OncoCilAir™ is a complex cellular model based on the co-culture at the air-liquid-interface of three different human components: bronchial cells, lung fibroblasts and NSCLC cell lines. After 30 days, the cells differentiate into a functional respiratory epithelium which comprises ciliated cells (pink), goblet cells (blue) secreting mucus (light blue), basal cells (yellow), fibroblasts (brown) and tumor nodules (green).

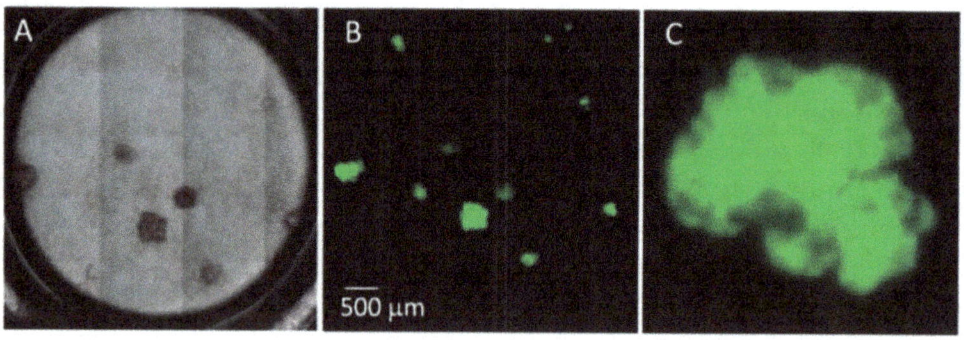


**Figure 3.** Cultured at the air-liquid interface in a convenient 24-wells format (A), the OncoCilAir™ model mimics the *in vivo* lung tissue of a patient with characteristic tumour lung nodules (B & magnification in C).

Several properties contribute to make OncoCilAir™ a relevant pre-clinical *in vitro* alternative: First, it is a 100% human three-dimensional model which summarizes human tumour-stroma interactions to assess therapies targeting host-tumor interactions (Fig.4). Second, it is a flexible system: depending on the cell line used to build its tumour component, OncoCilAir™ offers the possibility to recapitulate distinct molecular subsets of lung cancers (EGFR, KRAS, etc...) and thus to simulate patient stratification. Third, it is a bi-competency model: the fact that it includes both compromised and healthy tissues brings the possibility to experiment simultaneously drug efficacy and drug side-effect within a single culture. Lastly, its long lifespan (>3 months) allows to test chronic treatments and recurrence while reducing animal testing.

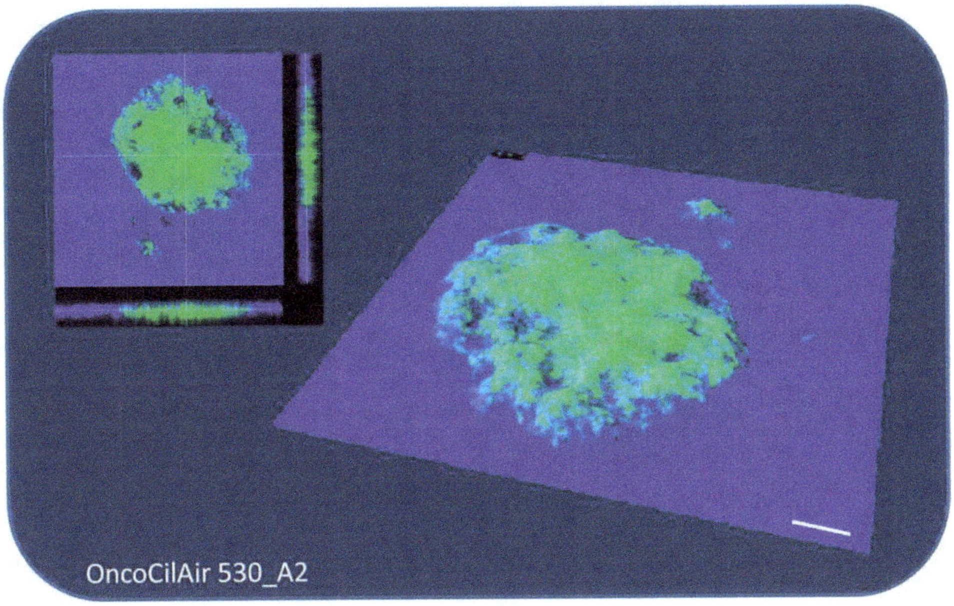


**Figure 4. A tumor nodule expanding within the OncoCilAir™ human airway epithelium.** Adenocarcima cells GFP+ (green) and human bronchial epithelial cells nuclei DAPI+ (blue) were visualized by confocal laser scanning microscopy. Scale bar represents 100 μm.

Accordingly, a dose response efficacy study with the investigational MEK inhibitors selumetinib and trametinib demonstrated that OncoCilAir™ showed responsiveness to anticancer drugs in agreement with previously reported data, and therefore can be used as a predictive tool for anticancer drug evaluation [82].

## 10. Future perspective

Hanahans and Weinberg highlighted six cancer hallmarks which provide us with a framework to understand this complex disease. These hallmarks include (i) sustaining proliferative signaling, (ii) evading growth suppressors, (iii) resisting cell death (iv) enabling replicative immortality, (v) inducing angiogenesis, and (vi) activating invasion and metastasis [83, 84]. However, in essence, cancer is a genetic disease with germ or autosomal mutations affecting genes implicated in cell division and/or in tissue integrity. These genetic alterations lead to unrestricted cell division and formation of a clone of cells which undergo further genetic changes. Some of these mutations promote features that endow cells with a selective advantage over normal cells, thus creating a more aggressive subclone with an even higher mutation rate, eventually leading to tumor formation [85]. The clonal theory has been corroborated by several decades of cancer researches: we now know that mutation in some specific genes, so-called oncogenes and tumor supressors, are primary cause for cancers. For lung cancers, the components of EGF signaling, such as EGF receptor and its downstream effectors (KRAS, BRAF, ALK, etc...) are the main drivers [33]. With the advance in biotechnology, it is now possible to rapidly identify the underlying mutations of the lung cancers for diagnostics and for personalized treatment.

<table>
<tr><th>Cancer hallmarks</th><th>Barriers</th><th>Appropiate in vitro models</th></tr>
<tr><td>Sustaining proliferative signal</td><td>Inadequate growth promotion</td><td rowspan="4">Cell lines<br>Spheroids<br>3D co-cultures<br>in vitro PnP</td></tr>
<tr><td>Evading growth suppressors</td><td></td></tr>
<tr><td>Resisting cell death</td><td>Apoptosis with loss of basement membrane</td></tr>
<tr><td>Enabling replicative immortality</td><td>Senescence</td></tr>
<tr><td>Inducing angiogenesis</td><td>Ischaemia</td><td rowspan="2">3D co-cultures<br>in vitro PnP</td></tr>
<tr><td>Activating invasion and metastasis</td><td>ECM and epithelial barrier</td></tr>
<tr><td>Deregulating cellular energetics</td><td>Acidosis</td><td>in vitro PnP</td></tr>
</table>

**Table 2.** Current and future *in vitro* lung cancer models sorted according to cancer hallmarks.

However, a genetic change is only one side of the same coin. It is generally recognized now that the microenvironment surrounding the cancer cells plays also a crucial role in cancer development [19, 83, 84]. Indeed, tumor cells have to overcome at least six barriers in order to become invasive [86]. The extracellular matrix, stroma cells, immune cells, etc... form an integral part of the tumor, therefore should be taken into account. In fact, not all the cancer cells can grow in standard cell culture conditions: out of 160 tumors, only 8 Chinese NSCLC cell lines have been established in culture [47].

Therefore, for tissue engineering, the most important, as well as the most challenging task is to recreate the *in vivo*-like tumor micro-environment.

Another important issue is to maintain the heterogeneity of the tumor populations. Despite of huge progresses made in cancer research, the toll cancer claims in both human lives and funds spent on health care has been only marginally reduced, and in some cases even increases [87, 88]. One of the reasons for this situation is the drug resistance. The underlying cause is the heterogeneity of the tumor cells: within a tumor several clones with different mutations may co-exist. Furthermore, another process termed the community effect may be involved. Studies have suggested that the ability of a cell to respond to a signal may be enhanced by, or even dependent on, other neighboring cells reacting in the same way at the same time [89]. This effect helps to explain the formation of blocks of tissue from sheets of cells, and could be of widespread occurrence and significance in various morphogenesis processes, including tumor development. The underlying mechanism of the community effect could be the autocrine or paracrine positive feedback loops, which have also been suggested and identified during tumor formation. Several studies have outlined the importance of autocrine IL-6 signaling in lung and breast cancers. For example, one group found a positive correlation between persistently activated tyrosine-phosphorylated STAT3, found in 50% of lung adenocarcinomas, and IL-6. Further investigation revealed that mutant EGFR could activate the oncogenic STAT3 pathway via upregulated IL-6 autocrine signaling [90].

The fact that most of the cancer cells, even the aggressive ones, cannot grow in culture once dissociated strongly supports this notion. In other words, all the cancer hallmarks are the hallmarks of the tumor as a whole, not that of individual cancer cells. This has to be taken into account during the development of *in vitro* cancer models.

| | Cell lines | Spheroids | 3D Co-culture Models | In vitro PnP |
|---|---|---|---|---|
| Pro | ▶ Appropriate for identifying the mutations and for elucidating the signalling pathways.<br>▶ High throughput screening of drug candidates. | ▶ Replicate only some features of cancer 3D environment (cell-cell interactions, community effect).<br>▶ Mechanistic studies.<br>▶ Drug screening and testing. | ▶ Reflect closely *in vivo* situations, having relevant cell-cell and cell-stroma interactions.<br>▶ Possibility to study cancer metastasis and tumor invasion.<br>▶ Allow testing the efficacy and toxicity simultaneously.<br>▶ Allow chronic treatments and resistance studies.<br>▶ Provide insight about mechanistic at all levels.<br>▶ Identification and validation of drug candidate.<br>▶ Suitable for personalized medicine. | ▶ An ideal model replicating most of the features of cancer development and cancer growth.<br>▶ Cell-cell and cell-stroma interactions, metastasis, immune responses, drugs circulation and metabolization, angiogenesis, etc... |
| Cons | ▶ Do not reflect the original *in vivo* situations, lack of relevant cell-cell and cell-stroma interactions.<br>▶ loss of relevant biomarkers.<br>▶ Lack of mechanical constraints from the adjacent healthy tissue. | ▶ Not cultured at ALI condition, these models are less relevant for lung cancers.<br>▶ Not possible to study metastasis.<br>▶ Lack of immune cells and no angiogenesis. | ▶ Lack of immune cells and no angiogenesis. | ▶ Could be difficult to standardize and to scale-up.<br>▶ Special expertise is needed. Often patent-protected. |

**Table 3.** Strengths and weaknesses of the different human *in vitro* models for lung cancer.

Ideally, *in vitro* lung cancer models should recapture all the hallmarks of human lung cancer. Each model has its own strength and weaknesses (Table 3). But depending on the application, simple models may be more relevant and sufficient. Models can therefore be sorted by complexity:

1. Cell lines

2. As simplest 3D model, the tumor spheroids represent already a progress with regarding to monolayer culture of tumor cell lines or primary tumor cells: the cell-cell interaction is restored. Stroma cells and or matrix could also be added to better mimic the *in vivo* situation.

3. Since the lung tumor cells are located at air-liquid interface, co-culture with the normal airway epithelial cells and fibroblast cells at air-liquid interface, illustrated by OncoCi-lAir™, is another realistic scenario for modeling the lung tumors.

4. *In vitro* PnP (Plug and Play) models with primary tumor derived from the patient.

In addition, Table 2 summarizes how the current, as well as the future *in vitro* cancer models can replicate some or all the cancer hallmarks, their use and limitations for drug development.

Finally, we would like to propose an ideal *in vitro* lung cancer model based on the above considerations, so-called *in vitro* PnP (Plug and Play) model (Fig.5).

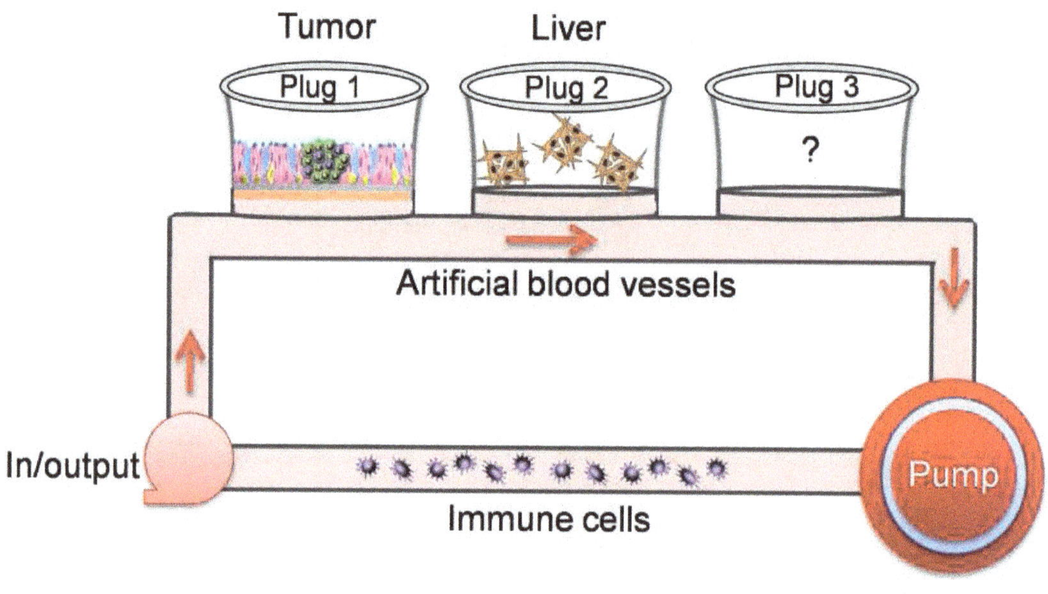


**Figure 5. Schematic representation of an ideal *in vitro* PnP (Plug and Play) lung cancer model.** A primary tumor derived from the patient is incorporated into a fully differentiated and healthy airway epithelium and cultured at air-liquid interface in a setting similar to OncoCilair™ (Mas et al., 2015); Then this co-culture model is plugged into a micro-fluidic device with artificial blood/or lymphatic vessels (pink color) containing circulating immune cells (blue color); liver cells (hepatocytes as spheroids, brown color) can also be integrated into the circuit through the plug number 2, providing metabolic capacity of drugs. If needed, other cells/organs can be further inter-connected in similar way. An input/output plug allows the addition of drug or the uptake of medium for analysis. The lung tissue culture remains accessible to apical exposure during all the experiment.

A primary tumor derived from the patient is incorporated into a fully differentiated and healthy airway epithelium and cultured at air-liquid interface, a setting similar to OncoCilair™ [82]. Then this co-culture model is plugged into a micro-fluidic device with artificial blood/or lymphatic vessels containing circulating immune cells; liver cells (hepatocytes as spheroids) can also be plugged into the circuit, providing metabolic capacity of drugs. If needed, other cells/organs can be further inter-connected in a similar way.

We are convinced that, with the development of new technologies such as microfluidic devices and 3D bio-printing, such models should quickly emerge and strengthen *in vitro* pre-clinical cancer research.

## Author details

Samuel Constant, Song Huang, Ludovic Wisniewski and Christophe Mas*

*Address all correspondence to: christophe.mas@oncotheis.com

OncoTheis Sàrl, Geneva, Switzerland

## References

[1] Malvezzi, M., et al., *European cancer mortality predictions for the year 2013.* Ann Oncol, 2013. 24(3): p. 792-800.

[2] Arrowsmith, J. and P. Miller, *Trial watch: phase II and phase III attrition rates 2011-2012.* Nat Rev Drug Discov, 2013. 12(8): p. 569.

[3] Scannell, J.W., et al., *Diagnosing the decline in pharmaceutical R&D efficiency.* Nat Rev Drug Discov, 2012. 11(3): p. 191-200.

[4] Rangarajan, A. and R.A. Weinberg, *Opinion: Comparative biology of mouse versus human cells: modelling human cancer in mice.* Nat Rev Cancer, 2003. 3(12): p. 952-9.

[5] Kung, A.L., *Practices and pitfalls of mouse cancer models in drug discovery.* Adv Cancer Res, 2007. 96: p. 191-212.

[6] Ruggeri, B.A., F. Camp, and S. Miknyoczki, *Animal models of disease: pre-clinical animal models of cancer and their applications and utility in drug discovery.* Biochem Pharmacol, 2014. 87(1): p. 150-61.

[7] Mak, I.W., N. Evaniew, and M. Ghert, *Lost in translation: animal models and clinical trials in cancer treatment.* Am J Transl Res, 2014. 6(2): p. 114-8.

[8] Odom, D.T., et al., *Tissue-specific transcriptional regulation has diverged significantly between human and mouse.* Nat Genet, 2007. 39(6): p. 730-2.

[9] Forsyth, N.R., W.E. Wright, and J.W. Shay, *Telomerase and differentiation in multicellular organisms: turn it off, turn it on, and turn it off again.* Differentiation, 2002. 69(4-5): p. 188-97.

[10] Rangarajan, A., et al., *Species- and cell type-specific requirements for cellular transformation.* Cancer Cell, 2004. 6(2): p. 171-83.

[11] Seok, J., et al., *Genomic responses in mouse models poorly mimic human inflammatory diseases.* Proc Natl Acad Sci U S A, 2013. 110(9): p. 3507-12.

[12] Dorman, G., et al., *Matrix metalloproteinase inhibitors: a critical appraisal of design principles and proposed therapeutic utility.* Drugs, 2010. 70(8): p. 949-64.

[13] Dong, X., et al., *Patient-derived first generation xenografts of non-small cell lung cancers: promising tools for predicting drug responses for personalized chemotherapy.* Clin Cancer Res, 2010. 16(5): p. 1442-51.

[14] Moro, M., et al., *Patient-derived xenografts of non small cell lung cancer: resurgence of an old model for investigation of modern concepts of tailored therapy and cancer stem cells.* J Biomed Biotechnol, 2012. 2012: p. 568567.

[15] Rong, S., et al., *Tumorigenicity of the met proto-oncogene and the gene for hepatocyte growth factor.* Mol Cell Biol, 1992. 12(11): p. 5152-8.

[16] Mestas, J. and C.C. Hughes, *Of mice and not men: differences between mouse and human immunology.* J Immunol, 2004. 172(5): p. 2731-8.

[17] Stratmann, A.T., et al., *Establishment of a human 3D lung cancer model based on a biological tissue matrix combined with a Boolean in silico model.* Mol Oncol, 2014. 8(2): p. 351-65.

[18] Lee, J.J., et al., *Stromal response to Hedgehog signaling restrains pancreatic cancer progression.* Proc Natl Acad Sci U S A, 2014. 111(30): p. E3091-100.

[19] Egeblad, M., E.S. Nakasone, and Z. Werb, *Tumors as organs: complex tissues that interface with the entire organism.* Dev Cell, 2010. 18(6): p. 884-901.

[20] Chen, W.J., et al., *Cancer-associated fibroblasts regulate the plasticity of lung cancer stemness via paracrine signalling.* Nat Commun, 2014. 5: p. 3472.

[21] Malvezzi, M., et al., *European cancer mortality predictions for the year 2014.* Ann Oncol, 2014. 25(8): p. 1650-6.

[22] Pesch, B., et al., *Cigarette smoking and lung cancer--relative risk estimates for the major histological types from a pooled analysis of case-control studies.* Int J Cancer, 2012. 131(5): p. 1210-9.

[23] Brambilla, E., et al., *The new World Health Organization classification of lung tumours.* Eur Respir J, 2001. 18(6): p. 1059-68.

[24] Ohe, Y., et al., *Randomized phase III study of cisplatin plus irinotecan versus carboplatin plus paclitaxel, cisplatin plus gemcitabine, and cisplatin plus vinorelbine for advanced non-small-cell lung cancer: Four-Arm Cooperative Study in Japan.* Ann Oncol, 2007. 18(2): p. 317-23.

[25] Reck, M., et al., *Tissue sampling in lung cancer: a review in light of the MERIT experience.* Lung Cancer, 2011. 74(1): p. 1-6.

[26] Nguyen, K.S., S. Kobayashi, and D.B. Costa, *Acquired resistance to epidermal growth factor receptor tyrosine kinase inhibitors in non-small-cell lung cancers dependent on the epidermal growth factor receptor pathway.* Clin Lung Cancer, 2009. 10(4): p. 281-9.

[27] Rosell, R., et al., *Screening for epidermal growth factor receptor mutations in lung cancer.* N Engl J Med, 2009. 361(10): p. 958-67.

[28] Sandler, A., et al., *Paclitaxel-carboplatin alone or with bevacizumab for non-small-cell lung cancer.* N Engl J Med, 2006. 355(24): p. 2542-50.

[29] Camidge, D.R., et al., *Activity and safety of crizotinib in patients with ALK-positive non-small-cell lung cancer: updated results from a phase 1 study.* Lancet Oncol, 2012. 13(10): p. 1011-9.

[30] Doebele, R.C., et al., *Mechanisms of resistance to crizotinib in patients with ALK gene rearranged non-small cell lung cancer.* Clin Cancer Res, 2012. 18(5): p. 1472-82.

[31] Shaw, A.T., et al., *Ceritinib in ALK-rearranged non-small-cell lung cancer.* N Engl J Med, 2014. 370(13): p. 1189-97.

[32] Chen, X., et al., *Clinical perspective of afatinib in non-small cell lung cancer.* Lung Cancer, 2013. 81(2): p. 155-61.

[33] Tsvetkova, E. and G.D. Goss, *Drug resistance and its significance for treatment decisions in non-small-cell lung cancer.* Curr Oncol, 2012. 19(Suppl 1): p. S45-51.

[34] Pao, W., et al., *Acquired resistance of lung adenocarcinomas to gefitinib or erlotinib is associated with a second mutation in the EGFR kinase domain.* PLoS Med, 2005. 2(3): p. e73.

[35] Engelman, J.A., et al., *MET amplification leads to gefitinib resistance in lung cancer by activating ERBB3 signaling.* Science, 2007. 316(5827): p. 1039-43.

[36] Katayama, R., et al., *Mechanisms of acquired crizotinib resistance in ALK-rearranged lung Cancers.* Sci Transl Med, 2012. 4(120): p. 120ra17.

[37] Ogawa, T., et al., *Methylation of death-associated protein kinase is associated with cetuximab and erlotinib resistance.* Cell Cycle, 2012. 11(8): p. 1656-63.

[38] Sequist, L.V., et al., *Genotypic and histological evolution of lung cancers acquiring resistance to EGFR inhibitors.* Sci Transl Med, 2011. 3(75): p. 75ra26.

[39] Yu, H.A., et al., *Analysis of tumor specimens at the time of acquired resistance to EGFR-TKI therapy in 155 patients with EGFR-mutant lung cancers.* Clin Cancer Res, 2013. 19(8): p. 2240-7.

[40] Mintz, B. and K. Illmensee, *Normal genetically mosaic mice produced from malignant teratocarcinoma cells.* Proc Natl Acad Sci U S A, 1975. 72(9): p. 3585-9.

[41] Mitra, A.K., et al., *MicroRNAs reprogram normal fibroblasts into cancer-associated fibroblasts in ovarian cancer.* Cancer Discov, 2012. 2(12): p. 1100-8.

[42] Sherman, M.H., et al., *Vitamin d receptor-mediated stromal reprogramming suppresses pancreatitis and enhances pancreatic cancer therapy.* Cell, 2014. 159(1): p. 80-93.

[43] Rowley, D.R., *Reprogramming the tumor stroma: a new paradigm.* Cancer Cell, 2014. 26(4): p. 451-2.

[44] Gazdar, A.F., et al., *Lung cancer cell lines as tools for biomedical discovery and research.* J Natl Cancer Inst, 2010. 102(17): p. 1310-21.

[45] Oboshi, S., et al., *A new floating cell line derived from human pulmonary carcinoma of oat cell type.* Gan, 1971. 62(6): p. 505-14.

[46] Sugaya, M., et al., *Establishment of 15 cancer cell lines from patients with lung cancer and the potential tools for immunotherapy.* Chest, 2002. 122(1): p. 282-8.

[47] Zheng, C., et al., *Establishment and characterization of primary lung cancer cell lines from Chinese population.* Acta Pharmacol Sin, 2011. 32(3): p. 385-92.

[48] Gazdar, A.F. and H.K. Oie, *Cell culture methods for human lung cancer.* Cancer Genet Cytogenet, 1986. 19(1-2): p. 5-10.

[49] Lam, D.C., et al., *Establishment and expression profiling of new lung cancer cell lines from Chinese smokers and lifetime never-smokers.* J Thorac Oncol, 2006. 1(9): p. 932-42.

[50] Aurisicchio, L., et al., *The promise of anti-ErbB3 monoclonals as new cancer therapeutics.* Oncotarget, 2012. 3(8): p. 744-58.

[51] Sekine, I., et al., *Emerging ethnic differences in lung cancer therapy.* Br J Cancer, 2008. 99(11): p. 1757-62.

[52] Zhang, J., et al., *Intratumor heterogeneity in localized lung adenocarcinomas delineated by multiregion sequencing.* Science, 2014. 346(6206): p. 256-9.

[53] Lee, J., M.J. Cuddihy, and N.A. Kotov, *Three-dimensional cell culture matrices: state of the art.* Tissue Eng Part B Rev, 2008. 14(1): p. 61-86.

[54] Matsusaki, M., C.P. Case, and M. Akashi, *Three-dimensional cell culture technique and pathophysiology.* Adv Drug Deliv Rev, 2014. 74: p. 95-103.

[55] Sant, S., et al., *Biomimetic Gradient Hydrogels for Tissue Engineering.* Can J Chem Eng, 2010. 88(6): p. 899-911.

[56] Margulis, A., W. Zhang, and J.A. Garlick, *In vitro fabrication of engineered human skin.* Methods Mol Biol, 2005. 289: p. 61-70.

[57] Huang, S., et al., *Potential of in vitro reconstituted 3D human airway epithelia (MucilAir) to assess respiratory sensitizers.* Toxicol *In vitro*, 2013. 27(3): p. 1151-6.

[58] Schaller, M., et al., *Models of oral and vaginal candidiasis based on in vitro reconstituted human epithelia.* Nat Protoc, 2006. 1(6): p. 2767-73.

[59] Even-Ram, S. and K.M. Yamada, *Cell migration in 3D matrix.* Curr Opin Cell Biol, 2005. 17(5): p. 524-32.

[60] Vacanti, J.P. and R. Langer, *Tissue engineering: the design and fabrication of living replacement devices for surgical reconstruction and transplantation.* Lancet, 1999. 354 Suppl 1: p. SI32-4.

[61] Bohari, S.P., D.W. Hukins, and L.M. Grover, *Effect of calcium alginate concentration on viability and proliferation of encapsulated fibroblasts.* Biomed Mater Eng, 2011. 21(3): p. 159-70.

[62] Godugu, C., et al., *AlgiMatrix based 3D cell culture system as an in-vitro tumor model for anticancer studies.* PLoS One, 2013. 8(1): p. e53708.

[63] Zhao, Y., et al., *Three-dimensional printing of Hela cells for cervical tumor model in vitro.* Biofabrication, 2014. 6(3): p. 035001.

[64] Djordjevic, B. and C.S. Lange, *Clonogenicity of mammalian cells in hybrid spheroids: a new assay method.* Radiat Environ Biophys, 1990. 29(1): p. 31-46.

[65] Ekert, J.E., et al., *Three-dimensional lung tumor microenvironment modulates therapeutic compound responsiveness in vitro--implication for drug development.* PLoS One, 2014. 9(3): p. e92248.

[66] Amann, A., et al., *Development of an innovative 3D cell culture system to study tumour--stroma interactions in non-small cell lung cancer cells.* PLoS One, 2014. 9(3): p. e92511.

[67] Thoma, C.R., et al., *3D cell culture systems modeling tumor growth determinants in cancer target discovery.* Adv Drug Deliv Rev, 2014. 69-70: p. 29-41.

[68] Huang, Y.J. and S.H. Hsu, *Acquisition of epithelial-mesenchymal transition and cancer stem-like phenotypes within chitosan-hyaluronan membrane-derived 3D tumor spheroids.* Biomaterials, 2014. 35(38): p. 10070-9.

[69] Huh, D., et al., *Reconstituting organ-level lung functions on a chip.* Science, 2010. 328(5986): p. 1662-8.

[70] Xu, Z., et al., *Application of a microfluidic chip-based 3D co-culture to test drug sensitivity for individualized treatment of lung cancer.* Biomaterials, 2013. 34(16): p. 4109-17.

[71] Ruppen, J., et al., *A microfluidic platform for chemoresistive testing of multicellular pleural cancer spheroids.* Lab Chip, 2014. 14(6): p. 1198-205.

[72] Ott, H.C., et al., *Regeneration and orthotopic transplantation of a bioartificial lung.* Nat Med, 2010. 16(8): p. 927-33.

[73] Mishra, D.K., et al., *Human lung cancer cells grown on acellular rat lung matrix create perfusable tumor nodules.* Ann Thorac Surg, 2012. 93(4): p. 1075-81.

[74] Mishra, D.K., et al., *Human lung cancer cells grown in an ex vivo 3D lung model produce matrix metalloproteinases not produced in 2D culture.* PLoS One, 2012. 7(9): p. e45308.

[75] Vaira, V., et al., *Preclinical model of organotypic culture for pharmacodynamic profiling of human tumors.* Proc Natl Acad Sci U S A, 2010. 107(18): p. 8352-6.

[76] Dong, M., et al., *Tissue slice model of human lung cancer to investigate telomerase inhibition by nanoparticle delivery of antisense 2'-O-methyl-RNA.* Int J Pharm, 2011. 419(1-2): p. 33-42.

[77] Atala, A., F.K. Kasper, and A.G. Mikos, *Engineering complex tissues.* Sci Transl Med, 2012. 4(160): p. 160rv12.

[78] Walles, T., et al., *The potential of bioartificial tissues in oncology research and treatment.* Onkologie, 2007. 30(7): p. 388-94.

[79] Wiszniewski, L., et al., *Long-term cultures of polarized airway epithelial cells from patients with cystic fibrosis.* Am J Respir Cell Mol Biol, 2006. 34(1): p. 39-48.

[80] Mas C, Huang S, Wiszniewski L, Constant S., *A new 3D human airway tissue model for in vitro lung cancer research (OncoCilAir™).* ALTEX Proceedings, 2014. 3(1/14): p. I-4-204.

[81] Mas C, Huang S, Wiszniewski L, Constant S., *In vitro Human Airway Tissue Model For Lung Cancer Research.* Am J Respir Crit Care Med 2014. 189: p. A3455.

[82] Mas C, Boda B, CaulFuty M, Huang S, Wiszniewski L and Constant S., *Antitumour efficacy of the selumetinib and trametinib MEK inhibitors in a combined human airway-tumour-stroma lung cancer model.* J Biotechnol., 2015. in press.

[83] Hanahan, D. and R.A. Weinberg, *The hallmarks of cancer.* Cell, 2000. 100(1): p. 57-70.

[84] Hanahan, D. and R.A. Weinberg, *Hallmarks of cancer: the next generation.* Cell, 2011. 144(5): p. 646-74.

[85] Nowell, P.C., *The clonal evolution of tumor cell populations.* Science, 1976. 194(4260): p. 23-8.

[86] Gatenby, R.A. and R.J. Gillies, *A microenvironmental model of carcinogenesis.* Nat Rev Cancer, 2008. 8(1): p. 56-61.

[87] Siegel, R., et al., *Cancer statistics, 2011: the impact of eliminating socioeconomic and racial disparities on premature cancer deaths.* CA Cancer J Clin, 2011. 61(4): p. 212-36.

[88] Malakoff, D., *Can treatment costs be tamed?* Science, 2011. 331(6024): p. 1545-7.

[89] Gurdon, J.B., *A community effect in animal development.* Nature, 1988. 336(6201): p. 772-4.

[90] Gao, S.P., et al., *Mutations in the EGFR kinase domain mediate STAT3 activation via IL-6 production in human lung adenocarcinomas.* J Clin Invest, 2007. 117(12): p. 3846-56.

# 9

# Current Management and Novel Therapeutic Strategies to Combat Chronic Delta Hepatitis

Hrvoje Roguljic, Sonja Sarcevic, Robert Smolic, Nikola Raguz Lucic, Aleksandar Vcev and Martina Smolic

## 1. Introduction

Forty years ago Mario Rizzeto's group identified a new antigen-antibody system (delta antibody and delta antigen (HDAg)) in HBsAg carriers with severe hepatitis [1, 2]. Further experiments in chimpanzees showed that this HDAg marked transmissible pathogen requires coexistence of HBV infection for its life cycle, proving its defective nature which requires HBsAg for transmission and replication [3]. As the cause of hepatitis D was identified, a virion particle (Figure 1.) composed of outer coat containing HBV envelope proteins (HBsAg) and inner nuclocapsid was described [4]. Internal nuclear like structure is comprised of single stranded, circular RNA molecule of 1700 nucleotides associated with two distinctive forms of hepatitis D antigen (HDAg), small and large subunit [5, 6]. Although HDV in its structure possesses HBsAg, HDV is classified as separate pathogen with own genus called *Deltavirus* [7]. This unusual virus is the smallest infectious pathogen in human virology, with unique replication cycle unknown to animal cells. During replication process a viral RNA is transcribed by hosts RNA polymerases [8], which usually transcribe DNA molecules, and after transcription HDV RNA is cleaved by its own ribozyme [9].

Dependence on the HBsAg presence results in two patterns of HDV infection. HDV can be transmitted simultaneously with HBV (co-infection pattern) or infection may occur at preceding HBV infected individual (super-infection pattern). Due to differences of HDV acquisition clinical course and outcome of HDV infection varies. However, many studies have shown that HDV infection causes more severe liver disease [10] and more rapid progression to cirrhosis [11] than HBV mono-infection alone.

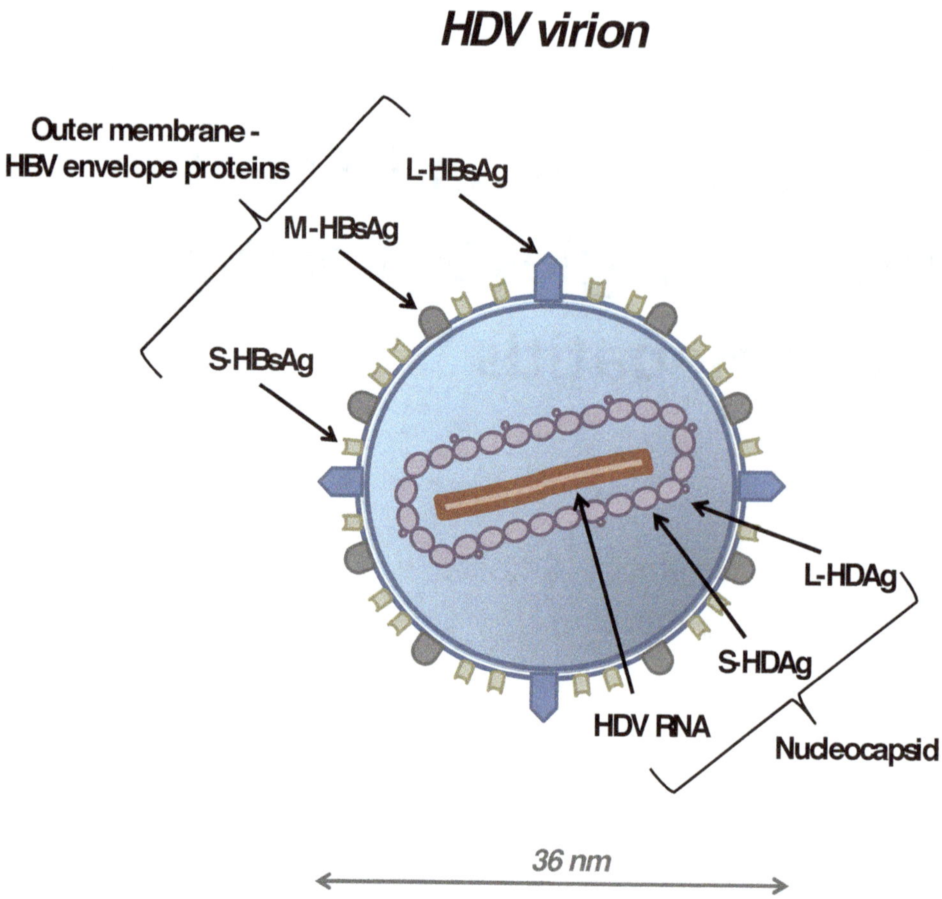


**Figure 1.** Structure of HDV virion. HDV is composed of outer membrane, HBV envelope proteins within a phospholipid bilayer, and inner nucleocapsid consisting of viral RNA and hepatitis delta antigens. L-HBsAg=large hepatitis B surface antigen. M-HBsAg=medium hepatitis B surface antigen. S-HBsAg=small hepatitis B surface antigen. HDV RNA=hepatitis D virus RNA. L-HDAg=large hepatitis D antigen. S-HDAg=small hepatitis D antigen.

Although many details regarding HDV viral cycle are revealed, therapy of HDV has not progressed. To date, treatment options of HDV infection are limited to interferon regimes with open issues about effectiveness of current approaches. Due to the unsatisfactory results further studies of novel drugs and therapy protocols are required. In this chapter current treatment procedures as well as novel therapeutic strategies to combat chronic HDV infection will be discussed.

## 2. Epidemiology

It is estimated that 15-20 million of HBsAg positive individuals are infected with HDV, but these numbers are not accurate because of absence of systematic screening in HBV infected individuals [12]. Interestingly, HDV infection is worldwide distributed; however the distribution is not uniform. Areas of HDV high prevalence are: Central Africa, Mediterranean countries, Middle East and South America, while in Western world HDV infection is limited to intravenous drug abusers [13]. Decrease of HDV incidence in industrialized world is caused by improvement of socioeconomic conditions such as implementation of HBV vaccination and systematic screening of blood and blood products. However, reduction in the number of infected individuals in developed countries has stopped, mainly due to the increased immigration from endemic areas [14]. Prevalence of anti-HD among HBsAg positive individuals in Western Europe has been stable during last decade ranging from 8.5 to 11.0 % [15, 16].

So far, eight HDV genotypes have been described. Most frequent is genotype 1 [17], which is prevalent worldwide, while genotypes 2 and 4 are mainly found in the Far East and genotype 3 is limited to Amazonian basin [18]. HDV genotypes 5-8 are found in patients originating from Africa [19]. Different HDV genotypes have impact on variations in clinical course of disease, thus genotypes 1 and 3 cause more severe disease, while genotype 2 is associated with milder form. Also, multiple genotypes of HDV can be found in high risk patients [20].

## 3. Transmission of HDV

HDV, as its helper HBV, is transmitted parenterally through the exposure to the blood and body fluids. In the developed countries the main route of transmission is by infected syringes among intravenous drug users. Although, there is an evidence for sexual transmission [21], it seems that HDV does not have the same rate of sexual transmission as HBV[22]. Due to the screening of the blood products, there is no more risk of HDV infections for the blood receiving patients. Despite the fact that HDV is parenterally transmitted, inapparent parenteral transmission within household [23] represents major route of transmission in the areas of the high prevalence. Therefore vaccination against HBV of all household members of infected individual is the crucial step in prevention of HDV infections. Vertical transmission from mother to the newborn is rare.

## 4. Clinical features

As defective virus, HDV replication depends on HbsAg synthesis, therefore HDV can be transmitted only in the presence of accompanied HBV infection. Based on the previous HBsAg status of the infected individual two major patterns of infection are distinguished: simultaneous HBV/HDV co-infection or superinfection by HDV of chronic HBsAg carriers [18].

In the simultaneous infection the fate of HDV depends on the host response to the HBV. When the expression of HBsAg is restrained, the HDV infection may result with abortive response, while abundance of HBsAg enables the full expression of HDV pathogenicity. As a result of this interaction between the two viruses, disease expression may vary. Clinically, HDV/HBV co-infection is usually similar to HBV mono-infection, although acute co-infection can be more severe and can be manifested as acute liver failure [24]. The rate of progression of HDV infection to chronic form is equal to that for acute hepatitis B, less than 5% [19].

Superinfection is defined as HDV infection of a chronically HBV infected individual. Preexisting chronic HBV infection represents perfect environment for replication of defective hepatitis D virus, resulting with abundant HDV expression and suppression of HBV replication. HBV suppression will become permanent, if HDV infection progress to chronic form [20]. Furthermore, superinfection is generally presented as severe acute hepatitis with shorter incubation time and will exceed to chronic HDV infection in high percentage of patients, up to 80% [25]. Clinically, HDV superinfection is manifested as a worsening of present HBV disease or as a new hepatitis in previously undiagnosed HBV infected individual. Along with detection of HDV serum markers, correct diagnosis of superinfection is clarified by negative IgM anti-HBc [21].

## 5. Symptoms and course

Symptoms of acute hepatits D infection are similar to the other forms of viral hepatitis. Initial phase of acute infection is characterized by nonspecific symptoms such as: fatigue, anorexia, nausea and lethargy accompanied with high increase of serum alanine aminotransferase and aspartate aminotransferase. Sometimes this phase is followed with icteric phase, characterized by jaundice, dark urine, clay-colored stools and elevated levels of serum bilirubin. Acute hepatitis is more severe in superinfection pattern, due to the fact that preceding HBV infection facilitates multiplication of HDV. Furthermore, acute disease can occur as fulminant hepatits, named as acute liver failure (ALF). ALF is a rare form of acute hepatitis; which is more often seen in acute hepatitis caused by HDV than other hepatothropic viruses. Clinically, ALF starts with nonspecific symptoms, such as fatigue and malaise followed by jaundice and hepatic encephalopathy and ultimately leading to coma. ALF is characterized by massive necrosis of hepatocytes, rapid clinical course; ultimately result with death of individual in 2-10 days. Without liver transplantation, ALF has lethal outcome in 80% of cases [26].

Choronic hepatitis D is the rarest form among chronic viral hepatitis, although it is the most severe and most progressive one. Chronic hepatitis D has three times higher risk for cirrhosis development than HBV chronic infection [27]. Clinically it is initially expressed as acute hepatitis in the half of the cases, probably due to initial acute superinfection [28]. However, symptoms of chronic hepatitis D are variable. Chronic hepatitis D can be manifested as fatigue, malaise and anorexia or its clinical course can be without any symptoms [9]. When cirrhosis is developed disease may be stable and asymptomatic for a long period or it can be manifested with complications related to the cirrhotic process. Once developed, a high number of patients with HDV cirrhosis will die of liver failure or hepatocellular carcinoma unless liver transplantation is performed [29].

## 6. Diagnosis

First step in diagnostic procedures is detection of HDV markers in the blood of HBsAg positive individual, due to the fact that HDV replication is possible only in the presence of HBV.

Actually, guidelines suggest that all HBsAg positive individuals should be screened for HDV infection, as well as members of high-risk group's like intravenous drug users, hemodialysis patients, health care and public safety workers. Also in the case of clinical deterioration of chronic HBV infection, superinfection with HDV should be considered.

Specific markers of HDV infection in serum are: Hepatitis D virus RNA, HDAg and anti-HDV. HDV RNA is detected in serum by molecular hybridization [30] or more sensitive RT-PCR [31], thus serum HDAg and anti-HDV are detected by enzyme-linked immunosorbent assay (ELISA) [32] and radioimmunoassay (RIA). During the diagnostic procedure, along with confirmation of HDV presence, it is necessary to clarify the stage of the infection due to the differences in clinical course and progonosis. Based on the interactions between two viruses, three patterns of HDV infections are distinguished: acute HDV/HBV co-infection, acute HDV infection of HBsAg positive carrier and chronic HDV infection.

Acute HBV/HDV co-infection is characterized with a high titre of IgM anti-HBc, a marker of acute HBV infection which enables to distinguishing confection from acute HDV superinfection. HDAg appears in the early phase of the acute infection and it is only transiently detectable in serum, unless patient is imunodeficient. Then HDAg can be detected for a longer period due to the weak immune system [33]. HDV RNA is also detectable in the early phase of acute infection [34] and represents a sensitive marker for virus replication present in 90% of patients. Nowdays, an active HDV infection is confirmed by detection of HDV RNA in the serum by sensitive real time PCR assays [35]. Although, HDV RNA test can be false negative due to the variability of the genome sequence, so that sero-conversion and detection of IgM anti-HDV is still helpful to establish diagnosis of acute infection.

In chronic HDV infection the high titre of IgG anti-HD antibodies persist even after viral clearance. Also, a large proportion of patients has positive IgM antiHD, a characteristic marker of acute infection. Persistence of anti-HD IgM antibodies indicates progression of disease to the chronic form. HDV RNA is present in the serum of chronically infected patients as HDAg.

Individual's positive for HDV serum markers should be subjected to the liver biopsy to determine histological stage of the liver disease, due to the fact that HDV serum markers or values of liver test do not reflect severity of liver damage [36]. Also, all the HDV positive patients should be tested for HCV and HIV because of the high frequency of co-infection with these parenterally transmitted viruses [37].

## 7. Treatment

Presence of HBsAg is necessary for the replication of the HDV, hence the therapeutic aim is to eradicate both pathogens. HDV is considered eradicated if HDV-RNA in serum and HDAg in the liver are negative 6 months after therapy [24]. Despite the sustained viral response, there is still a possibility of reactivation of HDV in HBsAg positive individual, due to the limitations of diagnostic procedures to detect a low level of HDV copies (1000 copies/ml). Experimentally in animal model, the posibillity to transfer HDV infection with serum diluted up to $10^{-11}$ was demonstrated [38]. Although HDV is considered eradicated when serum HDV RNA and HDAg in the liver are persistently undetectable, only eradication of HBsAg represents a complete cure and it is ultimate goal of HDV treatment. Eradication of virus results in normalization of ALT levels and stopping of liver fibrosis process, while developed anti HD antibodies will prevent re-infections [24].

So far only approved therapy for Hepatits D is standard interferon-$\alpha$ (IFN- $\alpha$). Long-term administration of high-dose standard IFN- $\alpha$, 5 million units daily or 9 million units three times per week for 12 months, results in normalization of alanine aminotransferase serum values, clearance of serum HDV RNA, and histological improvement in 50 percent of patients with chronic hepatitis D [39]. High-dose IFN therapy improves the long-term clinical outcome and survival rate of the patients, even if they have advanced disease and active cirrhosis before therapy induction [40]. There are still arguments going on with regard to duration of interferon treatment. Interferon therapy administered through 12 months has better results comparing to 6 months therapy [39], although prolongation of IFN therapy to 24 months does not result with increasing response to the treatment [41]. Unfortunately, large number of patients will appear relapse usually 2-6 months after termination of treatment [39]. Thus interferon therapy is insufficient for the majority of patients with chronic HDV, characterized with incomplete sustained viral response and common biochemical and virological relapses after cessation of treatment [42, 43]. Interferon treatment is often accompanied with numerous side effects, which requires a continuous supervision of the patients during treatment. Most common side effects are influenza like symptoms such as fatigue and weight loss [44]. Severe psychiatric disorders can appear as a result of prolonged high dose interferon therapy [42, 45], which disables interferon application to the certain number of patients. Another compulsory reason for cessation of interferon therapy is decompensation of liver disease, due to the fact that high number of patients has advanced disease and cirrhosis [46, 47].

Lately, pegylated form of interferon-$\alpha$ (Peg-IFN-$\alpha$) is introduced in therapy of HDV. It is characterized by longer half-life, which allows longer intervals between drug administrations. Treatment with Peg-IFN-$\alpha$ showed better response in naive patients and in previous nonresponders compared to standard IFN-$\alpha$ treatment [48, 49]. Patients not achieving SVR with standard interferon therapy, may eradicate serum HDV RNA after a 6-month treatment with Peg-IFN-$\alpha$ [50]. For the lowering of HDV RNA beyond detectable level, it is demonstrated that even standard doses of Peg-IFN- $\alpha$ are more successful than high doses of standard IFN- $\alpha$, although in that case seroconversion of HBsAg is not taken into consideration [51]. However, the rate of clearance of HBsAg is greater with Peg-IFN-$\alpha$, but overall clearance and seroconversion of HBsAg is low, only in 3-5% of cases [52]. Generally, it is difficult to assess the effectiveness of IFN-$\alpha$ therapy due to differences in study strategies that examined the effect of the treatment. Studies usually differ in forms of drugs, doses, duration of the treatment and patient follow-up period, making comparison of results a difficult task (Table 1.). Considering these differences in the previous studies, overall sustained viral response varies from 17 to 43 % [53]. Currently the largest hepatitis delta multicenter study is HIDIT I trial, which is carried out by the German Network of Competence for Viral Hepatitis (Hep-Net) in collaboration with centers from Turkey and Greece. In total of 90 patients with hepatitis D, the effect of Peg-IFN-α-2a in combination with adeofovir versus either drug alone was examined. Overall, 28% of the patients had sustained viral response after treatment with Peg-IFN-α-2a for 48 weeks, with no difference in efficacy between combined therapy compared with Peg-IFN-α-2a monotherapy [54]. From the results of current studies it is evident that treatment with Peg-IFN-α-2a has limited efficacy as a therpy of hepatitis delta, thus further investigations of potential tretment options are needed.

| Study and year | Patients (n) | Therapy | Duration (weeks) | Results |
|---|---|---|---|---|
| **Yurdaydin, 2008.** [74] | 39 | 1st group (n=14), Lamivudine (100mg/day) plus IFN-α-2a (9 MU/3x week) vs. 2nd group (n=8), IFN-α-2a vs. 3rd group (n=17), Lamivudine | 48 | BR: 1st(64%), 2nd(63%), 3rd(18%) EOTR: 1st(50%), 2nd(50%), 3rd(12%) SVR: 1st(36%), 2nd(50%), 3rd(12%) Combination treatment was not superior to IFN therapy. |
| **Gheorghe, 2011.** [75] | 49 | Peg-IFN-α-2b (1.5μg/kg/week) | 48 | BR: 50% EOTR: 33.3% SVR: 25% |
| **Ormeci, 2011.** [76] | 18 | Peg-IFN-α-2b (1.5μg/kg/week) | 96 weeks (n=11) and 48 weeks (n=7) | No significant difference between two groups in terms of HDV-RNA suppression and ALT normalisation. |
| **Wedemeyer, 2011.** [77] | 90 | 1st group (n=31) Peg-IFN-α-2a (180 μg/week) plus Adeofovir (10 mg/ daily) vs. 2nd group (n=29) Peg-IFN-α-2a vs. 3rd group(n=30) Adeofovir | 48 | BR: 1st(32%), 2nd(28%), 3rd(7%) EOTR: 1st(23%), 2nd(24%), 3rd(0%) SVR: 1st(26%), 2nd(31%), 3rd(0%) |
| **Karaca, 2012.** [78] | 32 | Peg-IFN-α-2a (180 μg) or Peg-IFN-α-2b (1.5 μg/kg) per week | 96 | EOTR: 50% SVR: 47% |
| **Kabaçam, 2012.** [79] | 13 | Entecavir (1 mg/day) | 48 | Ineffective in chronic hepatitis delta. |
| **Samiullah, 2012.** [80] | 238 | Peg-IFN-α-2b (1.5 μg/kg/week) | 48 | BR: 51.3% EOTR: 29.8% SVR: 29.4% |

**BR**: Biochemical response is determined by a normalization of ALT at the end of the treatment.

**EOTR**: The end of treatment response is defined by a HDV-RNA negative status.

**SVR**: A sustained virological response is defined by undetectable serum HDV-RNA at six months after the end of treatment.

**Table 1.** Recent studies for treatment of chronic delta hepatitis

Last 30 years many antiviral drugs are tested in the therapy of hepatitis D, but with limited succsess. Particulary it was tested efficiency of nucleoside and nucleotide analogues (NUCs) such as: lamivudine, adeofovir, famciclovir and entecavir; due to the fact that NUCs have some therapeutic efficancy against HBV. The effect of tenofovir was observed in a group of patients with concomitant presence of HCV, HBV and HDV infection. It seems that the prior long term treatment with lamivudine and tenofovir before introduction of IFN therapy might help fastering decline of HDV RNA copies in such patients. However, seroconversion of HBsAg was not observed. Patients who suffer from multiple infections with HCV, HBV and HDV present another group difficult to treat. Unfortunately, the consequence is a progressive liver fibrosis. It is shown that neither IFN monotherapy or combination therapy with NUCs and IFN are effective. Those patients are less sensitive to IFN therapy [55]. Babiker et al. report the case of successful depletion of serum HDV RNA in a patient with acute HDV superinfection due to 65 weeks treatment with tenofovir and lamivudine. But, after the cessation of the treatment HDV RNA levels began to increase [56]. Another combination therapy is the therapy with entecavir and PEG IFN$\alpha$-2a. In this case also, quantitative HBsAg was used as the treatment response guidance for dual infection with HBV and HDV. The seroconversion of HBsAg and undetectable HDV RNA levels were achieved after 35 months of such therapy. In this patient, the stage of liver fibrosis has also improved significantly. The consolidation therapy during next 12 months after the seroconversion was continued and the patient remained seronegative during 12 months after cessation of the therapy [57].

Possible new drug candidates for the therapy are the ones affecting the interaction between HD virion and HBsAg, as well as posttranslational modifications of HDV proteins, such as prenylation. Also, it seems IFN- $\lambda$ could be possible alternative for IFN-$\alpha$ because in the treatment of chronic hepatitis C, IFN- $\lambda$ proved to cause less side effects [53].

## 8. Liver transplantation in HDV patients

HDV infection is characterized with more severe disease than HBV monoinfection. Studies showed two times higher relative risk of cirrhosis and threefold risk increase of hepatocellular carcinoma in patients coinfected with HBV and HDV compared with HBV monoinfection [27, 58]. Consequently, liver transplantation (LT) represents only therapeutic option for the patients with end-stage liver disease, as well as for hepatocellular carcinoma and fulminant hepatitis due to the coinfection or superinfection with HDV and HBV.

Prevention of allograft reinfection is the main requirement for the long term survival. Major risk factor predicitng HBV-HDV recurrence after LT is a high level of HBV DNA (>$10^5$ copies/ml) at transplant, fortunately that is unusal feature of HDV disease course [59]. Therefore, patients coinfected with HBV and HDV generally do not require pretransplant antiviral B therapy. In case when pretransplant antiviral treatment is needed, entecavir or teneofovir are preferred rather than lamivudine, while IFN therapy is not recommended during the pre-transplant period. Other predictors of a low risk of HBV-HDV recurrence are low levels of HBV replication markers, HDV coinfection and fulminant hepatitis [60]. Coinfection with human immunodeficiency virus and recurrence of HCC represent a risk factors for HBV recurrence [61, 62].

The patient's prognosis and overall outcome after LT is on satisfactory level with current posttransplant therapy. Golden standard for prevention of recurrent disease is combination of hyperimmune serum against HBV(HBIg) and potent nucleoside analogue. Therapeutic strategy of low dose intramuscular HBIg in combination with lamivudine is the most cost-effective profilaxis [63], with the rates of the recurrence level as low as 4% at 4 years [64]. Therefore, the outcome of LT due to HDV related liver disease is similar to or better than in other indications of LT [65, 66].

Due to LT, HDV RNA becomes negative within the first days after transplantation, followed by a decline of HbsAg with almost identical pattern. However, HDVAg can be detected in the hepatocytes of the graft for several months after treatment [54]. This HDV latency in the graft represents a potential source of HDV recurrence, because of possible HBV superinfection and reexpression of HBsAg. Thus, transplanted patients should be monitored for HbsAG and HBV DNA every 3 months and for HDV RNA every 6 months.

## 9. Perspectives for a vaccine development against HDV

Since the details in pathophysiologic respose to HDV infection still aren't enlightened, there are difficulties in finding the effective vaccine against it. In the case of HDV infection, the antigen is nucleoprotein and the imunization means the activation of T cells (CD4+ and CD8+) which would destroy infected cells and prevent replication of the virus. Preclinical studies have been done on woodchuks. In this model of chronically infected woodchuks with woodchuck hepatitis virus (WHV), it is possible to achieve the superinfection with HDV. So far, T cell vaccine prevented the coinfection with WHV- HDV, but it failed to prevent the superinfection of chronic carriers of WHV. Further studies have to be done to resolve the problem of preventing the superinfection by stimulating T cells. This would mean that chronic carriers would have to be vaccinated frequently to activate a large number of T cells before the patient is exposed to HDV. [67]

## 10. Novel therapeutic strategies for future treatment

So far, the treatment outcome of hepatitis delta is not satisfactory. Thus, new therapy aproaches are necessary (Figure 2.). Interferon-$\alpha$ targets the HbsAg, whose depletion is crucial for succesful treatment of hepatitis delta. The major difficulty with such therapy are numerous adverse effects, since IFN-$\alpha$ receptors are also present in other tissues than hepatic. Additional problem is the necessity of long term application of IFN-$\alpha$ to achieve therapeutic response. Better candidate could be IFN- $\lambda$, since its receptors are present only on epithelial cells [68]. It has been shown that pegylated IFN- $\lambda$ used as monotherapy, or in combination with ribavirin, has significant antiviral activity against hepatitis C virus. Also, as expected, it causes less undesirable side effects. [69] Further studies must be done to evaluate the effectivness of IFN-$\lambda$ in treatment od chronic hepatitis delta.

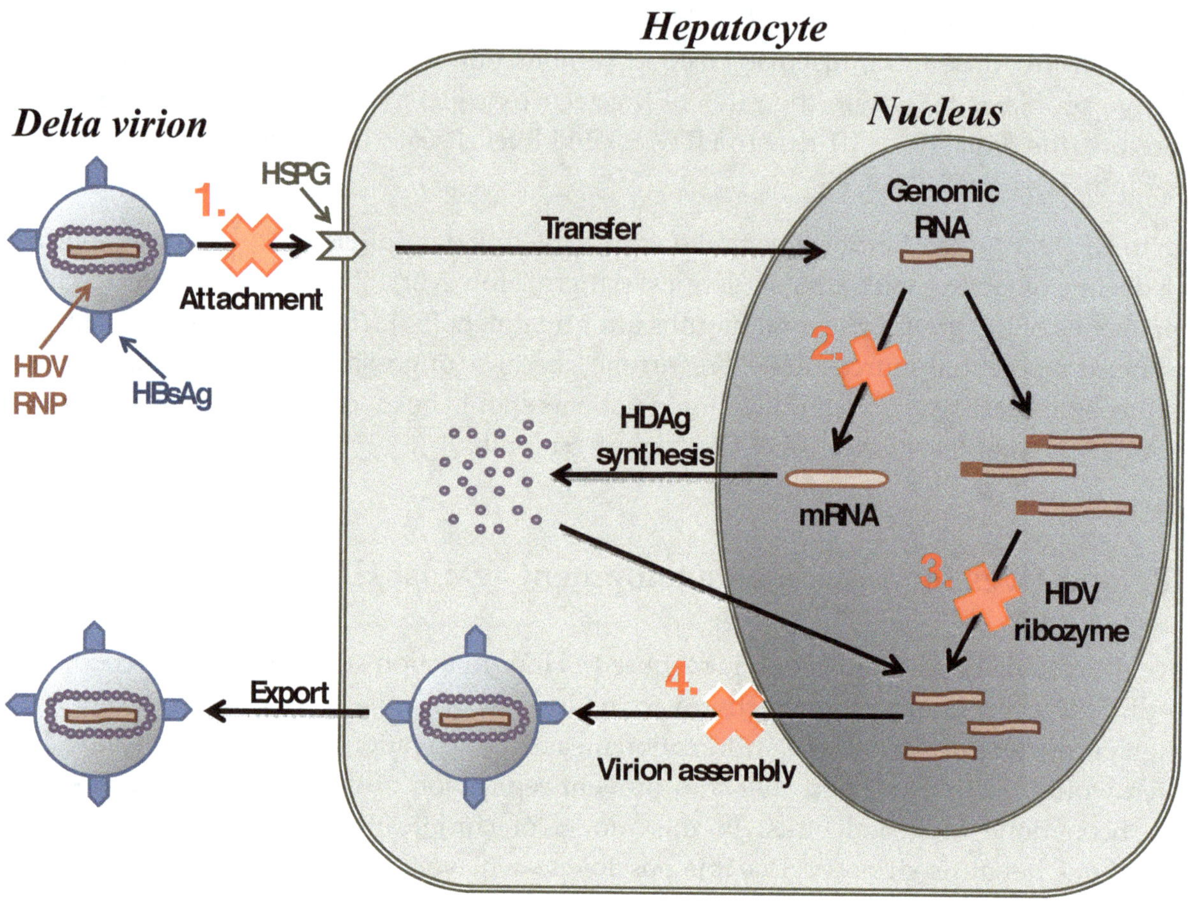


HDV RNP= hepatitis D virus ribonucleoprotein. HBsAg= hepatitis B surface antigen. HSPG=highly sulphated proteoglycans. HDAg=hepatitis D antigen.

**Figure 2.** Potential drug targets in HDV treatment. 1. Neutralizing of negativly charged HSPG may prevent HDV and HBV attachment to hepatocyte membrane. 2. Gene therapy targets genes which encode HDAg 3. Inhibition of HDV ribozymes would prevent virus replication, 4. Interferring with posttranslational modifications of HDVAg enables virion assembly.

Other strategy for therapy development is to interfere with posttranslational modifications of HDVAg. Such modifications are prenylation, acetylation, metylation and phosphorylation of HDVAg. Prenylation inhibitors proved effective in cell culture model and are currently in clinical studies. [54] Drugs interferring with other types of HDV posttranslational modifications haven't been developed yet. [70]

Since HDV genome is too small to code all the necessary particles for it's own replication, it almost entirely depends on the host's replication mechanisms. For example, it deceives host's RNA polymerases so they copy HDV genome. HDV replication is known as rolling replication mechanism, meaning that HDV circular genome is elongated into multimeric linear transcripts and than cleaved into multiple genome size monomers by it's own RNA. This type of RNA is known as ribozyme, which is actually HDV RNA with enzymatic activity.

Small interfering RNAs (siRNAs) are up to 25 nucleotides long double stranded RNAs which silence particular gene by binding to mRNA. After binding to target mRNA,siRNA causes it's degradation. In therapy of HDV infection, silencing gene which codes LHD-Ag would disable HD virion replication [16].

Ribozymes can also serve as target for therapy. It has been shown that amoxicillin, apramycin and ristomycin in complex with copper (II) bind to HDV ribozymes and inhibit them. [71] Further studies are necessary to investigate the therapeutic potential of such treatment.

Not only large HDAg (LHDAg) is important for the lifecycle of hepatitis delta virus, but also the small delta antigen protein (SHDAg). Therefore, it can also be the target for new drugs in development for HDV treatment.

It has been shown that the negatively charged highly sulphated proteoglycanes (HSPG) play a role in both HBV and HDV attachement to hepatocyte membrane. Those weak forces between opposite charged subjects enable virus attachment to the cell. [72] This kind of target could be good for developing the drug which would prevent binding of both HBV and HDV to hepatocyte surface by neutralizing the negative charge of HSPG.

Gene therapy would target HDVAg, which is proved to have crucial role in lifecycle of HDV. Design of specific molecule which binds to gene which encodes delta antigen is in progess. Some computational analyses have been done to simulate the silencing of target gene. [73]

## 11. Conclusions

HDV is an unusal, defective hepatotropic virus which causes severe acute hepatitis and most progressive chronic viral hepatitis. Despite the efforts in eradication of HDV, as its obligatory helper HBV, prevalence of HDV in developed countries remains stable and represents a relevant public health concern. Current conventional therapy of hepatitis delta is characterized with poor overall response, thus further investigations of novel treatment options are needed. Continuous research of virology and pathogenesis is necessary to provide fundamentals for development of novel approaches in treatment of HDV.

## Acknowledgements

The support of the J. J. Strossmayer University of Osijek research grant (to MS) and Ministry of science, education and sport research grant (to AV) are gratefully acknowledged.

## Author details

Hrvoje Roguljic[1], Sonja Sarcevic[2], Robert Smolic[1,2], Nikola Raguz Lucic[2], Aleksandar Vcev[1,3] and Martina Smolic[1,2*]

*Address all correspondence to: martina.smolic@mefos.hr

1 Department of Mineral Research, Faculty of Medicine, J. J. Strossmayer University of Osijek, Croatia

2 Department of Pharmacology, Faculty of Medicine, J. J. Strossmayer University of Osijek, Croatia

3 Department of Medicine, Faculty of Medicine, J. J. Strossmayer University of Osijek, Croatia

Authors declare no conflict of interest

## References

[1] Rizzetto M, Canese MG, Aricò S, Crivelli O, Trepo C, Bonino F, et al. Immunofluorescence detection of new antigen-antibody system (delta/anti-delta) associated to hepatitis B virus in liver and in serum of HBsAg carriers. Gut. 1977;18(12):997-1003.

[2] Rizzetto M, Shih JW, Gocke DJ, Purcell RH, Verme G, Gerin JL. Incidence and significance of antibodies to delta antigen in hepatitis B virus infection. Lancet. 1979;2(8150):986-90.

[3] Rizzetto M, Canese MG, Gerin JL, London WT, Sly DL, Purcell RH. Transmission of the hepatitis B virus-associated delta antigen to chimpanzees. J Infect Dis. 1980;141(5):590-602.

[4] Rizzetto M, Hoyer B, Canese MG, Shih JW, Purcell RH, Gerin JL. delta Agent: association of delta antigen with hepatitis B surface antigen and RNA in serum of delta-infected chimpanzees. Proc Natl Acad Sci U S A. 1980;77(10):6124-8.

[5] Gudima S, Chang J, Moraleda G, Azvolinsky A, Taylor J. Parameters of human hepatitis delta virus genome replication: the quantity, quality, and intracellular distribution of viral proteins and RNA. J Virol. 2002;76(8):3709-19.

[6] Ryu WS, Netter HJ, Bayer M, Taylor J. Ribonucleoprotein complexes of hepatitis delta virus. J Virol. 1993;67(6):3281-7.

[7] Alvarado-Mora MV, Locarnini S, Rizzetto M, Pinho JR. An update on HDV: virology, pathogenesis and treatment. Antivir Ther. 2013;18(3 Pt B):541-8.

[8] Lai MM. RNA replication without RNA-dependent RNA polymerase: surprises from hepatitis delta virus. J Virol. 2005;79(13):7951-8.

[9] Taylor JM. Structure and replication of hepatitis delta virus RNA. Curr Top Microbiol Immunol. 2006;307:1-23.

[10] Govindarajan S, Chin KP, Redeker AG, Peters RL. Fulminant B viral hepatitis: role of delta agent. Gastroenterology. 1984;86(6):1417-20.

[11] Fattovich G, Boscaro S, Noventa F, Pornaro E, Stenico D, Alberti A, et al. Influence of hepatitis delta virus infection on progression to cirrhosis in chronic hepatitis type B. J Infect Dis. 1987;155(5):931-5.

[12] Hadziyannis SJ. Review: hepatitis delta. J Gastroenterol Hepatol. 1997;12(4):289-98.

[13] Rizzetto M, Ponzetto A, Forzani I. Hepatitis delta virus as a global health problem. Vaccine. 1990;8 Suppl:S10-4; discussion S21-3.

[14] Wedemeyer H, Heidrich B, Manns MP. Hepatitis D virus infection--not a vanishing disease in Europe! Hepatology. 2007;45(5):1331-2; author reply 2-3.

[15] Heidrich B, Deterding K, Tillmann HL, Raupach R, Manns MP, Wedemeyer H. Virological and clinical characteristics of delta hepatitis in Central Europe. J Viral Hepat. 2009;16(12):883-94.

[16] Ciancio A, Rizzetto M. Chronic hepatitis D at a standstill: where do we go from here? Nat Rev Gastroenterol Hepatol. 2014;11(1):68-71.

[17] Shakil AO, Hadziyannis S, Hoofnagle JH, Di Bisceglie AM, Gerin JL, Casey JL. Geographic distribution and genetic variability of hepatitis delta virus genotype I. Virology. 1997;234(1):160-7.

[18] Ito T, Tahara SM, Lai MMC. The 3 '-untranslated region of hepatitis C virus RNA enhances translation from an internal ribosomal entry site. Journal of Virology. 1998;72(11):8789-96.

[19] Radjef N, Gordien E, Ivaniushina V, Gault E, Anaïs P, Drugan T, et al. Molecular phylogenetic analyses indicate a wide and ancient radiation of African hepatitis delta virus, suggesting a deltavirus genus of at least seven major clades. J Virol. 2004;78(5): 2537-44.

[20] Su CW, Huang YH, Huo TI, Shih HH, Sheen IJ, Chen SW, et al. Genotypes and viremia of hepatitis B and D viruses are associated with outcomes of chronic hepatitis D patients. Gastroenterology. 2006;130(6):1625-35.

[21] Wu JC, Chen CM, Sheen IJ, Lee SD, Tzeng HM, Choo KB. Evidence of transmission of hepatitis D virus to spouses from sequence analysis of the viral genome. Hepatology. 1995;22(6):1656-60.

[22] Weisfuse IB, Hadler SC, Fields HA, Alter MJ, O'Malley PM, Judson FN, et al. Delta hepatitis in homosexual men in the United States. Hepatology. 1989;9(6):872-4.

[23] Niro GA, Casey JL, Gravinese E, Garrubba M, Conoscitore P, Sagnelli E, et al. Intrafamilial transmission of hepatitis delta virus: molecular evidence. J Hepatol. 1999;30(4): 564-9.

[24] Pascarella S, Negro F. Hepatitis D virus: an update. Liver Int. 2011;31(1):7-21.

[25] Smedile A, Farci P, Verme G, Caredda F, Cargnel A, Caporaso N, et al. Influence of delta infection on severity of hepatitis B. Lancet. 1982;2(8305):945-7.

[26] Lee WM. Acute liver failure. N Engl J Med. 1993;329(25):1862-72.

[27] Fattovich G, Giustina G, Christensen E, Pantalena M, Zagni I, Realdi G, et al. Influence of hepatitis delta virus infection on morbidity and mortality in compensated cirrhosis type B. The European Concerted Action on Viral Hepatitis (Eurohep). Gut. 2000;46(3):420-6.

[28] Farci P, Niro GA. Clinical features of hepatitis D. Semin Liver Dis. 2012;32(3):228-36.

[29] Rosina F, Conoscitore P, Cuppone R, Rocca G, Giuliani A, Cozzolongo R, et al. Changing pattern of chronic hepatitis D in Southern Europe. Gastroenterology. 1999;117(1):161-6.

[30] Zignego AL, Dubois F, Samuel D, Georgopoulou U, Reynes M, Gentilini P, et al. Serum hepatitis delta virus RNA in patients with delta hepatitis and in liver graft recipients. J Hepatol. 1990;11(1):102-10.

[31] Wu JC, Chen TZ, Huang YS, Yen FS, Ting LT, Sheng WY, et al. Natural history of hepatitis D viral superinfection: significance of viremia detected by polymerase chain reaction. Gastroenterology. 1995;108(3):796-802.

[32] Shattock AG, Morgan BM. Sensitive enzyme immunoassay for the detection of delta antigen and anti-delta, using serum as the delta antigen source. J Med Virol. 1984;13(1):73-82.

[33] Grippon P, Ribiere O, Cadranel JF, Pelletier S, Pillot B, Emerit J, et al. Long-term delta antigenaemia without appearance of delta antibody in two immunodeficient patients. Lancet. 1987;1(8540):1031.

[34] Buti M, Esteban R, Roggendorf M, Fernandez J, Jardi R, Rashofer R, et al. Hepatitis D virus RNA in acute delta infection: serological profile and correlation with other markers of hepatitis D virus infection. Hepatology. 1988;8(5):1125-9.

[35] Mederacke I, Bremer B, Heidrich B, Kirschner J, Deterding K, Bock T, et al. Establishment of a novel quantitative hepatitis D virus (HDV) RNA assay using the Cobas TaqMan platform to study HDV RNA kinetics. J Clin Microbiol. 2010;48(6):2022-9.

[36] Zachou K, Yurdaydin C, Drebber U, Dalekos GN, Erhardt A, Cakaloglu Y, et al. Quantitative HBsAg and HDV-RNA levels in chronic delta hepatitis. Liver Int. 2010;30(3):430-7.

[37] Boyd A, Lacombe K, Miailhes P, Gozlan J, Bonnard P, Molina JM, et al. Longitudinal evaluation of viral interactions in treated HIV-hepatitis B co-infected patients with additional hepatitis C and D virus. J Viral Hepat. 2010;17(1):65-76.

[38] Ponzetto A, Hoyer BH, Popper H, Engle R, Purcell RH, Gerin JL. Titration of the infectivity of hepatitis D virus in chimpanzees. J Infect Dis. 1987;155(1):72-8.

[39] Farci P, Mandas A, Coiana A, Lai ME, Desmet V, Van Eyken P, et al. Treatment of chronic hepatitis D with interferon alfa-2a. N Engl J Med. 1994;330(2):88-94.

[40] Farci P, Roskams T, Chessa L, Peddis G, Mazzoleni AP, Scioscia R, et al. Long-term benefit of interferon alpha therapy of chronic hepatitis D: regression of advanced hepatic fibrosis. Gastroenterology. 2004;126(7):1740-9.

[41] Yurdaydin C, Bozkaya H, Karaaslan H, Onder FO, Erkan OE, Yalçin K, et al. A pilot study of 2 years of interferon treatment in patients with chronic delta hepatitis. J Viral Hepat. 2007;14(11):812-6.

[42] Gaudin JL, Faure P, Godinot H, Gerard F, Trepo C. The French experience of treatment of chronic type D hepatitis with a 12-month course of interferon alpha-2B. Results of a randomized controlled trial. Liver. 1995;15(1):45-52.

[43] Madejón A, Cotonat T, Bartolomé J, Castillo I, Carreño V. Treatment of chronic hepatitis D virus infection with low and high doses of interferon-alpha 2a: utility of polymerase chain reaction in monitoring antiviral response. Hepatology. 1994;19(6): 1331-6.

[44] Romeo R, Del Ninno E, Rumi M, Russo A, Sangiovanni A, de Franchis R, et al. A 28-year study of the course of hepatitis Delta infection: a risk factor for cirrhosis and hepatocellular carcinoma. Gastroenterology. 2009;136(5):1629-38.

[45] Lau JY, King R, Tibbs CJ, Catterall AP, Smith HM, Portmann BC, et al. Loss of HBsAg with interferon-alpha therapy in chronic hepatitis D virus infection. J Med Virol. 1993;39(4):292-6.

[46] Rizzetto M. Hepatitis D: thirty years after. J Hepatol. 2009;50(5):1043-50.

[47] Niro GA, Rosina F, Rizzetto M. Treatment of hepatitis D. J Viral Hepat. 2005;12(1): 2-9.

[48] Castelnau C, Le Gal F, Ripault MP, Gordien E, Martinot-Peignoux M, Boyer N, et al. Efficacy of peginterferon alpha-2b in chronic hepatitis delta: relevance of quantitative RT-PCR for follow-up. Hepatology. 2006;44(3):728-35.

[49] Erhardt A, Gerlich W, Starke C, Wend U, Donner A, Sagir A, et al. Treatment of chronic hepatitis delta with pegylated interferon-alpha2b. Liver Int. 2006;26(7): 805-10.

[50] Ferenci P, Formann E, Romeo R. Successful treatment of chronic hepatitis D with a short course of peginterferon alfa-2a. Am J Gastroenterol. 2005;100(7):1626-7.

[51] Alavian SM, Tabatabaei SV, Behnava B, Rizzetto M. Standard and pegylated interferon therapy of HDV infection: A systematic review and meta- analysis. J Res Med Sci. 2012;17(10):967-74.

[52] Li WC, Wang MR, Kong LB, Ren WG, Zhang YG, Nan YM. Peginterferon alpha-based therapy for chronic hepatitis B focusing on HBsAg clearance or seroconversion: a meta-analysis of controlled clinical trials. BMC Infect Dis. 2011;11:165.

[53] Rizzetto M. Current management of delta hepatitis. Liver Int. 2013;33 Suppl 1:195-7.

[54] Mederacke I, Filmann N, Yurdaydin C, Bremer B, Puls F, Zacher BJ, et al. Rapid early HDV RNA decline in the peripheral blood but prolonged intrahepatic hepatitis delta antigen persistence after liver transplantation. J Hepatol. 2012;56(1):115-22.

[55] Riaz M, Idrees M, Kanwal H, Kabir F. An overview of triple infection with hepatitis B, C and D viruses. Virol J. 2011;8:368.

[56] Babiker ZO, Hogan C, Ustianowski A, Wilkins E. Does interferon-sparing tenofovir disoproxil fumarate-based therapy have a role in the management of severe acute hepatitis delta superinfection? J Med Microbiol. 2012;61(Pt 12):1780-3.

[57] Chen GY, Su TH, Kao JH. Successful treatment of chronic hepatitis B and D with pegylated-interferon plus entecavir. J Formos Med Assoc. 2013.

[58] Fattovich G, Bortolotti F, Donato F. Natural history of chronic hepatitis B: special emphasis on disease progression and prognostic factors. J Hepatol. 2008;48(2):335-52.

[59] Samuel D, Muller R, Alexander G, Fassati L, Ducot B, Benhamou JP, et al. Liver transplantation in European patients with the hepatitis B surface antigen. N Engl J Med. 1993;329(25):1842-7.

[60] Degertekin B, Han SH, Keeffe EB, Schiff ER, Luketic VA, Brown RS, et al. Impact of virologic breakthrough and HBIG regimen on hepatitis B recurrence after liver transplantation. Am J Transplant. 2010;10(8):1823-33.

[61] Faria LC, Gigou M, Roque-Afonso AM, Sebagh M, Roche B, Fallot G, et al. Hepatocellular carcinoma is associated with an increased risk of hepatitis B virus recurrence after liver transplantation. Gastroenterology. 2008;134(7):1890-9; quiz 2155.

[62] Coffin CS, Stock PG, Dove LM, Berg CL, Nissen NN, Curry MP, et al. Virologic and clinical outcomes of hepatitis B virus infection in HIV-HBV coinfected transplant recipients. Am J Transplant. 2010;10(5):1268-75.

[63] Roche B, Samuel D. Liver transplantation in delta virus infection. Semin Liver Dis. 2012;32(3):245-55.

[64] Gane EJ, Angus PW, Strasser S, Crawford DH, Ring J, Jeffrey GP, et al. Lamivudine plus low-dose hepatitis B immunoglobulin to prevent recurrent hepatitis B following liver transplantation. Gastroenterology. 2007;132(3):931-7.

[65] Steinmüller T, Seehofer D, Rayes N, Müller AR, Settmacher U, Jonas S, et al. Increasing applicability of liver transplantation for patients with hepatitis B-related liver disease. Hepatology. 2002;35(6):1528-35.

[66] Kim WR, Poterucha JJ, Kremers WK, Ishitani MB, Dickson ER. Outcome of liver transplantation for hepatitis B in the United States. Liver Transpl. 2004;10(8):968-74.

[67] Roggendorf M. Perspectives for a vaccine against hepatitis delta virus. Semin Liver Dis. 2012;32(3):256-61.

[68] Donnelly RP, Dickensheets H, O'Brien TR. Interferon-lambda and therapy for chronic hepatitis C virus infection. Trends Immunol. 2011;32(9):443-50.

[69] Muir AJ, Shiffman ML, Zaman A, Yoffe B, de la Torre A, Flamm S, et al. Phase 1b study of pegylated interferon lambda 1 with or without ribavirin in patients with chronic genotype 1 hepatitis C virus infection. Hepatology. 2010;52(3):822-32.

[70] Hughes SA, Wedemeyer H, Harrison PM. Hepatitis delta virus. Lancet. 2011;378(9785):73-85.

[71] Stokowa-Sołtys K, Gaggelli N, Nagaj J, Szczepanik W, Ciesiołka J, Wrzesiński J, et al. High affinity of copper(II) towards amoxicillin, apramycin and ristomycin. Effect of these complexes on the catalytic activity of HDV ribozyme. J Inorg Biochem. 2013;124:26-34.

[72] Lamas Longarela O, Schmidt TT, Schöneweis K, Romeo R, Wedemeyer H, Urban S, et al. Proteoglycans act as cellular hepatitis delta virus attachment receptors. PLoS One. 2013;8(3):e58340.

[73] Singh S, Gupta SK, Nischal A, Khattri S, Nath R, Pant KK, et al. Identification and characterization of novel small-molecule inhibitors against hepatitis delta virus replication by using docking strategies. Hepat Mon. 2011;11(10):803-9.

[74] Yurdaydin C, Bozkaya H, Onder FO, Sentürk H, Karaaslan H, Akdoğan M, et al. Treatment of chronic delta hepatitis with lamivudine vs lamivudine + interferon vs interferon. J Viral Hepat. 2008;15(4):314-21.

[75] Gheorghe L, Iacob S, Simionov I, Vadan R, Constantinescu I, Caruntu F, et al. Weight-based dosing regimen of peg-interferon $\alpha$-2b for chronic hepatitis delta: a multicenter Romanian trial. J Gastrointestin Liver Dis. 2011;20(4):377-82.

[76] Ormeci N, Bölükbaş F, Erden E, Coban S, Ekiz F, Erdem H, et al. Pegylated interferon alfa-2B for chronic delta hepatitis: 12 versus 24 months. Hepatogastroenterology. 2011;58(110-111):1648-53.

[77] Wedemeyer H, Yurdaydìn C, Dalekos GN, Erhardt A, Çakaloğlu Y, Değertekin H, et al. Peginterferon plus adefovir versus either drug alone for hepatitis delta. N Engl J Med. 2011;364(4):322-31.

[78] Karaca C, Soyer OM, Baran B, Ormeci AC, Gokturk S, Aydin E, et al. Efficacy of pegylated interferon-$\alpha$ treatment for 24 months in chronic delta hepatitis and predictors of response. Antivir Ther. 2013;18(4):561-6.

[79] Kabaçam G, Onder FO, Yakut M, Seven G, Karatayli SC, Karatayli E, et al. Entecavir treatment of chronic hepatitis D. Clin Infect Dis. 2012;55(5):645-50.

[80] Samiullah S, Bikharam D, Nasreen. Treatment of chronic hepatitis delta virus with peg-interferon and factors that predict sustained viral response. World J Gastroenterol. 2012;18(40):5793-8.

# 10

# Intranasal Drug Administration — An Attractive Route for Some Drugs

Degenhard Marx, Gerallt Williams and
Matthias Birkhoff

## 1. Introduction

Intranasal drug administration has a long tradition and was and is still used for medical as well as recreational purposes. The most common use is for treatment of local symptoms e.g. nasal congestion in the course of a common rhinitis or inflammation linked to allergic rhinitis. The medications intended for local activity are well established and can be found across the globe in every pharmacy and drug store. Examples for topical treatment of rhinitis are decongestants (oxymetazoline, xylometazoline, naphazoline), anti-histamines (azelastine, levocabastine, olopatadine) and glucocorticoids (e.g. mometasone, budesonide, fluticasone). For this particular indication, drugs should act fast and only locally while systemic absorption should be as low as possible; this to avoid systemic side effects which are linked with typical oral formulations of comparable drug substances.

As described earlier [1] intranasal administration has much more potential. The nasal mucosa can be used for non-invasive systemic administration of drugs. The surface of the nasal mucosa in humans is around 150 cm$^2$, a tissue which is well supplied by blood vessels. This ensures a rapid absorption of most drugs, can generate high systemic blood levels and avoids the first pass metabolism which needs to be taken into account following oral administration. This bypassing of the gastrointestinal system even enables the delivery of peptide hormones [1]. Calcitonin and desmopressin are on the market for years now; insulin and glucagon were under clinical development for this administration route [2].

The rapid absorption of drugs via the nasal mucosa is also utilized for pain medications (e.g. fentanyl nasal sprays), rescue medications like naloxone for opioid overdosing or midazolam for seizures in children. An important aspect for such medications is that intranasal administration is considered a non-invasive administration route and easy to do for self-administration or for care-givers. It has a low potential for injuries or disease transmission (hepatitis B, HIV). This is of special importance if fast relief from severe symptoms is required and patient's ability to deal with injections is impaired. Intranasal triptanes for migraine treatment, fentanyl to stop cancer breakthrough pain and ondansetrone to relieve nausea are examples for this trend. For these indications, single dose systems or multi-dose pumps with counting or lock-out mechanisms are available to reduce the risk of unintended overdosing or misuse [1].

Vaccines may also benefit from the intranasal route. Existing vaccines commonly utilize the intramuscular and oral administration route. While the respiratory and gastrointestinal tract is very immune competent and fights with microbes permanently, the muscle is not the first choice. Intramuscular vaccination primarily induces systemic immune response, mainly via formation of vaccine-strain specific circulating antibodies. Injections of vaccines were done since the early days and they are indeed effective. So for most people today vaccination is equal to getting an intramuscular injection which is linked to pain. For the health care professional it is linked to fears of needle stick injuries, risk of disease transmission and dangerous medical waste.

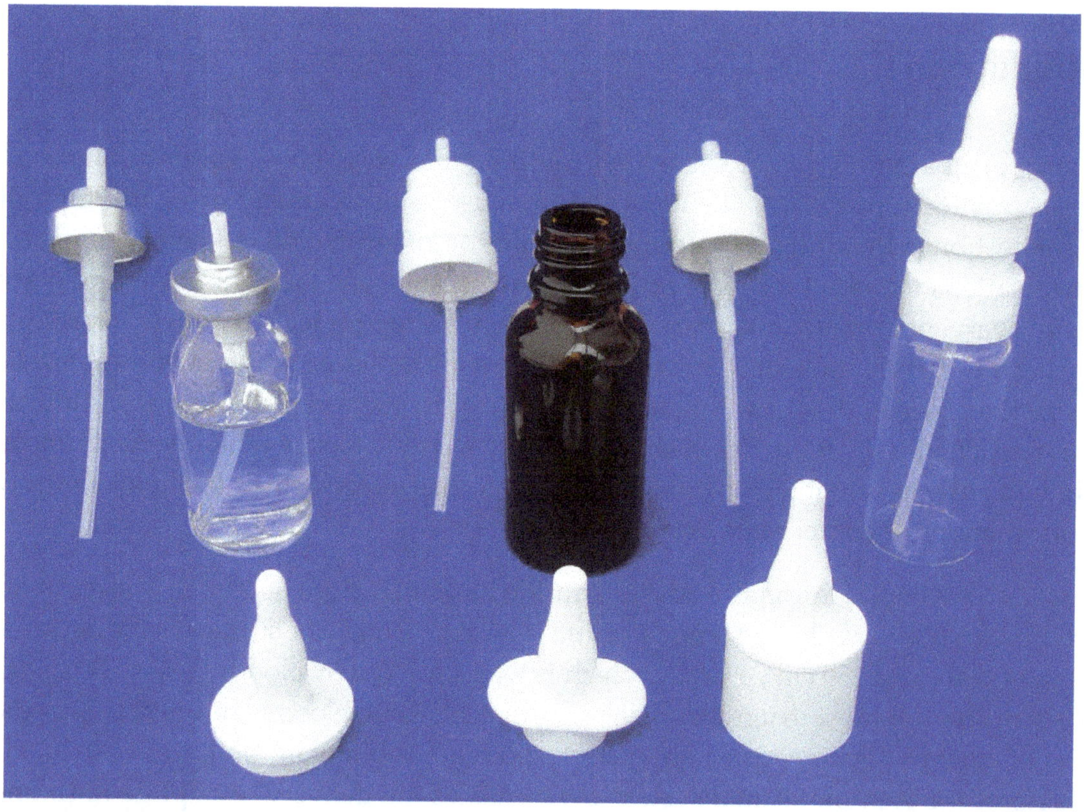

**Figure 1.** Multi-dose spray pumps can be fitted onto the bottles using a crimp ferrule, screwed-on or simply snapped on (from left to the right). In the forefront different types of nasal spray actuators.

Intranasal vaccination provides a promising non-invasive and gentle alternative. The nasal mucosa is continuously exposed to dust and microbes and therefore extremely immune competent. Due to the presence of the so called nasal-associated lymphoid tissue (NALT), intranasal vaccination elicits broader protection. It induces mucosal (protection at the site of infection) and systemic immunity, which includes antibody formation as well as activation of circulating immune cells. It has also been reported that the nasal route induces cross-protection against variant strains of e.g. influenza viruses, an observation which may contribute to the development of so-called "universal vaccines". There is also evidence that this administration route may enable the development of therapeutic vaccines for chronic, hard-to-treat diseases such as hepatitis B [3].

Intranasal administration is an attractive route for a wide range of drugs and indications. With this review we will try to provide some insight into this technology and some considerations for a successful development of such drugs.

## 2. Evolution of multi-dose spray pumps

Multi-dose spray pumps represent the highest share of delivery systems for intranasal administration. This type of pumps was developed some 50 years ago and ousted step by step droppers and pipettes. These multi-dose spray pumps now dominate the market because they are very cost effective and convenient. The technical solution is quite simple: drug formulation is filled into multi-dose bottles made of glass or different plastic materials, which are closed by attaching the nasal spray pump including a dip tube. Nasal spray pumps are displacement pumps and when actuating the pump by pressing the actuator towards the bottle, a piston moves downward in the metering chamber. A valve mechanism at the bottom of the metering chamber will prevent backflow into the dip tube. So the downward movement of the piston will create pressure within the metering chamber which forces the air (before priming) or the liquid outwards through the actuator and generates the spray. When the actuation pressure is removed, a spring will force the piston and actuator to return to its initial position. This creates an underpressure in the metering chamber which pulls the liquid from the container by lifting up the ball from the ball seat above the dip tube at the bottom of the metering chamber [1]. The metering chamber ensures the right dosing and an open swirling chamber in the tip of the actuator will aerosolize the metered dose. In these pumps systems no measures are taken to prevent microbial contamination when in use, thus the formulation must contain preservatives, in most cases benzalkonium chloride (BAC). To date, most of the medications administered nasally contain a preservative to support long storage times and proper in-use stability. For some years now, most manufacturers of delivery systems offer so called "preservative free systems" (PFS) which are designed in such a way that no preservatives have to be added. At least in Europe, authorities support the use of preservative-free nasalia and request it for children and adolescents [4]. A switch from preserved to unpreserved medications is also often used as a life-cycle management measure and the products are clearly labeled as "without preservatives" or "does not contain preservatives". Today, preservative free systems are most widely used to moisturize the nasal mucosa using saline solutions or for nasal decongestants.

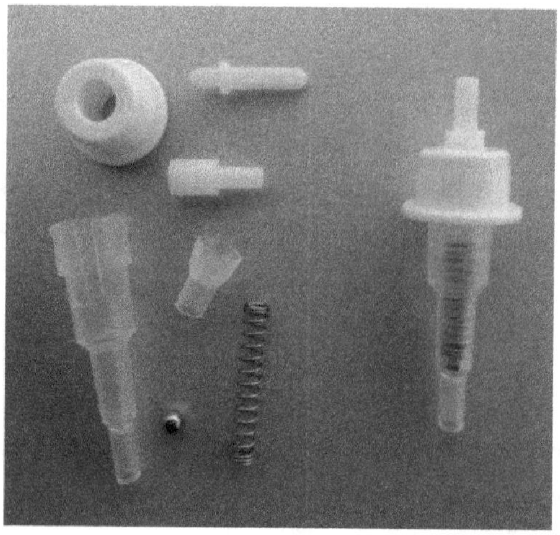

**Figure 2.** Components of a typical multi dose pump. For a fully functional system a dip tube, fixture and actuator need to be added.

In December 2012, the US Consumer Product Safety Commission (CPSC) issued a rule to require child resistant (CR) packaging for any over the counter or prescription product containing the equivalent of 0.08 milligrams or more of an imidazoline [5]. This class of drugs is widely used as decongestant for cough & cold medications. The reason for this request was the high number of accidental uptake of such medications by children and resulting serious health risks. The commission estimated that approximately 39 million units of nasal products containing imidazolines are sold annually in the US. A great proportion of the nasal products are presented with metering nasal spray pumps. In a comment [5] the CPSC stated that nasal spray pumps even when crimped onto the bottle are not considered CR and that either the pump action or the over cap must be child resistant. This forced the pharmaceutical industry to introduce child resistant features for nasal decongestants intended for the US market.

## 3. A short introduction on intranasal administration

Nasal sprays or drops are widely used and therefor easy-to-use and cost-effective solutions are already available for liquid or for dry powder formulated drug products. Also the basic requirements for the development of nasal sprays are well known. An important point when a development for nasal administration is considered: the product should have no unpleasant smell and should not be irritating or influence the sense of smell. There should be also no safety concern, if a dose is unintentionally shot into the eyes.

For most nasal spray pumps the dispensed volume per actuation is set between 50 and 140 µl, and an administered volume of 100 µl per nostril is optimum in adults. Higher volumes are prone to drip out immediately. So the anticipated dose should fit into a volume of roughly 100-200 µl when both nostrils are sprayed. Standard spray pumps will deposit most of the sprayed dose into the anterior region of the nasal cavity (see Fig. 3) [6]. Surface tension of the droplets and mucus layer will cause the immediate spread of the spray. Afterwards mucociliary clearance will distribute the liquid layer within the nasal cavity. Since the nasal mucus layer is continuously renewed and discarded into the throat, the nasal residence time of the administered drug depends on how fast it dissolves within the mucus layer and penetrates into the mucosa [7].

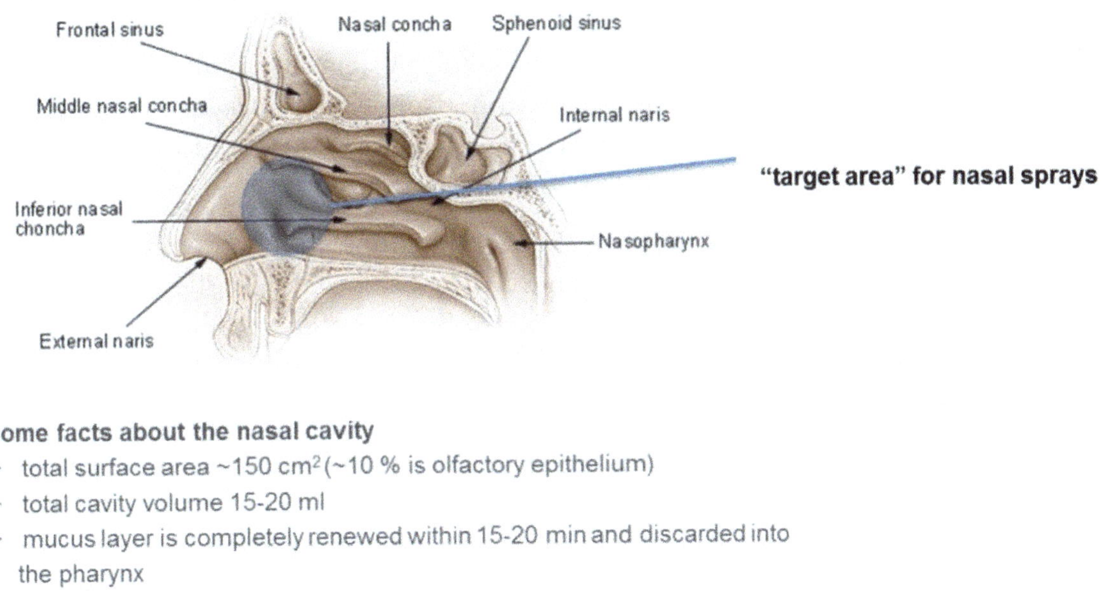


**Figure 3.** Anatomy of the nasal cavity.

If a nasal spray is considered, authorities will require a lot of data to describe the nasal spray pump and its performance as part of the container closure system [8, 9]. Most of these required parameters are used for quality control purposes. For nasal deposition efficiency, the spray plume angle and administration angle are critical factors, while many other spray parameters, including droplet particle size, have relatively minor influences on deposition within the nasal cavity [10].

The nose is a very effective filter and most particles and droplets will be caught within the nasal cavity. Only particles less than 10 μm median aerodynamic diameter, so called fine particles, can reach the lower airways during nasal breathing [11]. Most spray pumps will generate an aerosol with a mean particle size from 40-100 μm during the fully developed phase which is recognized as fine mist. Such an aerosol will deposit well in the nasal cavity.

To date, nearly all drugs for intranasal administration are liquids and just some recreational drugs are used as powders. Of course dry powder preparations can be used without the need for reconstitution to a liquid. The particle size should be in the same range as droplets from a nasal spray and fine particles should be minimized to avoid pulmonary deposition. The size and structure of the particles must be a compromise between safe administration (no fine particles, good deposition) and fast speed of dissolution of the particles within the mucus layer [3]. Powders for nasal administration will most likely need protection from moisture uptake though the moisture sensitivity may be formulation-dependent. Long term use of powder formulations may result in mucosal irritation and chronic use should be considered with caution, but single administration should be of much lower risk.

## 4. Which technology is on the market?

For intranasal administration of drugs a lot of delivery systems are available, simple and low cost as well as highly sophisticated. It ranges from droppers, to sprayers to be attached to a syringe, to so called unit- and bi-dose systems as well as multi-dose solutions for liquids. This wide range of available systems opens the door to tailored packaging.

There are some considerations to choose the right solution in a competitive environment. Convenient and safe use and cost of goods need to be balanced. Also the availability of high speed filling and packaging equipment for the selected presentation should be evaluated. There are of course some other considerations for the different types of systems which should be discussed here.

**Droppers** are the simplest and -just looking on packaging costs- the cheapest way to deliver medication into the nose. The blow-fill-seal (BFS) technology is widely used. The BFS droppers made of polyethylene or polypropylene are cheap but require special filling equipment. Also the material for the dropper (e.g. adhesion profile, evaporation rate) as well as processing temperatures during the BFS process may set some limitations. Splitting half doses from one single container may be a challenge and so for each nostril (if the medication requires this) one dropper needs to be considered. To deliver the right dose, some substantial overfilling is required which can be neglected for cheap formulations but may be important for expensive drugs.

Droppers for multi-dose presentations are still on the market but can be considered to be obsolete. A preserved formulation for multi-dose presentations is mandatory but preservatives will not solve all hygienic jaundices. Precise dosing is also close to impossible so that only drugs with a wide safety margin can be used with such systems. Intranasal administration using droppers is not very convenient. To get a good nasal deposition, the recipient should lie down or bend the head backwards to improve deposition.

For some rescue medications like naloxone or midazolam or some intranasal vaccines **spray tips** (see Fig. 4) attached to standard Luer-syringes are used to deliver the drug. The handling is somehow inconvenient, because in most cases the drug must be transferred from a vial into the syringe. Then the spray tip is attached and the system is ready for administration. The generated spray and the quality of the nasal deposition depend much on the characteristics of the spray tip and the smooth displacement movement of the plunger of the syringe. If no mechanical aid is employed (e.g. removable clips to split 2 half doses), it is difficult to separate doses for each nostril. Also, depending on the handling procedure, a dead volume of 70-130 µl for the spray tip + syringe combination must be considered. A concern for such kits may be a possible confusion of the administration route. The used syringes are easily fitted with a needle and there is some risk in real life, that the drug intended for intranasal administration is injected. Most of these disadvantages can be avoided if prefilled systems are used.

So called **unit/bidose systems** (see Fig. 5) for liquid formulations are state of the art for the intranasal administration of drugs requiring exact dosing. They have been on the market for more than 10 years for intranasal breakthrough pain and migraine management. The systems contain one or two separated half doses ready for administration. They are optimized for easy intuitive and safe handling. These systems will also ensure an optimal nasal deposition of the drug. These advantages are linked to a somehow higher price. The filling is similar to the procedure used for prefilled syringes and requires appropriate equipment.

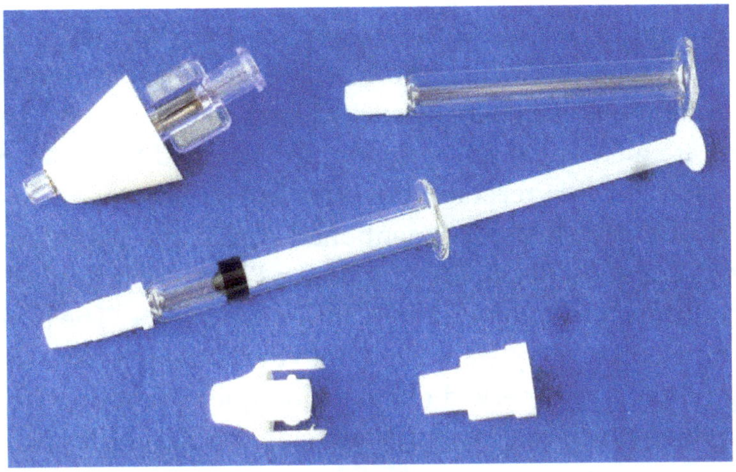

**Figure 4.** Spray tips for syringes which are used for the intranasal administration of naloxone, midazolam or some influenza vaccines.

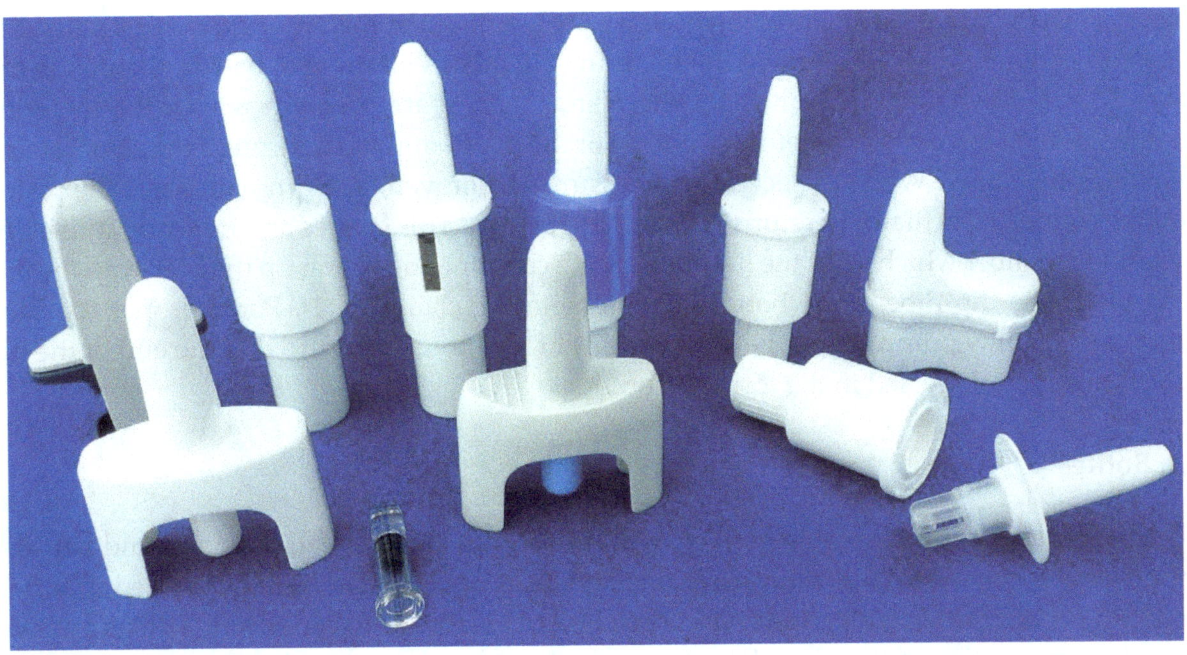

**Figure 5.** Examples of unit/bidose systems for liquids on the left with a glass vial which contains the one or two doses of the drug product and dry powder devices on the right.

**Dry powder systems**: In the near future, some drugs and vaccines will probably focus on dry powder formulations to take advantage of improved storage conditions. It may be a challenging task to generate a powder with the right particle size. As mentioned before, the particles must be designed for safe administration (no fine particle fraction), good deposition and fast dissolution within the mucus layer. For dry powders, electrostatic charge and moisture ingress must be considered. Systems which actively drive out the powder, using compressed air generated by a pump-like mechanism, seem to be better accepted than passive ones, where the powder is taken up by the nasal air flow. Dealing with dry powder needs of course different manufacturing and filling technologies, which are already available for other medications.

**Multi-dose solutions** are by far the most widely used package solution. In Asia, simple squeeze bottles are on the market which can be considered obsolete because exact dosing is not possible and during use mucus may be sucked back into the bottle. The current standard multi-dose solutions are metering nasal spray pumps attached to bottles containing 10-30 ml of a liquid formulation. For this reason we would like to provide a closer insight into the technology of spray pump systems. As mentioned earlier the manufacturer fills the drug formulation into multi-dose bottles made of glass or Pharma-grade plastic materials. These are then closed by attaching the spray pump including a dip tube. The pump may be fixed by a screw closure, crimped on or simply snapped onto the bottle [1]. Now the system should be tight and no leakage should be observed during subsequent handling. This filling process is done on high-speed lines which can easily fill and close 60-200 bottles per minute.

Before the system can be used, the pump must be primed. This is normally done by the patient just before first use. A number of priming strokes is required to purge the air off the system and dip tube and to deliver the product at the intended dose volume. Spray pumps are displacement pumps. When actuating the pump, a piston moves downward inside the metering chamber. A valve mechanism with a ball sealing the metering chamber against dip tube and container at the bottom of the metering chamber will prevent backflow into the dip tube. So the downward movement of the piston will create pressure within the metering chamber which forces the air (before priming) or the liquid outwards through the actuator and generates the spray. When the actuation pressure is removed, a spring will force the piston and the connected actuator to return to its initial position. This creates an underpressure in the metering chamber which pulls the liquid from the container by lifting up the ball from the ball seat above the dip tube at the bottom of the metering chamber [1]. For a proper repeated function the spray pump should be held in upright positions to ensure that the end of the dip tube is always submersed in the formulation.

### 4.1. Bottles

Bottles or containers are an integral part of multi-dose container closure systems and will also influence the general appearance of the final product. Special shapes may be used to differentiate a product from competitors. Glass bottles are less prone to cause interactions and will give good protection to the formulation even for long storage intervals. Sometimes the glass can influence the stability of the formulation (change in pH, release of trace metals). This depends of course on the quality of the glass which is described by its hydrolytic class (classes

I-III are normally used for pharmaceutical products). The disadvantages which glass bottles may have are the higher weight and the risk to breakage when dropped [1].

Bottles are also made of plastic material (e.g. polyethylene, polypropylene, polyethylene terephthalate). A pump supplier will most likely not manufacture these bottles because a complete different technology is used. Parts for spray pumps are quite exclusively made by injection moulding which gives high precision. Bottle manufacturers use a process referred to as blow-moulding. The general principle is to make a hollow raw part and then blowing up the material to the final dimensions. The most important disadvantage for all bottles made of plastic material is evaporation/weight loss during storage. Plastic materials are not a perfect barrier for gas or water evaporation. This problem can be tackled using laminated materials but these are more expensive. Another potential risk has to be considered: inks and adhesives from labels may migrate through the bottle wall and leach into the formulation [1].

Pure mechanics but critical for all types of bottles: the bottle opening must fit the pump exactly. It needs to be tested and dimensions need to be controlled because variations may cause leakages or damage the housing of the pump during final assembly. To avoid any issues, consultation of the pump system supplier is highly recommended as these companies are experienced in managing this interface. The pump supplier should be able to recommend a range of suited bottles from suppliers which provide reliable quality. Before switching to another bottle or bottle supplier, the compatibility with the pump system should be checked in advance [1].

## 5. First steps to identify the right delivery system

One of the first steps in approaching the development of an intranasal drug administration project is to select the appropriate system for delivering the drug formulation. The selection of the delivery system is strongly governed by the type of formulation envisaged for delivery. Most likely the formulation will be liquid (solution or suspension), but also powder or gel formulations are possible. Of course the dosing frequency as well as legal restrictions (e.g. for controlled substances) will influence the decision for a single or multi-dose presentation. Once the basic type of system has been selected, it is then prudent to do some basic compatibility investigation or studies in order to avoid any obvious incompatibilities between the components and the proposed active pharmaceutical ingredient (API) and any known excipients before moving on to the formulation development stage.

The materials used for the systems are selected by the manufacturer to warrant proper mechanical function and low likelihood of chemical interactions. In practice potential interactions between the formulation and parts of the spray pumps due to sorption or swelling should be excluded. Typical tests that could be considered at this stage include immersion tests of the functional parts of the pump in the formulation to detect swelling or discoloration. First tests with assembled pumps from this immersion test will provide data on potential effects on mechanical function (e.g. friction, metering).

| Material | Typical functions |
|---|---|
| Polyethylene (PE) | Functional parts of the pump, actuator and fixtures, dip tube, bottles |
| Polypropylene (PP) | Functional parts of the pump, actuator and fixtures, dip tube, bottles |
| Polyoxy methylene (POM) | Functional parts (may release formaldehyde!) |
| Rubber or elastomers | Gaskets, seals, stopper |
| Stainless steel | Springs, balls for valve mechanism |
| Aluminum | Ferrules for crimped connections |
| Glass | Bottles, vials, balls for valve mechanisms |

**Table 1.** Typical classes of materials used for nasal spray systems

A simple test for spray performance will assure that the formulation can be aerosolized by the considered pump and the delivered particle size is appropriate for effective nasal deposition. As mentioned earlier, the particle size should be in the range from at least 10 to a maximum of 150 µm. Particle sizes above 10µm assure that no product passes in to the lungs and impact in the nasal cavity. Droplets greater than 150 µl should be avoided as they are prone to run out of the nasal cavity immediately. It is not unwise to perform such preliminary compatibility tests with a certain range of different pumps to get an impression which may provide the best performance.

| Type of materials |
|---|
| Chemical name / identity of the material |
| Chemical name of any monomer used |
| Supplier name |
| Compliance with relevant standards in relation to their intended use (e.g. pharmacopeias) |
| Complete qualitative composition when: |
| The material is not described in the European or national pharmacopeias |
| The monography authorizes the use of several additives (from which the manufacturer may choose) |
| Specifications |
| Identification |
| Reference to European Pharmacopeia or Member State monographs or in-house monograph (if not described in EP or Member State monographs) |
| Non-compendial methods (with validation) should be included where appropriate |

**Table 2.** General information on the container closure system related to materials of construction which should be provided by the supplier of the system

At the end of the whole development process the requirements from authorities are straight forward: "For the final product (=formulation in combination with the whole container closure system) the suitability of the container closure system used for the storage, transportation (shipping) and use of the drug product should be discussed. This discussion should consider, e.g., choice of materials, protection from moisture and light, compatibility of the materials of construction with the dosage form (including sorption to container and leaching) safety of materials of construction, and performance (such as reproducibility of the dose delivery from the system when presented as part of the drug product)" [12].

## 6. Formulation development

Nasal drug formulations are broadly categorized into several types including solutions, suspensions, powders or gels. A key factor in selecting the type of nasal formulation to be developed is whether the therapy is intended for local or systemic application. Depending on the application, factors such drug absorption rate from the nasal mucosa into the systemic blood circulation and residence time in the nasal cavity become key elements in the formulation development process.

Taking as examples spray solutions and suspension type formulations, the following factors should be considered during nasal formulation development:

**Drug, particles:** consideration should be given to the desired therapeutic concentration for each dose, keeping in mind whether the total dose to the nasal cavity will be one (single nostril delivery) or two (one delivery into each nostril). For aqueous solutions and suspensions the typical dosing volume ranges are 50-140µl and for solution or suspension in pressurized metered dose inhalers (pMDIs) the typical delivery volumes are in the range of 25µl. The primary particle size of the API in suspension formulations also needs to be considered with regard to the droplet size delivered during dosing and any impact it may have on the dissolution of the particles once deposited in the nasal cavity.

**pH/buffers:** the pH inside the nasal cavity can influence the rate and extent of absorption of ionizable drugs. The average baseline human nasal pH is reported to be around 6.3 [13] and the pH of several commercially available nasal spray products are in the range of 3.5 to 7.0, and the optimal range for pH of these nasal formulations is suggested to be 4.5 to 6.5 [14]. The pH of the formulation can also affect the stability of the drug product during its shelf life so this also needs to be considered during development.

**Osmolality:** Studies have shown that hypotonic nasal spray formulations improve drug permeability through the nasal mucosa [15] and some marketed products report osmolality in the range 300-700mOsmol/K.

**Viscosity/surface tension:** the majority of commercially marketed products contain agents that modify the viscosity and surface tension of the formulations, they are included in order to manage factors such as thinning and thixotropic behavior and are key elements in the performance of the dispensed product such as drop particle size, spray angles and also influence the residence time of the product once delivered, in the nasal cavity.

| Ingredients | IIG limit for nasal route, %w/w | Function |
|---|---|---|
| Alcohol, 200 proof | 2 | Co-solvent |
| Anhydrous dextrose | 0.5 | tonicity |
| Anhydrous trisodiumcitrate | 0.0006 | buffer |
| Benzyl alcohol | 0.0366 | preservative |
| Benzalkonium chloride | 0.119 | preservative |
| Butylated hydroxyanisole | 0.0002 | antioxidant |
| Cellulose microcrystalline | 2 | Suspending agent, stabilizer |
| Chlorobutanol | 0.5 | preservative |
| Carboxymethyl cellulose Na | 0.15 | Suspending agent |
| Edetate disodium | 0.5 | Chelator, antioxidant |
| Hydrochloric acid | Not reported | pH adjustment |
| Methylparaben | 0.7 | preservative |
| Oleic acid | 0.132 | Penetration enhancer |
| PEG400 | 20 | Surfactant, co-solvent |
| PEG3500 | 1.5 | surfactant |
| Phenylethyl alcohol | 0.254 | Preservative, masking agent |
| Polyoxyl 400 stearate | 15 | surfactant |
| Polysorbate 20 | 2.5 | surfactant |
| Polysorbate 80 | 10 | surfactant |
| Propylene glycol | 20 | Co-solvent |
| Propylparaben | 0.3 | Preservative |
| Sodium chloride | 1.9 | tonicity |
| Sodium hydroxide | 0.004 | pH adjustment |
| Sulfuric acid | 0.4 | pH adjustment |

**Table 3.** Examples of key nasal formulation excipients and their inactive ingredient guidance (IIG) dosing levels

**Other excipients:** in addition to buffer salts several types of excipients may be required in order to develop a stable nasal spray formulation. These include solvents and co-solvents to keep the active pharmaceutical ingredient (API) in the dissolved or suspended state, as well as preservatives for non-sterile products. If the formulation is a suspension or emulsion, surfactants and/or emulsifying agents, stabilizers and suitable oil-phase components may be required. Although there are numerous surfactants, emulsifying agents, solvents, co-solvents, oils and preservatives available, only a limited number of excipients are listed in the US FDA inactive ingredient guide (IIG) for nasal products. Table 3 lists some key excipients and their IIG dosage levels, as reported in the FDA IIG database for nasal spray formulations [16].

**Controlling residence time in the nasal cavity:** increasing the residence time of the drug, once delivered on the nasal mucosa, can be beneficial especially for local applications and can aid drug absorption through the nasal mucosa. One approach is too increase the viscosity of the formulation but this should be balanced against any impact on droplet size distribution during delivery into the nasal cavity [17].

**Penetration enhancers:** these agents increase the penetration of drugs through the nasal mucosa. Typical penetration enhancing agents are solvents, co-solvents, ionic and some non-ionic surfactants, selected fatty acids, including oleic acid and certain lipids and cyclodextrin [18, 19].

**Powder and gel nasal formulations:** in formulating nasal powders the key elements to manage are controlling the primary particle size of the API as well as the excipients to get efficient nasal deposition, and selecting a system that provides acceptable protection of the powder during storage and efficient delivery to the nasal cavity during dosing. For nasal gel applications the formulations can be relatively simple and key elements will be stability and shelf-life and the selection of the dispensing system used to deliver the gel to the nasal cavity.

## 7. Performance parameters

Nasal drug product performance characterization is driven by regulatory requirements which allow for successful approval and marketing of these products. The most stringent regulatory standards for nasal drug products are issued in the USA [20] and in Europe [21]. During the development process information has to be documented on many factors in order to construct a regulatory dossier. Typical expectations for development characterizations in the US and Europe are detailed in Table 4.

Once approved and marketed these products have to be routinely controlled in order to assure ongoing performance and quality and the typical regulatory expectations for marketed nasal product specifications and testing are detailed in Table 5. The rationale behind these performance characterization tests are related to factors such as dosing accuracy, shelf life, product robustness and user safety, the key ones being as follows:

**Priming, re-priming:** most nasal spray pumps need to be primed in order to fill the dosing chambers before use and to assure full dosing of the product. In addition, some pumps do not retain the dose in the metering chamber when stored for longer periods, i.e. 7 days, 1 month etc. and may need to be re-primed before use after a specified period of non-use which will be defined in the patient leaflet.

| Characterization test | US | EU |
|---|---|---|
| Stability / shelf life | √ | √ |
| Temp. cycle testing | √ | √ |
| Priming re-priming | √ | √ |
| Micro/bioburden | √ | √ |
| Extractables | √ | √ |
| Leachables | √ | N/A |
| USP tests, 601, 87, 88, 661, 381... | √ | N/A |
| Drop testing, vibration, shipping, air transport tests | √ | √ |
| Effect of orientation | √ | √ |
| Plume geometry | √ | N/A |
| Profiling near exhaustion | √ | √ |
| Performance in the hands of different users | √ | √ |
| Particulates | √ | N/A |

**Table 4.** Examples of product characterization test during development of nasal spray products.

| Control test | US | EU |
|---|---|---|
| Priming, re-priming | √ | √ |
| Dose weight (through life) | √ | √ |
| Leakage | √ | √ |
| Dimensional, metrology | √ | √ |
| Droplet/particle size distribution | √ | √ |
| Spray pattern | √ | N/A |
| Extractables | √ | √ |
| Microbial limits | √ | √ |

**Table 5.** Examples of routine control testing for nasal spray products.

**Dose weight through life:** this test assures that the pump delivers the prescribed dose consistently throughout the use-life of the product, usually beginning middle and end of use. Regulatory requirements exist in most markets for limits on dosing accuracy and these can be found by referring to each country specific regulatory dosing limit specifications for nasal products.

**Leakage:** this assures that the product integrity is maintained throughout its proposed shelf life and that the contents are not lost during storage at various environmental conditions. The ICH stability test conditions [22] are the key reference with regard to stability testing.

**Dimensional/metrology measurements:** these assure that the spray pump meets specified critical quality dimensions in order to assure that the nasal product functions efficiently and meets the key performance tests assuring consistent quality.

**Particle size distribution:** this can refer to the primary particle size specification of the API itself in suspensions or to the droplet (liquid solution) or particle (powder) size distribution of the delivered spray. Specifications need to be put in place for this key parameter and the justified limits registered in the regulatory submissions as it is closely related to nasal deposition efficiency.

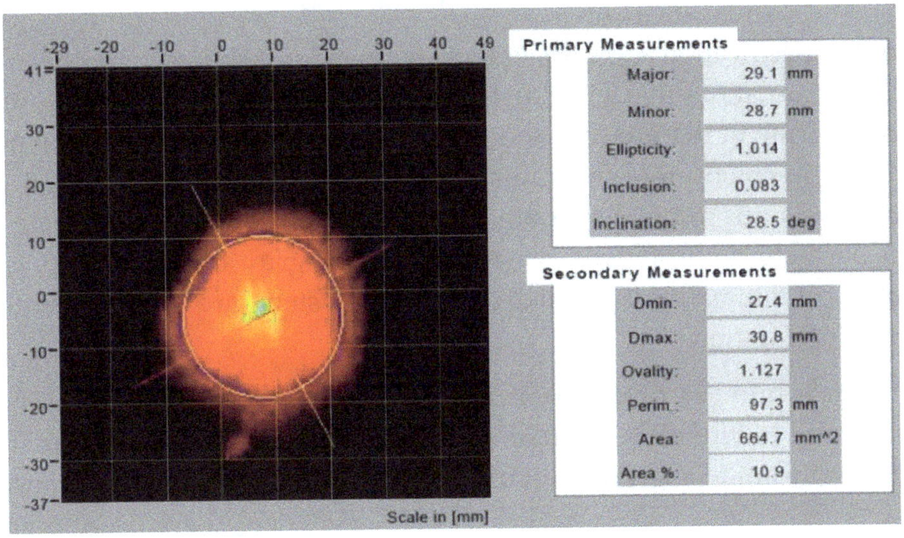


**Figure 6.** Typical display from a spray pattern test using laser imaging, which can give information about the ovality of the emitted spray.

**Spray pattern:** this is another test to assure consistent quality of the delivered nasal spray and characterizes parameters such as angle and plume shape, see Figures 6 and 7.

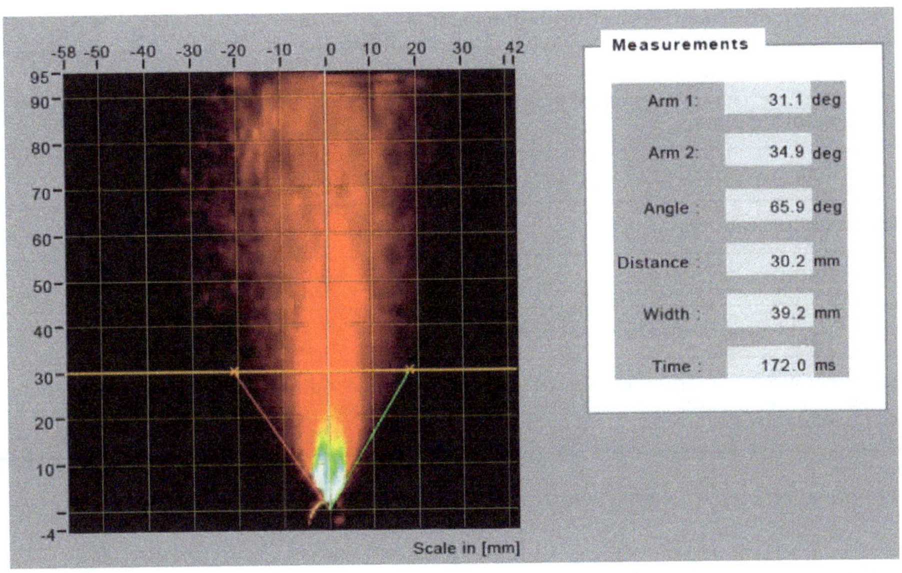


**Figure 7.** Typical display from a spray angle test using laser imaging, which can give information about the angle of the emitted spray.

**Extractables/leachables**: this test assures the safety of the product and specifically measures and controls the potential chemical contaminants which may come from the packaging or container closure system into the formulation and therefore be potentially toxic for the patients, if ingested. The PQRI [23] have issued detailed guidance documents on this subject in conjunction with the FDA which outline how to tackle this specific parameter.

**Particulates**: this test characterizes the contamination of the nasal formulation by any foreign particulates and is related to the overall safety of the product.

**Microbial limits**: specification and tests exist to measure and characterize this parameter, for preserved nasal formulations this will usually mean measuring the levels of preservatives, e.g. benzalkonium chloride in the product and during its proposed shelf life. The units of measurement are usually colony forming units (CFU's). For non-preserved nasal products the characterization tests are somewhat more complicated and include challenge testing with contaminated bacterial environments to assure the integrity of the system for protection against microbial contamination. Special drug delivery systems are needed in order to use non-preserved nasal formulations.

**Robustness**: here a number of different test are applied including dropping the whole packaging, exposure to vibration, simulation of shipping and transportation. These characterization tests are meant to assess the robustness of the product to normal transport and day to day use.

| |
|---|
| — Description of the assembled device and each individual component: |
| · Identification of the packaging component |
| — Product Name, Code / Item number |
| — Manufacturer |
| · Engineering drawings (with critical dimensions) |
| — Description of the manufacturing process |
| · Manufacturing process |
| · Operations performed after manufacture (washing, coating) |
| · Treatment procedures |
| — Description of the controls |
| · Incoming, in-process and release controls |
| · For materials of construction, the manufacturing process and the finished product (component or assembled device) |

**Table 6.** General information on the container closure system which should be provided by the supplier [8,9].

**User studies**: these tests look at the ergonomic and human factor aspects of the systems and include investigation and data generation on potential issues such as orientation, patient handling (young, old, comprised dexterity etc.), actuation forces and many other factors.

Regulatory Guidance's have appeared in the last few years outlining how to tackle these 'human factor' issues [24].

As can be seen from the above list of tests, the development process for a nasal drug product can be quite long, intensive, and costly and depending on the complexity of the product can take upwards of 18 months keeping in mind that suitable real time stability data also need to be generated for regulatory submissions.

## 8. Trends for nasal drug administration

### 8.1. Use of preservatives in multi-dose products

For some years now, so called "preservative-free multi-dose" systems ("PFMD") are on the market and gain share. Such systems are certainly appreciated by the growing number of patients who experienced discomfort with preserved formulations. The issue of significance for the patient and consumer, however, is the high incidence of local side effects attributed to preservatives. The discussion is controversial, and published preclinical and clinical studies are not always consistent. It seems to be clear that short-term use of preparations containing preservatives at low concentrations is well tolerated, but preservatives can cause serious inflammatory effects with long-term use [25]. The responses may include chemical irritation, hyperreactivity and true allergies [26]. The German Authorities (BfArM) addressed the use of benzalkonium chloride for nasal sprays in 2003 [27] which encouraged the preservative free systems for this administration route. Today a range of technical solutions is available to overcome this issue. The highest risk of contamination obviously comes from the orifice of the nasal spray system, because it may come in contact with skin and mucosa as well as with infected mucus in the nose. Some marketed systems use the oligodynamic activity of a silver wire in the tip of the actuator, a silver coated spring and ball [28]. Such systems are able to keep microorganisms down between long dosing intervals, even when the tip is immersed into bacterial contaminated fluid [29].

The most recent preservative free systems follow a purely mechanical approach to minimize interactions between parts of the device and the formulation. One technical solution to prevent contamination via the orifice is referred to as "tip seal technology" [25]. A spring loaded valve is located directly below the opening of the tip orifice and does not allow any microbes to migrate from any surfaces or contacted liquids into the system, the orifice is "sealed" under resting conditions. The tip seal keeps the system closed until a defined pressure (for nasal sprays it is more than 3 bar) is reached by pressing down the actuator. Then the system will open and the formulation is forced through the orifice with a higher pressure than needed to open the valve. When the pressure drops at the end of the actuation the tip seal will immediately close the orifice with an outward movement. So no backflow of potentially contaminated medication or other liquid is possible. Depending on the pump system, the fluid path may even be "metal-free", which means the springs needed for the device operation do not come in contact with the formulation [25].

To avoid contamination of the formulation via venting air different technical solutions are used. The simplest way is sterile filtration of the venting air using separate filters or filter gaskets. For oxygen-sensitive formulations, so called collapsing bags or depressed systems are used. The formulation is filled in a special, microbial tight bag which is protected by a surrounding bottle. When dispensing the product, the bag collapses with the content not coming in contact with the ambient air. Some pumps are constructed in such a way, that the whole system is air-tight and during use some vacuum (up to -300 mbar) is generated within the bottle. Those systems allow even a purging with inert gases to reduce oxygen content in the container head space [25].

These described technical solutions to make the use of preservatives obsolete are well established and mature technologies.

### 8.2. Non-aqueous nasal formulations

The majority of prescription nasal spray products on the market are aqueous formulations. Just recently some so called "dry mist" nasal sprays (e.g. QNASL®, ZETONNA™) were introduced. For these products the technology of the pressurized metered dose inhalers (pMDI's) is utilized which are well established for the treatment of asthma bronchiale and chronic obstructive pulmonary disease. The active ingredient is dissolved or suspended into hydrofluoroalkane (HFA) propellant and typical delivery volumes are in the range of 25μl. Non-aqueous nasal spray formulations are suspected to have increased levels of safety risks due to the fact that they use excipient such as propylene glycol, isopropyl alcohol and PEG400, which are known to cause local irritation particularly for chronic use [30]. Nasal steroids such as beclomethasone and ciclesonide are formulated in such non-aqueous HFA propellants and in this case it is the same formulation approach as is used for inhalation suspension products using pressurized metered dose inhalers (pMDI's).

### 8.3. Side actuated spray pumps

An innovative development in nasal spray pumps are side actuated nasal spray devices designed to help improve patient compliance due to their reduced dependence on patient actuation force or speed. These devices are intended to be compact, ergonomic with intuitive design and have short and motionless nasal nozzles where the fingers are no longer in contact with the nostrils. They have softer actuation and are suitable for a wide range of applications including pediatrics and elderly patients who may have compromised dexterity.

### 8.4. Unit- and bi-dose sprayer

Unit dose devices can also be considered attractive options for certain types of therapy, especially for all kinds of rescue medications. The ready to use packaging will reduce stress (e.g. no fear for injuries, disease transmission) and handling errors which may happen in such situations. Such kind of packaging also limits the amount of drug which needs to be handled which is important for controlled substances.

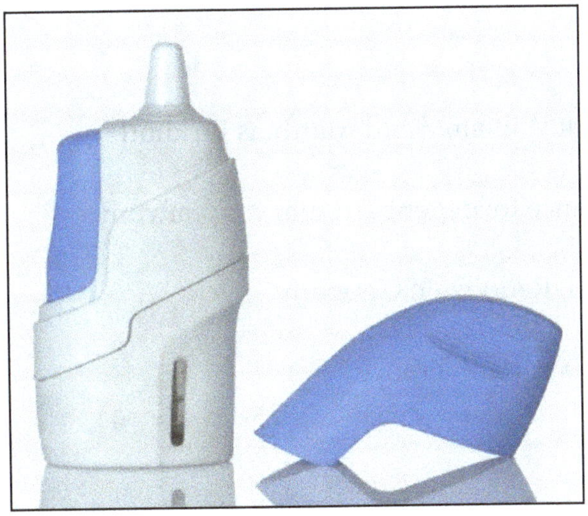

**Figure 8.** Example of a side actuated multi-dose spray pump

**a.** Pain management, e.g. migraine or cancer breakthrough pain episodes, here the molecules are often potent and the amount of dose should be limited in order to avoid any undesirable side-effects or risks of diversion or misuse.

**b.** Vaccines are often one-off treatments and they can be formulated in powder forms so as to avoid the cold chain logistics difficulties associated with liquid vaccines and can easily be used out the hospital environment, such as field vaccination stations.

By using such unit dose or single throw away devices, one can avoid many of the issues outlined above for pain or vaccination therapies.

## 9. Conclusion

Intranasal drug administration is a technology with an interesting past and a fascinating future. In only a few fields cooperation between developers of novel pharmaceutical remedies on one side and manufacturers of sophisticated delivery systems on the other side is equally essential. Precise metered dosing, maximum flexibility, product protection and, last not least, patient adherence are the key areas to work on. The increasing use of unpreserved formulations in both prescription and OTC (over the counter) products establishes additional challenges. Patients and consumers appreciate the convenient and intuitive handling of modern nasal delivery systems, properties which are important for further and sustainable success of nasal administration in general. However, with regulatory demands increasing, professional guidance is needed and should be provided by manufacturers of nasal drug delivery systems to support pharmaceutical companies in finding the optimum configuration. Even though such support can not exempt marketers form performing proper due diligence on the finished product, it is obvious that time to market can be reduced substantially if available resources are utilized in a proper cooperation mode.

## Author details

Degenhard Marx[1*], Gerallt Williams[2] and Matthias Birkhoff[1]

*Address all correspondence to: degenhard.marx@aptar.com

1 Aptar Radolfzell GmbH, Radolfzell, Germany

2 Aptar France SAS, Le Vaudreuil, France

## References

[1] Marx D and Birkhoff M (2011). Multi-Dose Container for Nasal and Ophthalmic Drugs: A Preservative Free Future?, Drug Development - A Case Study Based Insight into Modern Strategies, Dr. Chris Rundfeldt (Ed.), ISBN: 978-953-307-257-9, InTech, DOI: 10.5772/27767. Available from: http://www.intechopen.com/books/drug-development-a-case-study-based-insight-into-modern-strategies/multi-dose-container-for-nasal-and-ophthalmic-drugs-a-preservative-free-future

[2] Leary AC, Dowling M, Cussen K, O'Brien J, Stote RM. Pharmacokinetics and pharmacodynamics of intranasal insulin spray (Nasulin) administered to healthy male volunteers: infuence of the nasal cycle. J Diabetes Sci Technol. 2008, 2(6): 1054-60

[3] Marx D, Leitz M, Fagot C. Do We Need New Devices for Intranasal Vaccination? Drug Development & Delivery. 2011, 11 (3): 54-59

[4] Guideline on pharmaceutical development of medicines for paediatric use, 3 January 2013, EMA/CHMP/QWP/805880/2012 Rev. 2

[5] Consumer Product Safety Ccommission 16 CFR Part 1700, CPSC Docket No. 2012–0005, Requirements for child-resistant packaging: Products containing imidazolines equivalent to 0.08 milligrams or more. December 12, 2012

[6] Fagot Ch and Marx D. Intranasal vaccines -a platform technology for an innovative vaccine industry. December 2011, Express Pharma India, access at http://archive.expresspharmaonline.com/20111231/research02.shtml

[7] Suman JD, Laube BL, Lin TC, Brouet G, Dalby R. Validity of in vitro tests on aqueous spray pumps as surrogates for nasal deposition. Pharm Res. 2002;19(1): 1-6

[8] Guidance for Industry: Nasal Spray and Inhalation Solution, Suspension, and Spray Drug Products - Chemistry, Manufacturing, and Controls Documentation. US Department of Health and Human Services, Food and Drug Administration, Center for Drug Evaluation and Research (CDER). Rockville, MD; 2002

[9] Committee for medicinal products for human use (CHMP). Guideline on the pharmaceutical quality of inhalation and nasal products. London: European Medicines Agency; 2006

[10] Foo MY, Cheng YS, Su WC, Donovan MD. The influence of spray properties on intranasal deposition. J Aerosol Med. 2007, 20(4): 495-508

[11] Stuart BO. Deposition and clearance of inhaled particles. Environ Health Perspect. 1984; 55: 369-390

[12] ICH Harmonised Tripartite Guideline: Pharmaceutical Development Q8; Step 4 version, November 2005

[13] Washington N., et al, 'Determination of baseline human nasal pH and the effect of intranasally administered buffers', Int. J. Pharm. 198:139-146 (2000)

[14] Aurora R., et al, 'Development of nasal delivery systems: a review', Drug Del. Tech. 2(7), 70-73 (2002)

[15] Farina D., 'Regulatory aspects of nasal and pulmonary spray drug products', published in handbook of non-invasive drug delivery systems, Ed. V.Kulkarni, Elsevier, Oxford, UK, 247-290 (2010)

[16] FDA IIG (Inactive Ingredient Guidance), http://accessdata.fda.gov/scripts/cder/iig/index.cfm

[17] Dayal P., et al, 'Evaluation of different parameters that effect droplet size distribution from nasal sprays using the Malvern Spraytech, J. Pharm. Sci., 93: 1725-1742 (2004)

[18] Law S.L., et al, 'Preparation of desmopressin-containing liposomes for intranasal delivery', J. Control. Rel., 70: 375-382 (2001)

[19] Davis S., et al, 'Absorption enhancers for nasal drug delivery', Clin. Pharm., 42(13), 1107-28 (2003)

[20] Nasal Spray and Inhalation Solution, Suspension, and Spray Drug Products Chemistry, Manufacturing and Controls Documentation, U.S. Department of Health and Human Services, Food and Drug Administration, Center for Drug Evaluation and Research (CDER), May 1999

[21] EMEA-Heath Canada: Joint Guideline on the Pharmaceutical Quality of Inhalation and Nasal Products EMEA/CHMP/QWP/49313/2005

[22] Stability testing of new drug substances and products Q1A, ICH harmonized tripartite guideline, 6 February 2003

[23] Safety thresholds and best practices for extractables and leachables in orally inhaled and nasal drug products, PQRI Leachables and Extractables Working Group, 8 Sep 2006

[24] Human factors engineering—Design of medical devices, ANSI/AAMI HE75, 2009/(R)2013

[25] Marx D and Birkhoff M. Will the future be preservative-free? Manufacturing Chemist Pharma, published 17th May 2013, access at

[26] http://www.manufacturingchemist.com/technical/article_page/Will_the_future_be_preservativefree/88155

[27] Hong J, Bielory L. Allergy to ophthalmic preservatives. Curr Opin Allergy Clin Immunol.

[28] 2009;9(5):447-453.

[29] Bescheid des Bundesinstitut für Arzneimittel und Medizinproduke für benzalkoniumchlorid-haltige Arzneimittel zur Anwendung in der Nase, A 37489/38186/03 Bonn, Dezember 2003

[30] Groß D. The COMOD-System – a preservative free drug therapy against glaucoma. 321-328, in Orgül/Flammer (Editors): Pharmacotherapie in glaucoma, Bern 2000

[31] Bagel S, Wiedemann B. Extension of in-use stability of preservative-free nasalia. Europ J Pharmaceutics and Biopharmaceutics. 2004, (57): 353–358

[32] Kibbe A.H., (Ed), Handbook of pharmaceutical excipients, 3rd Edition, Am. Pharm. Asso., 392-398, 442-444 (2000)

# Permissions

All chapters in this book were first published in DDDFMM, by InTech Open; hereby published with permission under the Creative Commons Attribution License or equivalent. Every chapter published in this book has been scrutinized by our experts. Their significance has been extensively debated. The topics covered herein carry significant findings which will fuel the growth of the discipline. They may even be implemented as practical applications or may be referred to as a beginning point for another development.

The contributors of this book come from diverse backgrounds, making this book a truly international effort. This book will bring forth new frontiers with its revolutionizing research information and detailed analysis of the nascent developments around the world.

We would like to thank all the contributing authors for lending their expertise to make the book truly unique. They have played a crucial role in the development of this book. Without their invaluable contributions this book wouldn't have been possible. They have made vital efforts to compile up to date information on the varied aspects of this subject to make this book a valuable addition to the collection of many professionals and students.

This book was conceptualized with the vision of imparting up-to-date information and advanced data in this field. To ensure the same, a matchless editorial board was set up. Every individual on the board went through rigorous rounds of assessment to prove their worth. After which they invested a large part of their time researching and compiling the most relevant data for our readers.

The editorial board has been involved in producing this book since its inception. They have spent rigorous hours researching and exploring the diverse topics which have resulted in the successful publishing of this book. They have passed on their knowledge of decades through this book. To expedite this challenging task, the publisher supported the team at every step. A small team of assistant editors was also appointed to further simplify the editing procedure and attain best results for the readers.

Apart from the editorial board, the designing team has also invested a significant amount of their time in understanding the subject and creating the most relevant covers. They scrutinized every image to scout for the most suitable representation of the subject and create an appropriate cover for the book.

The publishing team has been an ardent support to the editorial, designing and production team. Their endless efforts to recruit the best for this project, has resulted in the accomplishment of this book. They are a veteran in the field of academics and their pool of knowledge is as vast as their experience in printing. Their expertise and guidance has proved useful at every step. Their uncompromising quality standards have made this book an exceptional effort. Their encouragement from time to time has been an inspiration for everyone.

The publisher and the editorial board hope that this book will prove to be a valuable piece of knowledge for researchers, students, practitioners and scholars across the globe.

# List of Contributors

**Mark Voskoboynik**
Sarah Cannon Research Institute UK, London, UK
Department of Medical Oncology, Guy's Hospital, London, UK

**Hendrik-Tobias Arkenau**
Sarah Cannon Research Institute UK, London, UK
University College London, London, UK

**Charles J. Malemud**
Department of Medicine, Division of Rheumatic Diseases, Case Western Reserve University, School of Medicine, Cleveland, Ohio, USA

**Ken Yasukawa**
School of Pharmacy, Nihon University, Funabashi, Chiba, Japan

**Ibrahim Jantan, Syed Nasir Abbas Bukhari, Lam Kok Wai and Mohammed Ahmed Mesaik**
Drug and Herbal Research Center, Faculty of Pharmacy, Universiti Kebangsaan Malaysia, Jalan Raja Muda Abdul Aziz, Kuala Lumpur, Malaysia

**Mohamed Ali Seyed Mohamed**
Drug and Herbal Research Center, Faculty of Pharmacy, Universiti Kebangsaan Malaysia, Jalan Raja Muda Abdul Aziz, Kuala Lumpur, Malaysia
School of Life Science, B.S. Abdur Rahman University, Seethakathi Estate, Vandalur, Chennai, India

**Simon A. Young and Terry K. Smith**
Biomedical Sciences Research Complex, The North Haugh, The University, St. Andrews, Fife Scotland, U.K

**Adriana Ceci and Viviana Giannuzzi**
Fondazione per la Ricerca Farmacologica Gianni Benzi onlus, Valenzano, Italy

**Donato Bonifazi, Mariagrazia Felisi and Fedele Bonifazi**
Consorzio per Valutazioni Biologiche e Farmacologiche, Pavia, Italy

**Lucia Ruggieri**
Gruppo Italiano per gli Studi di Farmacoeconomia, Pavia, Italy

**Elizabeth Hong-Geller and Sofiya N. Micheva-Viteva**
Los Alamos National Laboratory, Bioscience Division, Los Alamos, NM, USA

**Samuel Constant, Song Huang, Ludovic Wisniewski and Christophe Mas**
OncoTheis Sàrl, Geneva, Switzerland

**Hrvoje Roguljic**
Department of Mineral Research, Faculty of Medicine, J. J. Strossmayer University of Osijek, Croatia

**Sonja Sarcevic and Nikola Raguz Lucic**
Department of Pharmacology, Faculty of Medicine, J. J. Strossmayer University of Osijek, Croatia

**Robert Smolic and Martina Smolic**
Department of Mineral Research, Faculty of Medicine, J. J. Strossmayer University of Osijek, Croatia
Department of Pharmacology, Faculty of Medicine, J. J. Strossmayer University of Osijek, Croatia

**Aleksandar Vcev**
Department of Mineral Research, Faculty of Medicine, J. J. Strossmayer University of Osijek, Croatia
Department of Medicine, Faculty of Medicine, J. J. Strossmayer University of Osijek, Croatia

**Degenhard Marx and Matthias Birkhoff**
Aptar Radolfzell GmbH, Radolfzell, Germany

**Gerallt Williams**
Aptar France SAS, Le Vaudreuil, France

# Index